Evaluating International Public Health Issues

Mbuso Precious Mabuza

Evaluating International Public Health Issues

Critical Reflections on Diseases and Disasters, Policies and Practices

Springer

Mbuso Precious Mabuza
Johns Hopkins University
Baltimore, MD, USA

ISBN 978-981-13-9786-8 ISBN 978-981-13-9787-5 (eBook)
https://doi.org/10.1007/978-981-13-9787-5

This Springer imprint is published by the registered company Springer Nature Singapore Pte Ltd.
The registered company address is: 152 Beach Road, #21-01/04 Gateway East, Singapore 189721, Singapore

To my family, here is to posterity!

Foreword

Health is a state of complete harmony of the body, mind and spirit. When one is free from physical disabilities and mental distractions, the gates of the soul open. (**BKS Iyengar**)

In any society, the survival of human beings is determined by bridging factors within the healthcare environment. The dynamics of culture is one factor that is dominant in this equation where it is seen as the way of life of a particular group of people, especially as shown in their ordinary behaviour and habits, their attitudes towards each other and their moral and religious beliefs. It should be borne in mind that individuals within a culture have basic needs to satisfy and their higher-order needs will only be addressed if the situation and circumstances are conducive. The economic environment is shaped by the gross national income per capita which is determined by income growth, inflation, exchange rates and population change which guide the level and quality of existence of individuals. It is against this background where policy and programme challenges in low-, middle- and high-income countries have to function and address the concerns of all the role players on the healthcare stage.

The health sector can be placed in the framework of a revised economic model where there is careful management of wealth (finance, funding) and resources (employees, clients and facilities) and a concerted effort is made to avoid waste through careful planning and thrifty use of all the elements. The factors contributing towards the efficiency of a revised health sector economy are in the first instance labour represented by intellectual contributions, including experience in and out of education, training, skills and natural abilities. In order to remain competitive, health places a premium on the care providers who bring these soft skills to the workplace. Many of the advances in the world today are the result of the application of intellectual human resources. In South Africa, however, this is translated in a negative sense where the general public is increasingly becoming disillusioned with the poor clinical quality of care in many public health sector clinics and hospitals.

There is a need for political commitment to provide a legal and institutional framework to support quality assurance in healthcare, encompassing a connection between the functions of the health value chain. Retaining healthcare providers hinges on two factors that ultimately affect behaviour, namely, extrinsic motivation and intrinsic motivation. Extrinsic motivation relates to financial rewards for the provision of a service. Intrinsic reward or motivation in the opposite spectrum can be in the form of encouraging the satisfaction of higher-order needs through positive feedback and reinforcement to repeat behaviour achieving the set goals. Strong and appropriate leadership together with effective planning and more engagement between the actors in the heath sector are vital to ensure incentive policies are appropriately implemented and maintained.

A further factor in the health economic forum is capital that has been acquired, and the objective is to employ it to deliver services to clients together with building and maintaining related infrastructures. Capital is a scarce resource, and budgeting and financing issues are some of the main challenges facing the health system in a shrinking economy where the demand for services is overshadowed by the lack and quality of supply. The following of strategic policies to ensure successful implementation of the procedures to ultimately deliver health services to clients is questioned in many sectors of the healthcare environment, and there is a lack of transparency and accountability of the control function.

A factor completing the equation of the adapted health economic model is entrepreneurship where it is represented by a person who organises and manages an enterprise with a dominant trait of initiative. In the twenty-first century, the demands for health services have increased due to the spreading of diseases, considering improved transport links between communities. Although the mobility of low-income communities is restricted, there is, however, an increase in passing trade, bringing external health issues with them. The healthcare profession needs to create new and reliable models through their entrepreneurs to bridge the gap between the different levels of income groups by providing health services and infrastructure through a transformation ranging from the old to contemporary.

In the future, the focus on health will be directed towards low-income countries where it is unlikely they will all enter the realms of their prosperous opposite counterparts. The world of health will have to continue facing crucial challenges of aging populations, continuous prevalence of non-communicable diseases and the tendency of urbanization, leaving rural areas vulnerable. The social gap between wealthy and poor communities where health inequalities are prevalent will have to be addressed by the application of contemporary policies related to available funding and appropriate research. The contrary is still prevalent in some world regions with young population groups where communicable diseases control the direction of healthcare, thus creating an imbalance in providing services to clients by addressing non-communicable maladies.

The setting of priorities and policies for public health interventions forms the background of an ever-increasing concern of the burden related to diseases that cause the most morbidity or mortality in a population.

"The physician must be able to tell the antecedents, know the present and foretell the future and they should mediate these things and have two special objectives in view with regard to disease, namely, to do good or to do no harm" (Hippocrates).

Economic and Management Sciences
Stellenbosch University
Stellenbosch, South Africa

Elza Thomson

Preface

International health is a field which deals with health across regional or national boundaries. In some quarters, international health is sometimes referred to as global health, geographic medicine or international medicine. While it is possible that there may be common health issues affecting many countries, it is a truism that the health terrain is not level within and between low-, middle- and high-income countries. There is a vast gap that exists between the rich and the poor in terms of inequitable healthcare access. Whether or not that gap is narrowed is dependent on the rate at which it is narrowed which is largely dependent on the commitment and effective action by all stakeholders and in particular the heads of state and government, policy makers, health professions and agencies for delivering healthcare. The great unmet health need, the serious deficiencies in health systems and the most telling country-specific inadequacies cluster around the single but painfully complex question of how to provide equitable care for large numbers of people on limited resources, particularly in the low- and middle-income countries.

The changes that are needed require effective and accountable leadership, new approaches to addressing health challenges, new forms of professional capability, new attitudes of professional and academic people, provision of quality and equitable services for all, meaningful engagement and involvement of all stakeholders and integration of indigenous and modern knowledge systems. Generally, there is a need for a paradigm shift that embraces sustainability well beyond the immediate piecemeal changes. As such, effective and efficient approaches towards finding sustainable solutions to the unique challenges should be context-specific.

The issue of financing is one of the main challenges affecting the health systems of most low- and middle-income countries. Much as the health agenda of low- and middle-income countries is largely driven by international development agencies or international funding agencies, such an approach is not sustainable. Effective leadership, governance, homegrown health solutions and locally generated funding should be prioritised as a matter of urgency if low- and middle-income countries are to win the battle against the heavy disease burden they carry. While most high-income countries have been largely challenged by the epidemic of chronic non-communicable diseases, and other issues related to aging, as more and more of their populations live longer, low- and middle-income countries face a multiple burden of the burgeoning epidemic of chronic non-communicable diseases and communicable diseases.

One wonders if the greater focus and investment on fighting the HIV and AIDS pandemic over the past few decades has had detrimental effects on the opportunity cost of addressing other serious public health issues including the surge in non-communicable diseases, such as cancers, diabetes mellitus, cardiovascular diseases and co-morbidities, in low- and middle-income countries. It is a cause for concern that globally, non-communicable diseases (NCDs) such as diabetes mellitus, heart disease, stroke and cancer account for approximately 70 per cent of all deaths and the impact is more pronounced in those younger than 60 years of age. While it is at least encouraging that the United Nations Sustainable Development Goals (SDGs) commit countries to reduce premature mortality from NCDs by a third, there are lessons to be learned from the strengths and weaknesses of implementing the United Nations Millennium Development Goals (MDGs). The impact on health of climate change cannot be ignored as this is touted as the biggest global health threat of the twenty-first century. It is also important not to ignore the impact on health of globalisation, environmental degradation, pollution, wars, disasters, genetically modified food, lifestyle, substance misuse, overuse of therapeutic agents and exposures to occupational hazards. There is no doubt that a radical and sustainable course correction is required as a matter of urgency if the global goal of controlling some of the biggest killers in the world is to be achieved.

It is against this backdrop that this book presents critical discussions and reflections on international health, policies, strategies, programmes, systems, diseases and public health issues in low-, middle- and high-income countries. Some of the intriguing discussions in this book are centred around the following main topics: international public health and the burden of diseases; inequity in low- and middle-income countries and the colonial history of public health; health systems; the UN millennium development goals and sustainable development goals; diseases control and the promotion of public health equity; adolescents, sexual reproductive health and equity; and globalisation, climate change and disasters.

Baltimore, MD, USA Mbuso Precious Mabuza

Contents

Abbreviations and Acronyms

ACA	Affordable Care Act
AIDS	Acquired Immunodeficiency Syndrome
ART	Antiretroviral Therapy
ARV	Antiretroviral Drug
CC	Climate Change
CD	Communicable Disease
CDC	Centers for Disease Control and Prevention
DDT	Dichlorodiphenyltrichloroethane
DFID	Department for International Development
DOTS	Directly Observed Treatment Short Course
EHP	Essential Health Package
EMA	European Medicines Agency
EPI	Expanded Program on Immunization
GAVI	Global Alliance for Vaccines and Immunisation
GDP	Gross Domestic Product
GF	Global Fund
GFATM	The Global Fund to Fight AIDS, Tuberculosis and Malaria
GHWA	Global Health Workforce Alliance
GMAP	Global Malaria Action Plan
GOBI-FFF	Growth Monitoring, Oral Rehydration, Breast Feeding, Food Supplementation and Female Literacy
HHS	US Department of Health and Human Services
HIV	Human Immunodeficiency Virus
HNP	Health, Nutrition and Population
IDA	International Development Association
IFIs	International Financial Institutions
IMF	International Monetary Fund
MDGs	Millennium Development Goals
MDR-TB	Multidrug-Resistant Tuberculosis
NCD	Non-communicable Diseases
NHI	National Health Insurance

NHP	National Health Policy
NHPS	National Health Protection Scheme
ODA	Official Development Assistance
OSD	Occupation-Specific Dispensation
PHC	Public Healthcare
RBM	Roll Back Malaria
SADC	Southern African Development Community
SARS	South African Revenue Service
SDGs	Sustainable Development Goals
SUN	Scaling Up Nutrition
SWAp	Sector-Wide Approach
TA	Technical Assistance
TAC	Treatment Action Campaign
TB	Tuberculosis
UN	United Nations
UNAIDS	Joint United Nations Programme on HIV/AIDS
UNFCCC	United Nations Framework Convention on Climate Change
UNHCR	United Nations High Commissioner for Refugees
UNICEF	United Nations Children's Fund
USA or US	United States of America
USAID	United States Agency for International Development
VCT	Voluntary Counselling and Testing
WB	World Bank
WHPA	World Health Professions Alliance
WHO	World Health Organization
WTO	World Trade Organization
XDR-TB	Extensively Drug-Resistant Tuberculosis

Chapter 1
International Public Health and the Burden of Diseases

Abstract Tackling the global disease burden is paramount in the context of the burgeoning epidemic of communicable and non-communicable diseases, especially in low- and middle-income countries. While most high-income countries have successfully implemented cost-effective interventions to tackle their burden of non-communicable diseases, low- and middle-income countries have to prioritise cost-effective interventions to tackle the multiple burden of communicable and non-communicable diseases and to strengthen their efforts to effectively address other key issues of public health concern. The irony is that while low- and middle-income countries carry the heaviest burden of disease, such countries have a minor share of the total global health spending, yet their economies are severely challenged and their populations are the most affected by poverty which has a negative impact on health. This chapter gives a critical overview on the following topics: What is International Public Health? Epidemiology and the burden of diseases; Understanding the magnitude of the disease burden.

Keywords Ambient air pollution · Burden of disease · Cancer · Cardiovascular diseases · Chronic respiratory conditions · Communicable diseases · Demographic transition · Diabetes · Disability-adjusted life year · Cholera · Ebola · Epidemic · Epidemiological transition · Epidemiology · Global health · Hepatitis · HIV and AIDS · Incidence · Injuries · International public health · Malaria · Mental health · Mortality · Non-communicable diseases · Prevalence · Quality-adjusted life years · Tropical diseases · Tuberculosis

1.1 What is International Public Health?

Although there may be similarities between International public health and Global health, these disciplines should not be confused as there are some fundamental differences between the two. Some of the more appealing definitions of international public health are:

M. P. Mabuza, *Evaluating International Public Health Issues*,
https://doi.org/10.1007/978-981-13-9787-5_1

International public health can be defined as the area of study, research, practice and art of collective efforts to prevent disease, promote health, and prolong quality of life that places a priority on improving health and achieving equity in health for all people worldwide.

International public health is a combination of sciences, skills and beliefs that is directed to the maintenance and improvement of the health of all the people through collective social actions, internationally.

On the other hand, "Global health includes public health, but also strives to use many other diverse disciplines, such as public policy, engineering, law, psychology, history, complementary medicine, anthropology, journalism, among others."

1.2 Epidemiology and the Burden of Diseases

Epidemiology is not about individuals, but it is a population science in the sense that it deals with the study of the distribution and determinants of health-related states or events in specific populations, and application of this study to the control of health problems (Mabuza 2018). Burden of disease includes the diseases which cause the most morbidity (illness or disability) and mortality (death) in a population. Burden of disease can be measured in 'disability-adjusted life year' or DALY. One DALY is one year of healthy life lost, for example, one year with blindness or loss of hearing, or one healthy year lost due to premature death as compared to full life span. There are major variations in the burden of disease by age, sex, and world region.

In public health, there is need to find the facts of the problem and also use statistics and epidemiological data to understand the problem at population level before deciding on a solution. It is worth highlighting that there are limitations in calculating the disease burden because the assumption is that the best data will be available, yet in reality the availability of data is patchy in other parts of the world. Ideally, it would be better to include an assessment about how people perceive their quality of life, and so calculate 'quality-adjusted life years'.

1.2.1 Descriptive and Analytical Epidemiology

The distinction between descriptive and analytical epidemiology is that:

Descriptive epidemiology describes the occurrence of disease and other health-related characteristics in human populations in terms of person (the "who": age, sex, social class), the place (the where: geographic location), and time (the when: season, time of day/week). Analytical epidemiology investigates the association between a given disease or health status and possible causative or protective factors. Analytical epidemiology attempts to explain why health-related outcomes occur and whether interventions work.

1.2.2 Epidemic

An epidemic is defined as the rapid increase in the level of a disease or occurrence in a community or region of a group of illnesses of similar nature, clearly in excess of normal expectancy, derived from a common source.

1.2.3 Epidemiological Transition

The change in disease patterns and causes of death is known as the epidemiological transition, such as a shift from a high burden of communicable diseases to a high burden of non-communicable diseases (Sarukhan 2018). The speed of the epidemiological transition brings with it, huge challenges for both domestic policymakers and the international organisations that distribute aid and run health programmes (Economist 2018).

1.2.4 Demographic Transition

Demographic and epidemiological transitions are of significance in terms of being a guide about the type of interventions that need to be prioritised for that particular setting. For example, very early in the demographic transition, countries experience high birth and death rates, which implies that the proportion of younger people in the population is higher while the proportion of older people is smaller, suggesting that communicable diseases might be a big issue as compared to chronic non-communicable diseases (Walley and Wright 2010). For the demographic transition to be a dividend, it is paramount that issues of policy, access to prevention, testing, treatment and care, and quality of service delivery are promptly addressed. Otherwise, both the demographic transition and the epidemiological transition will lead to more chronic diseases.

1.2.5 Prevalence and Incidence

Prevalence focuses on existing cases at a specific time. Prevalence cases include new cases (incident cases) and cases which occurred any time previously as long as they still have the condition at the time of the assessment. Cases who have died or recovered by the time of assessment are excluded. Incidence is the number of new cases of a specific disease occurring during a certain period.

The apparent contradiction between the higher incidence of myocardial ischaemia among men and a higher prevalence of this disease among women older than 70 may be as a result of a higher number of men than women who suffer from myocardial ischaemia for the first time, and most of these men suddenly die from this disease. A study reveals that men have a higher incidence of sudden cardiac death than women, with the ratio of 3:1. This implies that women have a higher probability to live longer with the disease than men, hence the higher prevalence of myocardial ischaemia among women older than 70.

Influenza and haemorrhagic fever (Ebola fever) are two examples of diseases that have a high incidence but low prevalence. There are many new cases of influenza especially during the winter season, and each case of influenza usually lasts for a short period because most of the patients recover within one or two weeks. During an outbreak of haemorrhagic fever (Ebola fever) there are many new cases that are reported, and yet the total number of cases of haemorrhagic fever at a particular point in time regardless of the disease onset is low because most of the patients die within a short period of time (for example within a week) due to fatal haemorrhage.

Rheumatoid arthritis (RA) and Asthma are two examples of diseases that have a low incidence but a relatively high prevalence. Generally, there are not many new cases of rheumatoid arthritis, and yet the total number of existing cases of rheumatoid arthritis is relatively high due to the fact that patients suffering from rheumatoid arthritis tend to live with the disease for a long time if the disease is properly managed. There are also not many new cases of asthma, and yet the total number of existing cases of asthma is high because patients tend to live with asthma for a long time if the disease is properly managed.

1.2.6 Incidence Rate, Mortality Rate, and Prevalence Rate

(a) The incidence rate, sometimes referred to as incidence density takes into account the length of disease-free time each individual in the at-risk population remained under observation. Incidence rate can be expressed as follows:

    Number of new cases of a disease during a specified period/Total person-time of observation

(b) Mortality rate, sometimes referred to as death rate is the number of deaths relative to the population over a defined period of time. A mortality rate can be calculated only if the death data as well as the population figures are reliable (Joubert and Ehrlich 2007).

(c) According to Joubert and Ehrlich (2007), Prevalence rate, sometimes referred to as prevalence is:

    Number of existing cases at a specific point in time / Number of people in the at-risk population at that time.
    Strictly speaking, this should be referred to as Prevalence rather than Prevalence rate, because it is not expressed per unit of time (Joubert and Ehrlich 2007).

1.2.7 Proportion and Ratio

The difference between a proportion and a ratio is that a proportion tells us what fraction of the population is affected. A ratio is an expression of the quantity of one entity in relation to that of another. For example, if 10 boys and 30 girls are born, the ratio of boys to girls is 10:30 or 0.33 (Joubert and Ehrlich 2007).

1.2.8 Crude Rates

The advantages of using crude rates are that they are actual summary rates, and they are readily calculable for comparison.

Disadvantage of using crude rates is that age composition introduces distortion into a crude rate. Since populations vary in composition (most notably, age) differences in crude rates are difficult to interpret.

1.3 Understanding the Magnitude of the Disease Burden

It is important to know and to have detailed reliable information from a statistical and epidemiological perspective about the burden of disease or the diseases that cause the most morbidity or mortality in a population, as this would inform priorities and policies for public health interventions (Murray and Lopez 1997).

Developing countries contribute approximately 80% to the global mortality due to non-communicable diseases (Alwan and MacLean 2009). This is a very huge point, and it makes one realise the magnitude of the challenge that low- and middle-income countries are faced with, in addition to the already huge burden of communicable diseases such as HIV and AIDS, tuberculosis (TB), and malaria. In fact, the magnitude of such a challenge ceases to be just a low- and middle-income countries' issue, but it now becomes a global challenge that requires urgent coordinated international interventions.

It is of concern that there is so much focus on some diseases such as HIV and AIDS, malaria and tuberculosis, and dragging of feet in dealing with non-communicable diseases, injuries, emerging and re-emerging communicable diseases, and the impact of climate change and air pollution on health. Such an approach can be detrimental because if there is no immediate action, the problem of non-communicable diseases, injuries, emerging and re-emerging communicable diseases, and the health impact of climate change will spiral out of proportion and become such a huge and costly problem to address. On the other hand, it cannot be generalised that tackling other diseases such as HIV and AIDS, malaria and tuberculosis first and dealing with non-communicable diseases, injuries, emerging and re-emerging communicable diseases, later, would not be beneficial, because the burden of disease varies between regions and between men, women and children (Walley and Wright 2010).

Even though there have been enormous gains in the fight against HIV and AIDS, TB, and malaria, there is an upsurge of these diseases in some parts of the world. This upsurge in cases of HIV and AIDS, TB and malaria, is possibly due to a number of reasons such as complacency, ineffective leadership, ineffective and inefficient interventions, unsustainable financing and programmes, weak health systems, globalisation, and drug resistance, among others. Climate change is also playing a part in the upsurge of malaria even in parts of the world which were considered malaria-free zones.

TB is the top infectious killer in the world. With ten million new TB infection in 2017, and the World Health Organization's End TB strategy having a $1.3 billion annual shortfall, the much-anticipated September 2018 high-level meeting on tuberculosis came and went without governments laying out any specific or new funding pledges. As such, the meeting was characterised as a failure of global leadership to make TB a priority.

In 2018, the global AIDS response had reached a precarious point as the gains that had been achieved were beginning to be compromised by complacency, stigma and discrimination, prevention crisis, funding crisis, and leaving other population groups such as children and young people behind. Although the number of new HIV infections continued to decline in 2017, the global rate of new HIV infections was not falling fast enough to reach the 2020 milestone. Globally, there were approximately 980,000 new HIV infections in 2017, and women continued to account for a disproportionate percentage of new infections in sub-Saharan Africa as they represented approximately 59% of the global new HIV infections in the same year. As deaths declined faster than new HIV infections, the number of people living with HIV had grown to 36.9 million [31.1–43.9 million], globally.

> *It is distressing that, in 2017, 180 000 children became infected with HIV, far from the 2018 target of eliminating new HIV infections among children.* ***(Michel Sidibe, Executive Director).***

Eastern and southern Africa has only 6.2% of the world's population but it is home to half of the world's people living with HIV. An estimated 800,000 people in eastern and southern Africa acquired HIV in 2017, and an estimated 380,000 people died of AIDS-related illness. Mozambique, South Africa and the United Republic of Tanzania accounted for more than half of new HIV infections and deaths from AIDS-related illness in the region in 2017.

Both the rate of new HIV infections and burden of HIV remain high in western and central Africa. The incidence to prevalence ratio in the region has changed little since 2010: it stood at 0.06, twice as high as the epidemic transition benchmark of 0.03. Cameroon, Cote d'Ivoire and Nigeria together accounted for approximately 71% of new HIV infections in the region in 2017. Nigeria alone accounted for more than half of new infections and deaths from AIDS-related illness, in part reflection its large population size compared to other countries in the region.

Asia and the Pacific has the second highest number of people living with HIV in the world, and, the region's HIV epidemic is concentrated among key populations and their intimate partners. Progress in reducing new HIV infections has slowed in recent years, and there are rising epidemics in some countries. Insufficient coverage of harm reduction services threatens further progress. Condom use was low among gay men and other men who have sex with men in several countries, and across the region among people who inject drugs. Prevention programmes often struggle to reach young key populations. Other challenges include the criminalisation and incarceration of key populations, stigma and discrimination (particularly in health-care settings), lack of innovation in service delivery models, slow pace of introducing new technologies, and strong dependence on international financing for effective prevention measures.

The region's strong performance along the 90-90-90 continuum of services saw deaths from AIDS-related illness decline by 12% from 2010 to 2017. Although there has been little change in the number of new HIV infections in Latin America over the previous 15 years, high treatment coverage and low AIDS-related mortality has driven a gradual decline in the region's incidence to prevalence ratio, which was 0.06 in 2017. Gay men and other men who have sex with men accounted for 41% of HIV infections in 2017, and key populations and their sexual partners represented more than three quarters of new infections overall.

There has been moderate progress on both prevention and treatment in the Caribbean, and the annual number of new HIV infections among adults in the Caribbean declined by 18% from 2010, from 19,000 to 15,000. Deaths from AIDS-related illness declined by 23% over the same period. As a result, the region's incidence to prevalence ratio is edging towards the 0.03 epidemic transmission benchmark, reaching 0.05 in 2017.

Although the Middle East and North Africa was the region with the lowest HIV prevalence, at 0.1% among adults aged 15–49 years, there were an estimated 18,000 new HIV infections in 2017, 12% more than the 16,000 in 2010. Annual deaths from AIDS-related illness have stabilised at nearly 10,000 since 2015, but the trend since 2010 has been an 11% increase. The region's incidence to prevalence ratio has hovered around 0.08 for much of the previous decade, far from the 0.03 epidemic transition benchmark.

Eastern Europe and central Asia is the only region in the world, where the HIV epidemic continued to rise rapidly, and the epidemic is concentrated predominantly among key populations, and in particular people who inject drugs. A 30% increase in new HIV infections since 2010 has the region falling behind in its efforts to reach the target of reducing new HIV infections by 75%. The HIV incidence to prevalence ratio of 0.09 is three times higher than the 0.03 epidemic transition benchmark. National HIV surveillance data in several countries also indicate that HIV infections are growing among the general population, particularly urban residents and labour migrants. High coverage of HIV services for much of the last two decades has resulted in steady progress towards ending the AIDS epidemic in the region, hitting the epidemic transition benchmark of 0.03 in 2017. Already low rates of HIV incidence and AIDS-related mortality have declined even further since 2010: in 2017, they reached about 70,000 and 13,000, respectively.

Whilst there has been so much focus on HIV/AIDS/TB and malaria, most recent studies have continued to identify ambient air pollution as one of the most important risk factors contributing to death and disability. Some of the air pollution-related health effects include lower respiratory infections, cancers, cardiovascular diseases, chronic respiratory diseases, increased hospitalisations, and reduced life expectancy from heart and lung disease.

Worldwide exposure to ambient particulate matter contributed to 4.1 million deaths from heart disease and stroke, lung cancer, chronic lung disease, and respiratory infections in 2016.

It is highlighted in the State of Global Air Report 2018 that 95% of the world's population lives in areas exceeding World Health Organization (WHO) Guideline for healthy air, and that nearly 60% lives in areas that do not meet even the least-stringent air quality target from WHO.

According to the World Health Organization, non-communicable diseases (NCDs) account for approximately 71% of the 57 million global deaths. While NCDs are often associated with high income countries which are going through epidemiological transitions whereby there is a higher proportion of older people and a smaller proportion of younger people in the population, the reality is that there is a surge in chronic non-communicable diseases in low- and middle-income countries which already carry a high burden of diseases (Alwan and MacLean 2009). The rapid surge in chronic non-communicable diseases such as diabetes, cardiovascular diseases, cancer, tobacco-related morbidities and mortality, and mental health issues such as depression, has largely been ignored, or not prioritised, particularly in many developing countries. This has been largely due to the fact that there has been so much focus on the other high priority areas such as HIV and AIDS, tuberculosis and malaria, yet it should feature at the top of the global burden of disease, as an estimated 72.3% (39.5 million) of all deaths in 2016 were from non-communicable diseases. The negative socio-economic impacts of this oversight are enormous, because this exacerbates poverty and widens inequalities (International Federation of Medical Students 2018). It is forecast that in 2040, ischaemic heart disease, stroke, and respiratory infections will remain among the top 3 global causes of premature death (Institute for Health Metrics 2018).

To the government leaders gathered in New York, 27 September 2018, for the third UN high-level meeting on non-communicable diseases (NCDs), Michael R. Bloomberg brought a positive message. The 41 million annual deaths from NCDs are largely preventable. What's needed to save millions of lives is political will.

Many of the most effective measures to fight NCDs don't require a lot of money. They do require political will. (***Global Health Now, September 26, 2018***).

Cities can be the engines of change beyond their borders. When policies work at a local level, national governments are more likely to adopt them. ***(Global Health Now, September 26, 2018)***.

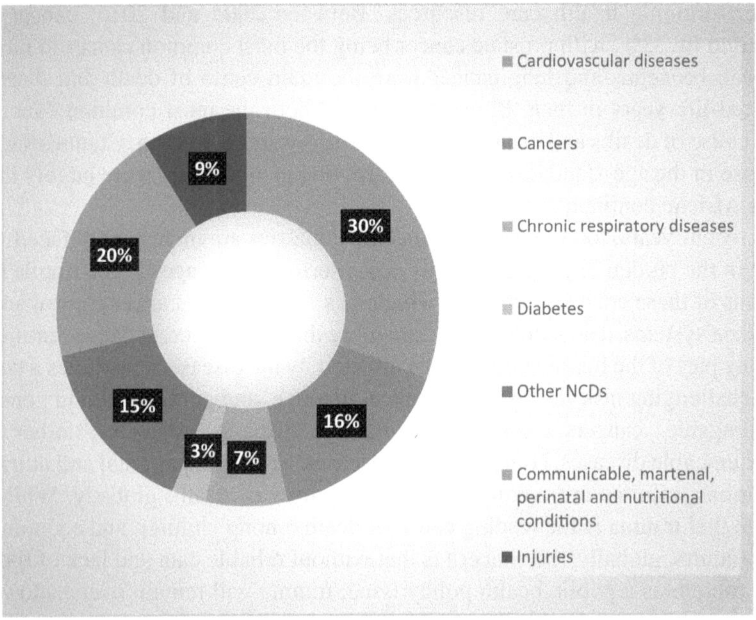

Fig. 1.1 Global mortality (% of total deaths), all ages, both sexes, 2016

Special interests will always push back against policies that impact their bottom line, but the number one responsibility of government is to protect people's well-being. (***Global Health Now, September 26, 2018***).

Figure 1.1 highlights that, globally, cardiovascular diseases were the main cause of death in 2016. In the past, the main non-communicable diseases such as cancer, cardiovascular diseases (such as stroke, hypertensive heart disease, peripheral vascular disease, among others), and diabetes mellitus were generally considered to be diseases of the affluent such as in the high-income countries. In recent times, cancer, cardiovascular diseases, and diabetes mellitus have exploded to the level of 'epidemics' in low- and middle-income countries. The reasons for this explosion are varied, but evidence shows that this is heavily linked with inequities largely perpetrated by globalisation and rapid urbanisation. This has increasingly widened the gap between non-communicable diseases health outcomes of those people who are advantaged and those who are disadvantaged or marginalised. The health disparities are not unique to low- and middle-income countries, but they are striking even in high-income countries such as the United States of America where there is a glaring gap along racial and ethnic lines.

Cancer is a worldwide burden, and its occurrence has a broad geographical diversity and variations in the magnitude and profile of the disease between and within world regions (World Health Organization 2018). Globally, there were approximately 18.1 million new cancer cases and around 9.6 million cancer-related deaths in 2018. Cancer ranks among the leading causes of death worldwide, and as part of the epidemiological transition, cancer incidence is expected to increase in the future, further straining health care resources. Between 2005 and 2015, cancer cases increased by 33%, with prostate cancer being the most common cancer in men, but tracheal, bronchus and lung cancer were the main cause of death and disability-adjusted-life-years in men. Breast cancer was both the most common cancer and main cause of deaths and disability-adjusted-life-years in women. Countries with an increase in the age-standardized deaths rates due to all cancers were largely located in the African continent.

In recent years, low- and middle-income countries are increasingly faced with a surge in the burden of cancer, and this poses serious challenges to the fragile health systems of these countries, most of which lack or have poor cancer control and surveillance systems. The fact that there are more than 200 different cancer entities and that any part of the human body can be affected by the disease, constitutes a particularly challenging task for research, clinical practice, and public health in general.

Alongside cancers, chronic respiratory diseases, diabetes, other non-communicable diseases, communicable diseases, maternal, perinatal and nutritional conditions, injuries are among the leading causes of death, globally. While it is known that trauma is the leading cause of death among children and economically active adults, globally, the concern is that without reliable data and lack of focus on this problem as a public health policy issue, trauma will remain overshadowed by well-known health crises.

Diabetes, particularly Type 2 diabetes is fast becoming a worldwide emergency as it seriously challenges the health systems of both developed and developing countries (Animaw and Seoum 2017). Type 2 diabetes is increasingly appearing not only in overweight or obese people, but also in thin people and in children across all ethnic groups (Narayan 2016). Of the estimated 400 million people with diabetes, approximately 300 million are in low- and middle-income countries. There is a disparity between developed and developing countries in terms of the prevention of diabetes and the management of diabetes complications such as cardiovascular diseases (Brookman-May et al. 2017). Diabetes exerts a significant burden resulting in increased morbidity and mortality, decreased life expectancy, reduced quality of life, and reduced individual and national income losses (Mohan et al. 2013). Although some of the regions with the heaviest burden of diabetes are the Western Pacific, South East Asia, Europe, Middle East, and North America, the sub-Saharan Africa region is showing a dramatic increase in the rate of diabetes.

The soaring rate of diabetes throughout the world is one of the biggest catastrophes the world has ever seen. While the equally increasing rate of obesity is an associated risk of type 2 diabetes, such an association is not that simplistic as an increase in type 2 diabetes is also seen among people who are thin (Colagiuri et al. 2015).

Chronic viral hepatitis is a major global public health threat, with some 500 million people worldwide estimated to be currently infected with hepatitis B or C. These two diseases are the cause of significant global morbidity and mortality with their sequelae, liver disease and primary liver cancer. There is an estimated 350 million people worldwide who are chronic hepatitis B carriers, with a disproportionately high burden (>8% prevalence) in Africa, Asia and the Western Pacific, where there is generally a high burden of infectious diseases and poor infection protection measures. Given the magnitude of the global burden of hepatitis, it is encouraging that the World Health Organization has seen it proper to develop and implement the Global Hepatitis Strategy, towards elimination of Hepatitis B and C, by 2030 (World Health Organization 2017a, b).

The sporadic outbreaks of emerging and re-emerging communicable diseases such as Ebola, Pandemic influenza, cholera, diphtheria, dengue fever, among others, cannot be overlooked, as the rapid and intense transmission of such diseases carries risks beyond the settings in which they occur. Such outbreaks have often caught many health systems ill-equipped to deal with, particularly in the developing regions. In fact, the outbreak of Ebola which spread to a number of West African countries between 2013 and 2015, was the most severe, largest and longest lasting of any outbreak of the virus since its discovery. Even international health organisations such as the World Health Organisation were ill-prepared to deal with that particular Ebola outbreak. The World Health Organization acknowledged that the sporadic outbreak of Ebola in the Democratic Republic of Congo, in 2018 and 2019, was a big challenge to contain due to the wide geographic range, unlike previous Ebola outbreaks in the country. The puzzle is further complicated by the complexity of accessing conflict zones where the Ebola outbreak could spiral out of proportion, and potentially pose a global public health threat. The question is, are countries, health systems and global public health ready to handle Ebola outbreaks, and other severe disease outbreaks, now, and in the future?

Much as it is laudable that up to 20 countries have eliminated cholera as a public health threat, and that African governments have committed and endorsed strategies set out in the Global Roadmap aimed at reducing cholera deaths by 90% by 2030, the reality is that cholera continues to be a major public health issue, particularly in settings with unsafe drinking water sources. The issue is compounded by the fact that cholera is a disease of poor and vulnerable populations, notably in conflict situations and where sanitation and hygiene are inadequate. The bottom line is that cholera is still a threat to human health, and it marks a failure of global health as the disease still kills more than 107,000 people per year, despite having the knowledge and means to hand to effect change (GBD Diarrhoeal Disease Collaborators 2018).

The global burden of neglected tropical diseases (such as, Buruli ulcer, Chaga's disease, cysticercosis/taeniasis, dengue fever, dracunculiasis, food-borne trematodiasis, human African trypanosomiasis, leishmaniasis, leprosy, lymphatic filariasis, rabies, schistosomiasis, onchocerciasis/river blindness, and trachoma) cannot be overlooked as it is estimated that more than a billion people, mostly in the developing countries, are infected with one or more of this group of bacterial, parasitic, viral, and fungal infections. For example, dengue, a rapidly spreading mosquito-borne viral disease carried by the *Aedes aegypti* and *Aedes albopictus* mosquitos, can affect people of all ages, and half of the world's population is at risk of contracting dengue. Approximately 400 million dengue infections occur globally on an annual basis, and there are more than 20,000 dengue-related deaths each year around the world. Dengue outbreaks are observed in tropical and sub-tropical areas and have recently caused outbreaks in parts of mainland United States of America and Europe (Murray et al. 2013; World Health Organization 2017a, b). Dengue has expanded in recent years due to urbanisation, air travel, population growth and climate change (Murray et al. 2013; World Health Organization 2017a, b).

There is no doubt that the burden of communicable diseases continues to be high, and at the same time there is a dramatic increase in the burden of non-communicable diseases, particularly in low- and middle-income countries. This implies that improving international public health should no longer primarily be on communicable diseases (as it has been for many years), but more focus should also be on non-communicable diseases. Although this may strike some health experts as premature, such an epidemiological transition or change in disease patterns and causes of death, implies that policymakers will have to think carefully about which health services to prioritise, and how best to supply them, and ensure that ever more resources will be consumed by chronic conditions (Economist 2018). As such, it may be necessary to prioritise a holistic approach in implementing interventions that will tackle communicable diseases and non-communicable diseases based on the most common causes of morbidity and mortality affecting that particular population (Economist 2018).

It is crucial to get reliable statistical and epidemiological information about the burden of disease as this will inform the policies and interventions for tackling these diseases, and that such interventions should be relevant for that particular context and setting (Walley and Wright 2010). It is usually cost-effective to holistically tackle disease burdens early than to have a fragmented approach or to wait for later (Liese et al. 2010).

References

Alwan, A., & MacLean, D. R. (2009). A review of non-communicable disease in low- and middle-income countries. *International Health, 1*(1), 3–9.

Animaw, W., & Seoum, Y. (2017). Increasing prevalence of diabetes mellitus in a developing country and its related factors. *PLoS One, 12*(11), e0187670. https://doi.org/10.1371/journal.pone.0187670.

Brookman-May, S. D., et al. (2017). Challenges, hurdles and possible approaches to improve cancer in developing countries – A short breakdown of the status quo and future perspective. *Advances in Modern Oncology Research, 3*(5), 205–212. https://doi.org/10.18282/amor.v3.i5.221.

Economist. (2018). *The epidemiological transition is now spreading to the emerging world.* https://www.economist.com/special-report/2018/04/26/the-epidemiological-transition-is-now-spreading-to-the-emerging-world

GBD Diarrhoeal Disease Collaborators. (2018). Ending cholera for all. *Lancet of Infectious Diseases*, (18) October 2018. Available from www.thelancet.com/infection. Accessed 1 Oct 2018.

Institute for Health Metrics and Evaluation (IHME). (2018). *The power of models*. Seattle: Institute for Health Metrics and Evaluation.

International Federation of Medical Students. (2018). *Non communicable diseases and the 4 most common shared risk factors*. Adopted at the IFMSA General Assembly March Meeting 2018 in Hurghada, Egypt.

Joubert, G., & Ehrlich, R. (2007). *Epidemiology: A research manual for South Africa*. New York: Oxford.

Liese, B., Rosenberg, M., & Schratz, A. (2010). Programmes, partnerships, and governance for elimination and control of neglected tropical diseases. *The Lancet, 375*(9708), 67–76.

Mabuza, M. P. (2018). *Epidemiology and statistics for public health research: Concepts, applications and critical perspectives*. Beau Bassin: Lambert Academic Publishing.

Mohan, V., Seedat, Y. K., & Pradeepa, R. (2013). The rising burden of diabetes and hypertension in Southeast Asian and African Regions: Need for effective strategies for prevention and control in primary health care settings. *International Journal of Hypertension, 2013*, 1–14. https://doi.org/10.1155/2013/409083.

Murray, C. J. L., & Lopez, A. D. (1997). Mortality by cause for eight regions of the world: Global burden of disease study. *The Lancet, 349*(9061), 1269–1276.

Murray, N.E., et al. (2013) *Epidemiology of dengue: Past, present and future prospects*. Available from https://www.ncbi.nlm.nih.gov/pmc/articles/PMC3753061/. Accessed 25 Sept 2018.

Narayan, V. (2016). The mysteries of type 2 diabetes in developing countries. *Bulletin of the World Health Organization, 94*, 241–242. https://doi.org/10.2471/BLT.16.030416.

Sarukhan, A. (2018) *The epidemiological transition (or what we died, die and will die from)*. Available from https://www.isglobal.org/en/healthisglobal/-/custom-blog-portlet/la-transicion-epidemiologica-o-de-que-moriamos-morimos-y-moriremos-/3098670/0. Accessed 27 Nov 2018.

Walley, J., & Wright, J. (2010). *Public health: An action guide to improving health*. New York: Oxford.

World Health Organization. (2017a). *Dengue and severe dengue*. Available from http://www.who.int/mediacentre/factsheets/fs117/en/. Accessed 26 Sept 2018.

World Health Organization. (2017b). *Towards the elimination of hepatitis B and C by 2030*. The draft WHO Global Hepatitis Strategy, 2016–2021 and global elimination targets. Geneva. Available from www.who.int/hepatitis. Accessed 1 Oct 2018.

World Health Organization. (2018). *Global mortality of TB*. Geneva.

Chapter 2
Inequity in Low- and Middle-Income Countries and the Colonial History of Public Health

Abstract The political power and influence of the medical model and issues of ethnicity and socio-economic status continue to influence current attitudes to and practices in public health programmes and contribute to continuing health inequalities and inequities in low- and middle-income countries. Poverty is a major public health issue in many low- and middle-income countries and the inequalities and inequities that exacerbate it. The gap between the rich and the poor still gets wider and wider all the time and deepens the inequalities. Unlike the rich, those who live in poverty continue to bear the brunt of poor health and discrimination. A potential solution to address poverty is to have the highest calibre of political leadership that will show commitment and vision to meaningfully and sustainably address the issue of poverty. This chapter gives a critical overview on the following topics: Historical influence on current policies and practices in public health; Poverty as a public health issue; Impact of inequalities and inequities in public health.

Keywords Colonial history of public health · Ethnicity in public health · Inequality · Inequity · Medical model · Political power in public health · Poverty · Socioeconomic status in public health

2.1 Historical Influence on Current Policies and Practices in Public Health

> *Examination of historical documentation of the early exploration and trading voyages through which Europeans introduced the seeds of devastating epidemics to the peoples of the Americas; of the multitude of deaths caused by the slave trade; and of the growth of the industrial revolution which saw the poor of Britain migrating to live in cities in crowded and insanitary slums, riven by TB, typhoid and diarrhoea, all leave little doubt that the quest for economic and political power drove the expansion of research and development in public health and provided the conditions for paradigmatic shifts in science and medicine.* ***(Doyal, Sanders)***.

The past has been characterised by paradigm shifts that have resulted in huge gains for some people and huge losses for other people, and many of the consequences of such shifts have continued to have an influence in many aspects of life even to this

M. P. Mabuza, *Evaluating International Public Health Issues*,
https://doi.org/10.1007/978-981-13-9787-5_2

day. This discussion identifies ways in which examples of policy and practice from the past continue to influence current attitudes to and practices in public health programmes and contribute to continuing health inequalities and inequities in low-income countries.

Political power and the past successes of medical science and technology provided leverage for policy makers to implement health systems that were largely centred around the medical model because even the early public health movement employed a medical scientific model to justify its cause (Naidoo and Wills 2009). Although the new public health movement is trying to project a broader scope particularly encompassing the social determinants of health, the power and influence of the medical model is not that easy to untangle because it influences attitudes to many current public health programmes.

Having lived in previously colonised countries such as the Kingdom of Eswatini and South Africa, one realises that there are still ramifications of the colonial past in the health systems of these two countries, despite the fact that, on paper, the health systems of these two countries are considered to be comprehensive. For example, the health system of apartheid South Africa provided separate services for white people and for people of colour, whereby, the advantaged minority population of European origin had access to bigger and better health services in the urban areas, and the disadvantaged majority population of African origin only had access to poor health services (Dennill and Vasuthevan 2005). In post-apartheid South Africa, things have not changed much because the bigger and well-resourced private health sector is largely accessed by those who can afford, whereas the poor majority who cannot afford expensive private sector healthcare are still trapped in the poorly resourced and deteriorating public health sector and are disadvantaged.

As such, this contributes to continuing health inequalities and inequities in low- and middle-income countries such as in sub-Saharan Africa, South America, South East Asia, among others. In terms of inequalities, there is a widening gap between the rich and the poor to such an extent that some of the low- and middle-income countries are even considered among the most unequal societies in the world. Inequalities in income and health continue to be a challenge not only in low- and middle-income countries but in high-income countries as well (Walley and Wright 2010). Although there are different perspectives about the concept of inequalities, some studies suggest that there appears to be consensus that widening inequalities are a recipe for disaster and are very dangerous for health (Scambler 2008).

In terms of inequities, there is still a marked difference between the disease profiles of the urban areas and the rural areas, whereby morbidity and mortality are higher in the rural areas than in the urban areas due to disparities in quality of life and healthcare (Dennill and Vasuthevan 2005).

The political power and influence of the medical model and issues of ethnicity and socioeconomic status continue to influence current attitudes to and practices in public health programmes and contribute to continuing health inequalities and inequities in low- and middle-income countries.

2.2 Poverty as a Public Health Issue

Poverty is a major public health issue in sub-Saharan Africa, Asia and the Americas, and the inequalities and inequities that exacerbate it. One is confronted with issues of abject poverty on a daily basis in countries such as South Africa, and this issue appears to be widespread and much deeper than initially thought. Interestingly, South Africa is considered to be one of the biggest economies in Africa, and yet it has health outcomes that are worse than those of smaller economies (Coovadia et al. 2009).

Could the deepening poverty in South Africa be due to the legacy of apartheid whereby people of African origin were discriminated against and the wealth was in the hands of the minority population of European origin (Coovadia et al. 2009)? One would say, maybe yes, maybe no. Maybe yes, in the sense that in South Africa, the majority of people of African origin are still very poor, and the wealth is still largely in the hands of people of European descent, and, of course, a handful of the elite previously disadvantaged people. Maybe no, in the sense that sometimes there is the tendency to blame the past even long after the political power has been taken away from the hands of the colonisers. Much as it has to be acknowledged that it may take time to address the imbalances of the past, it is still believed that the South African democratic government which has been in power for over two decades should at least have covered some ground by now in terms of effectively addressing the issue of poverty.

Unfortunately, the reality is that even after the new government's policy to remove discrimination and to promote wealth redistribution to try and address the imbalances of the colonial past, this has not really been successful because the wealth is still concentrated among the few at the top including the new African millionaires, as there is an emergence of a new elite group in South Africa (Chopra et al. 2009). The gap between the rich and the poor still gets wider and wider all the time, and deepens the inequalities as already mentioned in an earlier discussion. Unlike the rich, those who live in poverty continue to bear the brunt of poor health and discrimination. Such inequalities and inequities have exacerbated the poverty situation in South Africa.

A potential solution to address poverty is to have the highest calibre of political leadership that will show commitment and vision to meaningfully and sustainably address the issue of poverty (Sewankambo and Katamba 2009). This should ensure that the whole population, and particularly the poor or disadvantaged have the highest attainable standard of health which encompasses medical care, access to safe drinking water, adequate sanitation, education, health-related information, and other underlying determinants of health, and freedoms such as the right to be free from discrimination (Backman et al. 2008). The poverty reduction strategy should focus also on empowering people and to create self-employment opportunities in their own communities to ensure self-sustainability (Dennill and Vasuthevan 2005).

2.3 Impact of Inequalities and Inequities in Public Health

There is emergence, persistence and even worsening inequalities, in spite of growing worldwide attention to health, and the influence of capitalism thereto (Birn et al. 2009). There is no doubt that our world seems to be dominated by profiteering and financial markets, underpinned by the concept of capitalism which seems to have entrenched the inequalities and inequities in our society.

Marxist theorists and other theorists have noted the close connection between the economy and the welfare state, and that if money is to be spent on welfare, the first thing that has to be established is economic prosperity, and this suggests that the welfare state ensures that it justifies the inequalities of capitalism (Scambler 2008).

South Africa has somewhat become a welfare state, because, post-apartheid South Africa's government policy to remove discrimination and promote wealth redistribution has led to initiatives that include improved pensions, a burgeoning number of social grants, and a social expenditure programme to build houses, and provide clean water, sanitation, and electricity (Chopra et al. 2009). The expenditure programme of building of houses, provision of clean water, sanitation, and electricity, though implemented to some degree in the rural areas, is more concentrated in the peri-urban, urban and industrial areas where there is also widespread expansion of informal settlements. All these initiatives require a lot of money to be pumped in, and such money must come from somewhere, otherwise, these initiatives cannot be sustained. It is therefore hardly surprising that there is such a huge tax that the South African population has to pay through the South African Revenue Service (SARS). Such tax seems to take away whatever little income the poor can get, thus perpetuating the cycle of poverty and the deepening inequalities. Could this be a justification of the inequalities of capitalism by the welfare state?

Merson et al. (2012) see this as globalisation-driven, foremost, by the formation of larger social groupings such as megacities. These megacities are often coupled with a culture of consumerism, whereby, people end up spending beyond their means. Even the private health sector and the pharmaceutical industry are having an influence on or are influenced by capitalism as they are driven by profit making. The cycle of poverty also gets perpetuated in this way as people end up having to live on credit, and those who earn little are even more vulnerable.

Merson et al. (2012) are interesting when they posit that no viable alternative to capitalism is possible and that the end of history has been reached as far as ideological development is concerned. Could this be an indication that a point of no return has been reached as far as the inequalities and inequities are concerned? There is no doubt that capitalism is having a huge influence in terms of the perpetuation of inequalities and inequities.

An article about the socioeconomic disparities in breast cancer treatment among older women, highlights that those who are at the bottom end of the scale, in terms of socioeconomic status, are often at a disadvantage, especially when it comes to access to healthcare (Dennill and Vasuthevan 2005). This issue is so widespread that it does not only affect low- and middle-income countries but it also affects high-income countries. Studies show evidence of the existence of, and even increases in socioeconomic inequalities in health, and that this continues to mount in most countries (Birn et al. 2009).

The article about the socioeconomic disparities in breast cancer treatment among older women, though not conclusive, suggests that there was no racial difference with regard to breast cancer treatment received by older white and black women in Alabama, but there were differences by area-level socioeconomic status (White et al. 2013). In sub-Saharan Africa, low socioeconomic status is generally synonymous with the rural areas where there generally are poor living conditions, lack of available services which results in poor sanitation and poor access to safe water, fewer educational and employment opportunities, there are fewer medical care services available and often they are inaccessible because transport is inadequate. White et al. (2013) highlight almost similar low socioeconomic conditions in the state of Alabama to the ones that have been highlighted about the rural areas of the sub-Saharan Africa region.

There is no doubt that something needs to be done to address the situation of socioeconomic disparities as such disparities exacerbate health inequalities. Health inequality refers to differences in health between different individuals, and it is seen as primarily the consequence of individual biological differences (Merson et al. 2012). While it is not easy to address the biological differences, a suggestion to bridge the health inequalities is to address health inequity because health inequity is seen as something on which it is possible to act and change because its origins are the consequences – albeit directly – of human actions in the first place through the social determinants (Merson et al. 2012). One would, therefore, encourage that the solution aimed at bridging the health inequalities be based on the recognition that relationships exist between a variety of economic, political, legal, social, and physical factors and health.

Promoting equal access to the social, economic, political, and cultural resources necessary to promote health or prevent diseases, would be very crucial. In the context of inequalities and inequities, one would suggest that there be equal access to employment and educational opportunities, provision and adherence to the highest standards of sanitation and hygiene, provision and access to the best healthcare services and adequate transport services across the board.

References

Backman, G., Hunt, P., Khosla, R., Jaramillo-Strouss, C., Fikre, B. M., Rumble, C., Pevalin, D., Paez, D. A., Pineda, M. A., Frisancho, A., Tarco, D., Motlagh, M., Karcasanu, D., & Vladescu, C. (2008). Health systems and the right to health: An assessment of 194 countries. *The Lancet, 372*(9655), 2047–2085.

Birn, A., Pillay, Y., & Holtz, T. H. (2009). *Textbook of international health: Global health in a dynamic world.* New York: Oxford.

Chopra, M., Lawn, J. E., Sanders, D., Barron, P., Abdool-Karim, S. S., Bradshaw, D., Jewkes, R., Karim, Q., Flisher, A. J., Mayosi, B. M., Tollman, S. M., Churchyard, G. J., & Coovadia, H.

(2009). Achieving the health millennium development goals for South Africa: Challenges and priorities. *The Lancet, 374*(9694), 1023–1031.
Coovadia, H., Jewkes, R., Barron, P., Sanders, D., & McIntyre, D. (2009). The health and health system of South Africa: Historical roots of current public health challenges. *The Lancet, 374*(9692), 817–834.
Dennill, K., & Vasuthevan, S. (2005). *The health of southern Africa*. Cape Town: Juta.
Merson, M. E., Black, R. E., & Mills, A. J. (2012). *Global health: Diseases, programs, systems, and policies*. London: Jones & Bartlett.
Naidoo, J., & Wills, J. (2009). *Foundations for health promotion*. London: Elsevier.
Scambler, G. (2008). *Sociology as applied to medicine*. London: Elsevier.
Sewankambo, N. K., & Katamba, A. (2009). Health systems in Africa: Learning from South Africa. *The Lancet, 374*(9694), 957–959.
Walley, J., & Wright, J. (2010). *Public health: An action guide to improving health*. New York: Oxford.
White, A., Richardson, L. C., Kronitras, H., & Pisu, M. (2013). Socioeconomic disparities in breast cancer treatment among older women. *Journal of Women's Health, 0*(0), 1–7.

Chapter 3
Health Systems

Abstract The first step towards health systems strengthening is to understand that a health system is a dynamo of interactions and synergies between the building blocks, namely, leadership and governance, health financing, medicines and technologies, health information, health workforce, and service delivery. Effective leadership and governance are the cornerstone and important entry point for discussions of health policy, design, implementation, and for raising performance in healthcare delivery. Human resources for health are a vital building block of a health system, and they are central towards the attainment of better health outcomes. In recent times, disease-focused multi-billion-dollar health initiatives have emerged in the landscape of public health, and governments of many low- and middle-income countries have increased their spending on health. However, in the absence of systematic evidence, there is ongoing debate about the merits of the global aid architecture and aid effectiveness in health. It is argued that technical assistance is often tied to and driven by donors and is not appropriate for the local setting of low- and middle-income countries. Recognising the reality of limited resources and flatlining of international donor funding, it is important for low- and middle-income countries to be efficient by meeting priority health needs or follow the approach of defining and providing a context-specific minimum service package or essential health package (EHP) of high quality.

Keywords Consumers of healthcare services · Essential health packages · Global aid architecture · Governance · Healthcare financing · Healthcare providers · Health systems strengthening · Human resources for health · International health consultancy · Knowledge management · Leadership · Medical malpractice · Monitoring performance · National health insurance · Health policies · Policymakers · Public-private partnerships · Quality improvement in health · Sector-wide approach · Technical assistance

M. P. Mabuza, *Evaluating International Public Health Issues*,
https://doi.org/10.1007/978-981-13-9787-5_3

3.1 Health Systems and Health Sector Reform

Health systems encompass all the entities and means whose primary goal is to improve the health of individuals and the population (World Health Organization (WHO) 2000). Crucially, health systems carry out service provision, resource generation, financing and stewardship, with the overall goals of achieving good health, responsiveness to the expectations of the population, and fairness of financial contribution (World Health Organization (WHO) 2000).

Although health systems vary greatly from country to country, many poor countries have weak health systems which become a major barrier in terms of the delivery of essential health services (Merson et al. 2012).

Lack of meaningful community engagement has been one of the major downfalls in the implementation of health policies and programmes in many countries. Much as some of the vertical funders of global health initiatives have played an important role in disease control, particularly in disease burdened settings, the truth is that the negative consequences of such initiatives are often overlooked.

The governments of the recipient countries often find themselves in a predicament, because on the one hand, they urgently need the financial support to address the disease burdens in their respective countries, and on the other hand they are unable to confront the vertical funders about their concerns, largely due to fear of losing the financial support. As such, the reality is that since the international vertical funders have the financial power, they end up driving the disease response agenda in the recipient countries. Such an agenda tends to be largely medicalised and overlooks the other main tenets of health and sustainability.

Some of the international vertical funders do focus on addressing aspects such as poverty as an important element of health. In such cases, the poverty alleviating interventions and programmes are designed and implemented according to the so-called evidence-based international standards and measures. However, such measures fall short of understanding the context of how the recipient populations see themselves and what solutions they think will work and be sustained. Recipient governments themselves tend to follow a similar posture to that of the international vertical funders by designing and implementing health policies without having meaningfully engaged with the population.

Marginalisation of the Indigenous People of Bolivia, Honduras and Nicaragua
In the cases of Bolivia, Honduras and Nicaragua (some of the poorest countries in South America), indigenous people are largely absent or marginalised from the planning, design and implementation of policies and programmes that directly affect their lives and communities (Feiring 2003). The negative consequence of the marginalisation of indigenous people can undermine sustainable development as the needs of indigenous people are unique and they vary from setting to setting. As such, poverty reduction strategies should take into account indigenous people's values and their own concept of poverty and wealth, and to involve them in the planning, design, implementation and monitoring of policies and programmes (Feiring 2003).

The unsuccessful universalistic implementation of the conditional cash transfer programme, aimed at improving primary school enrolment and access to healthcare services in Bolivia (one of the most diverse countries in South America), can be attributed to a number of factors, including lack of meaningful engagement of the entire population, from the beginning (McGuire 2013).

The Denmark-Bolivia Country Policy Paper 2013–2018 is interesting based on Denmark's vision for continued partnership with Bolivia and to contribute towards poverty reduction, sustainable development, green growth and promotion of human rights in Bolivia (Ministry of Foreign Affairs of Denmark 2013). In the document, it is also mentioned that there will be commercial business opportunities for Denmark and the potential for Danish enterprises to use Bolivia as an entry point to other South American markets (Ministry of Foreign Affairs of Denmark 2013). Was there any meaningful engagement with the population of Bolivia in the context of such a partnership? Who is bound to benefit the most from the Denmark-Bolivia international development partnership?

It is interesting that many countries have already implemented or are striving towards implementing a national health insurance (NHI) or national health protection scheme (NHPS) in one form or another, largely to address issues of inequalities in healthcare access. There is no doubt about the merit of an NHI or NHPS, however, an NHI or NHPS should not be seen as a quick fix or an immediate piece-meal change without planning for the consequences and the future. The planning, design, implementation, monitoring and evaluation of an NHI or NHPS should be viewed from a broader scheme of things, through effective leadership, management, governance and context.

National Health Policy and National Health Protection Scheme in India
It is interesting that the thrust of the National Health Policy (NHP) announced by the government of India, in March 2017, has adopted an insurance-based health protection model, whereby the government strategically purchases secondary and tertiary healthcare services from the private sector in order to fill critical gaps in the public health sector (Ahuja 2017). While the NHP emphasises universal health access, evidence shows that when the state purchases services from the private sector, it does not reduce the out-of-pocket health expenditure by the poor (Mishra and Agarwal 2017). The question is, how this is going to be sustained, bearing in mind that the India government's current expenditure on health is approximately 1.2% of GDP versus the global average level of 5.4%, and that India's basic health services is among the worst in the world as it is ranked 112 out of 190 countries (Sahoo 2018)? Another concern is India's unfinished agenda of the Millennium Development Goals (MDGs), and the many challenging targets that still need to be met towards achieving the Sustainable Development Goals (SDGs) by 2030 (Kumar et al. 2016). Some commentators feel that the implementation of India's National Health Protection Scheme (NHPS) was rushed. The concern is that while the public health system is not in a good state, and there are challenging SDGs to achieve, the government appears to be pulling out of providing health services and allowing the private sector to play a dominant role (Mishra and Agarwal 2017).

National Health Insurance in Afghanistan

Interestingly, the government of Afghanistan took a more cautious approach by conducting a feasibility study to determine the needs for health insurance, readiness for health insurance, and preparation for health insurance and roadmap, by engaging all stakeholders (Health Policy Project 2015). The findings of the feasibility study show that there is need for health insurance in Afghanistan, but there is need to first address structural issues related to sources of funding as there is currently heavy reliance on donor funding. It is acknowledged that despite the urgent need for health insurance in Afghanistan, there are legal barriers, lack of understanding and awareness of health insurance at community and government levels, lack of technical capacity, current quality of care, a large informal work sector, and inability to pay among members of the public (Health Policy Project 2015). Strong political commitment is required to address such challenges, and, as such, until all the challenges are addressed, Afghanistan is not in a position to establish health insurance schemes in the short term (Health Policy Project 2015).

Healthcare Issues of Indigenous and Senior Populations of Canada and USA

In the case of Canada, since the late 1940s, health insurance models were created to eliminate the financial barriers to care, and the intention was to follow this with reform of health service delivery models and social determinants of health with emphasis on population health needs. While the government has achieved the goal of establishing the health insurance, reform of health service delivery is still a challenge, and, for this to be achieved, it requires bold political vision and leadership, and joint effort by the government, healthcare providers and the public. All along, the government has involved prominent stakeholders and experts in policy development for health, and it is only recently that the role of citizens as individuals or groups is beginning to be defined and understood (Ham 2001). It is considered sound leadership to ensure that all stakeholders at all levels are involved in policy development for health, rather than the vertical or top-down approach that is often seen in many countries.

In Canada, the issue of lack of meaningful involvement of seniors and indigenous people is still rearing its head, from time to time. As such, the Commonwealth Fund's 2017 International Health Policy Survey of Seniors aimed at providing perspectives on how well health systems in Canada are meeting the needs and expectations of seniors, was necessary, even though this survey benchmarked with experiences of seniors from ten other high-income countries (Canadian Institute for Health Information 2018). It was encouraging to see that 80% of Canadian seniors rated their health as excellent, very good or good, which is a higher proportion than the international average (Canadian Institute for Health Information 2018). Although Canada's health system is viewed among the best in the world, it is of concern that Canada continues to perform below the international average in terms of Canadian citizens being unsatisfied with the quality of healthcare they receive, and being unable to get a same-day or next day appointment in primary healthcare (Evans 2018; Canadian Institute for Health Information 2018).

It is equally concerning to see from the survey results that the USA seniors are sicker, more economically vulnerable, and face greater financial barriers to medical care and social care as compared to seniors in the ten other countries (Osborn 2017).

The Health System of Cuba – A Good Model

The case of Cuba's health system is a beacon of hope as it is regarded as a good model from which many low-, middle- and high-income countries can learn. Over the years, Cuba's economic and political isolation has been challenging and painful, and yet, in the midst of such pain, one of the best health systems in the world was developed, through great leadership and political will by the government of Cuba. Lessons learnt from the flourishing health system of Cuba are that building an effective and strong health system is not spontaneous; it is systematic, consistent and sustainable; it requires political will, commitment and accountability; it is embedded in sound principles of public and social nature, preventive orientation, accessibility, free of cost, legitimate and meaningful community participation, inter-sector approach, international cooperation, adequate application of technological innovations, and availability and use of tools for monitoring and evaluation (Serrate et al. 2007).

Challenges and Opportunities of the Health System of Cambodia

If Cuba can do it, there is definitely hope for many other countries such as Cambodia whose health systems had been crippled by history of war, lack of financing, inequitable access, shortage of healthcare workers, and poor healthcare service delivery in the public sector. It is encouraging to see that Cambodia's government has been showing political will and commitment in recent times, evidenced by the concrete health policy initiatives to improve accountability, coordination, equity, accessibility of basic health services, affordability, efficiency, quality of care, protection of the poor, and to ensure sustainable development (Suy et al. 2017).

Challenges and Opportunities on Health Policies of the Western Balkans

The case of the Western Balkans countries such as Bosnia and Herzegovina, Serbia, Kosovo, Montenegro, Croatia, and The Former Yugoslav Republic of Macedonia, is an interesting one from the perspective of their health policies at national and European level, and the fact that some of these countries are relatively new. While the Western Balkans countries have made notable progress in their respective healthcare reforms and in line with the European Union requirements, there are still many challenges (Hodzic 2017). The challenges are mainly related to poorly organised and unsustainable healthcare financing; poor implementation of policy and legislative documents; poor monitoring and evaluation of policies and strategies nor analysis for impact; lack of involvement of patients in the development of health policies; and lack of regulations to prevent the misuse of public powers, especially with regard to public procurement (Hodzic 2017). Much as it is encouraging that the Swiss government is well positioned and already putting special emphasis on supporting Kosovo to address the health policy and programme challenges, there is urgent need for political will and governance in Kosovo and the rest of the Western Balkans to address the challenges (Swiss Agency for Development and Cooperation (CDC) 2016).

Internationally and intra-nationally, the days of business as usual are over, as health leaders, policy makers and governments have tried a countless number of times to implement fixes which have not had much impact (Porter and Lee 2013). In healthcare, the focus must shift to a fundamental change "value agenda" which at its core is maximising value for consumers of healthcare services (Porter and Lee 2013).

Governments across the world will fall short of meeting the Sustainable Development Goals (SDGs) unless they drastically change gear and take urgent action. It cannot be business as usual if many countries are experiencing an explosion of communicable and non-communicable diseases (NCDs), if the agenda of dealing with environmental degradation and climate change and its health effects is being glossed over, if man-made humanitarian crises still persist, if inequalities on healthcare access between the rich and the poor are not improving, if unsustainable healthcare financing is still a major issue in many low- and middle-income countries, if there is still polarisation and lack of meaningful integration between the so called "mainstream" and "non-mainstream" health systems, if many health systems are so fragile that they are on the brink of collapse, if effective leadership for health is still a "scarce commodity" in many countries.

Birn and Richter (2017) make an interesting observation about the international health agenda being largely driven by capitalist and philanthrocapitalist fundamentals and narrow medicalised understanding of disease and its control. The questions are: how ethical is the capitalist driven international health agenda, who really benefits, what are the consequences for recipient governments and the health of their populations, and how can capitalism and the predatory market logic to support human equity and ecological survival into the future be tamed or transformed (Van de Pas 2017)?

Ultimately, Heads of State and Government, and not Ministers of Health, must take decisive action for ownership in the best interest of their populations and for future generations, through political will, accountability, effective and efficient implementation of context-specific health policies and programmes, and sustainable investment (Nishtar et al. 2018).

Whilst it should be recognised that each country's health system is unique, reforms should aim to address the main challenges that typically face health systems which include issues of poor usage and inequitable access of services in the poorest countries, inefficiency, and consumer dissatisfaction (Merson et al. 2012). The key health sector reform areas that policymakers should consider in order to address the health systems challenges are regulation, financing, resource allocation and provision (Merson et al. 2012).

Regulation is crucial because it ensures that minimum quality standards are set and enforced, and it also encourages efficient and equitable health care financing and delivery of services (Merson et al. 2012). The unfortunate reality is that many poor countries do not have the capacity to enforce regulation effectively, largely because of the numerous small-scale health providers particularly in the private sector, and also due to competing interests (Merson et al. 2012).

Financing should feature prominently on the policy agenda for health reforms because most health systems in the poor countries are poorly funded, which exacerbates inequitable access to and delivery of services and impedes the achievement of Development Goals (Fryatt et al. 2010). As such, policymakers of countries such as South Africa are seriously engaged with the process of implementing a National Health Insurance (NHI) to try and address the issue of inequitable access to health services. Some suggestions are that policymakers should implement policies that will make it compulsory for those who are rich to pay tax such as in the better-off countries and to target public funding at the poorest sectors of society (Merson et al. 2012).

Resource allocation has to take into consideration the reforming of payment systems and the mechanisms by which payments between providers and purchasers of service are made, bearing in mind the contractual agreements (Merson et al. 2012). Governments should make allocations for specific packages of essential health services such as family planning, vector control, clinical services, monitoring and surveillance, among others (Merson et al. 2012).

Provision of services should be considered in terms of decentralisation of services, competition between providers as means to improve efficiency, and improvement of primary health care services (Merson et al. 2012). Policies need to be implemented to address the issue of capacity of health human resources. Other key areas of consideration should include evidence-based healthcare, increasing the influence of users over health providers so that the providers are held accountable for their performance, and to ensure that there is quality improvement (Merson et al. 2012).

Whilst policymakers are better positioned to influence reforms for strengthening health systems, the challenge is to know and understand what the specific health system requires, as each health system is unique and sometimes unpredictable. As such, the reforms should be context-specific (World Health Organization (WHO) 2007a, b, c).

Health care reform offers both promising opportunities and formidable risks for both service suppliers and consumers. Many health systems are using market mechanisms, competition, and incentives as a way of driving reform. The benefits of this are seen as increased responsiveness to the needs of patients and payers, and the ability to increase and reduce supply quickly when required, greater efficiency, innovation such as the development of new and effective pharmaceuticals, and less unhelpful meddling in provider management by central authorities.

The increased responsiveness to the needs of patients, the ability to increase supply when required, the great efficiency and innovation, would be a factor in allowing the family to obtain medication that would be more effective in bringing the child's fever down. Through managed care, and through the medical aid schemes, in South Africa and the Kingdom of Eswatini, medication can also be delivered for example by motorcycles or speed delivery to where patients live. For example, if the medication is brought to the family, it would help so that the mother does not have to travel far to get treatment for the child. These advantages are potentially important but come with some problems and costs. The policy question is, at what point the costs exceed the expected benefits?

It is worth remembering that health care market operates differently from the more familiar market of goods and services where transactions are based on supply and demand. In health care markets, suppliers such as providers, facilities and doctors create their own demands, making for a complicated and imperfect relationship with the consumers or patients (Birn et al. 2009). As such, unregulated health markets are unlikely to provide equitable health care because they put the consumer or the patient at a disadvantage while the providers reap benefits. Government's intervention in health markets is therefore practical, necessary, and morally sound to ensure that there is equitable access to healthcare. The government does not need to be the only instrument in this regard, but market forces can also do the same thing by making government a partner – not a prosecutor.

Although market mechanisms are undoubtedly effective in terms of increasing responsiveness and efficiency, some caution is required as much of the evidence is debatable or unclear and little of it comes from systems with fixed administratively set prices. Market mechanisms have limitations as a method for shaping the system and should be seen as part of a mix of policies rather than a magic bullet solution.

Nonetheless, the dominant international health actors insist on a market approach to health services especially in low- and middle-income country settings, where donors are instrumental in health financing (Birn et al. 2009).

3.2 Health Systems Strengthening and the Role of Knowledge Management and Leadership

The WHO (2000) acknowledges that leadership or stewardship is ultimately concerned with the oversight of the entire health system, and that healthcare financing is the main challenge facing low- and middle-income countries. It can be deduced that the main channels through which the health system is affected are through leadership and its impact on healthcare financing and related effects such as multi-stakeholder harmonisation and service delivery.

Fragmented and poorly-led health systems are a silent killer as they cause more sickness and disproportionate numbers of deaths within populations just as in epidemics (Dwyer and Wilhelmsen n.d.). Although it is often technically and medically known what is required to reduce illness and to save lives, but what is often lacking is the dearth of knowledge and skills to lead and manage the complexities of health systems (Dwyer and Wilhelmsen n.d.).

Evidence shows that there is lack of an enabling environment for health systems leadership to flourish, particularly in the low- and middle-income countries such as in sub-Saharan Africa, and this calls for a disruption in the status quo (Gilson and Agyepong 2018). Typically, current leadership practices are a barrier to health systems strengthening as they tend to show features of authoritarian rather than participatory leadership style, decision-making is largely centralised or individualised, and the dominance of medical professionals is an impediment to progress (Gilson and Agyepong 2018). Such a status quo is a recipe for disaster because it could exacerbate the fragility of the other key building blocks of health systems.

"Knowledge management (has potential for maximising results through continuous assessment, capture, synthesis, generation, and sharing of relevant information and knowledge) – connecting the right people to the right data, information, and knowledge at the right time – is increasingly being considered as an effective approach to help strengthen health systems" (USAID 2012). For example, in the finance building block of the health system, knowledge management ensures that a health system has adequate funds and can potentially help identify barriers to service access. As such, the management of this knowledge will affect individual lives, whole communities, and, ultimately, the health, social, and economic status of the entire world. "Studies show that global health organisations that adopt knowledge management strategies and practices can strengthen the performance of health care workers and programmes, and, therefore, leveraging the power of knowledge management can transform global health and development" (Sullivan et al. 2015).

Leadership literature identifies leadership as a central pillar for health systems strengthening, in terms of improving the priority areas of access, quality and utilisation, to ensure sustainability and positive impact (Alva et al. 2009; Opio et al. 2010). As such, there has been a growing realisation that all leaders in healthcare should have the skills and competency to lead. This includes the ability to scan for opportunities and resources, focus on priority areas, alignment and mobilisation, inspiring, planning, organising, implementing, monitoring and evaluation.

Effective leadership is the sine qua non for achieving maximum impact from health investments at global, national and local levels, yet, this vital pillar is often missing (Quick 2011). Much as it is laudable that the World Health Organization (WHO) recently issued a statement calling all countries to make three specific commitments to universal health coverage, and be prepared to announce them at the World Health Assembly scheduled for 21 May 2018, such commitments are not enough, unless health systems are strengthened (Eghan 2018).

An eight-year retrospective study aimed at evaluating the leadership training program within the Centres for Disease Control and Prevention, revealed that such a program had a positive impact on the participants' leadership effectiveness (Woltring et al. 2003). However, it can be argued that such leadership effectiveness was more about how the participants felt after the training process rather than the impact of their leadership, in practice. It can also be argued that with the rapidly changing healthcare environment, leadership skills and competencies, alone, do not guarantee better health outcomes (Jooste 2009).

In that regard, the WHO (2007a, b, c) suggested a framework that included leadership competencies, adequate numbers of trained leaders, an enabling working environment, and functional support systems. The good thing about having such a framework is that it provides a structure of what needs to be done so that there could be accountability of leadership's implementation of policy.

However, the WHO framework for leadership and management strengthening in health systems appears to overlook the contextual factors such as how to deal with unique complexities of each specific environment. The application of such a framework and the impact of leadership in specific settings could be a challenge. In most instances, leaders know what to do, in theory, but the application or implementation is always a challenge.

The leadership theories, models or frameworks have been criticised because they are generic instead of being context-specific, bearing in mind that regions, countries and districts are unique, and one glove does not fit all. Theories, models or frameworks are useful as a point of reference, but they should not be prescriptive and static, they should be relevant and evolving, in line with the constantly changing healthcare landscape.

Heading (2009) puts it succinctly in a discussion paper which highlights that the changing health systems environment requires more than a mechanistic approach, but a consideration of broader influences and local issues. As such, leadership strengthening of health systems should consider a mix of leadership traits, behaviours, tools, and contextual factors (Heading 2009).

Global Health Leadership

The Report of the G8 Health Experts Group acknowledges the global health leadership mandate that the WHO has, as well as the financial global health dominance of the World Bank. The strength of the report is that it highlights the need to reposition and strengthen global health leadership, in line with the changing landscape of global health architecture, bearing in mind the limitations of WHO and the World Bank.

The WHO, operating within the United Nations, responsible for global health leadership and governance, produced a report with comparisons and rankings of different health systems (Smith and Papanicolas 2012). The comparison and ranking of health systems serves the purpose of benchmarking so that strengths and weaknesses could be highlighted from which lessons could be learnt for better performance (Kumar and Ozdamar 2004). However, the weaknesses of such comparisons were the methodological challenges that were inherent in such comparisons as health systems differ from a contextual and cultural perspective (Kelley et al. 2006). There was also the dilemma of how the findings should be communicated to the policymakers, and how such findings should be used by the policymakers of the different countries (Kelley et al. 2006).

The World Health Report 2000 acknowledges that leadership or stewardship is ultimately concerned with the oversight of the entire health system, and that healthcare financing is the main challenge facing low- and middle-income countries (WHO 2000). The World Health Report placed leadership on the lap of national authorities or policy makers to ensure that policies are implemented and that there are specific indicators for better performance of health systems (WHO 2000). It also placed the responsibility on leadership to ensure that there is effective healthcare financing to enable equitable healthcare access by all (WHO 2000). However, the WHO report was oblivious of the uniqueness of each country and the complexity of the roles that multiple stakeholders such as the private sector, NGOs, and development or donor agencies could play in the health system. In an assessment of the

World Health Report 2000, it is argued against the report's mechanistic view of health systems strengthening. Such mechanistic view focused on the "conventional wisdom" of "magic bullets" to fix the health systems challenges from a government's perspective, and overlooked the social, economic, and political dynamics of each country. There is need to have a better understanding of leadership's successes and challenges in the health sector so that context-specific solutions could be developed, bearing in mind the multiple stakeholders in the context of each setting.

A summary of the debate at the Special Session on Future Directions in Health Care Financing held at the 6th Congress of the International Health Economics Association (iHEA) highlighted the knowledge gap pertaining to healthcare financing in low- and middle-income countries (Danish Ministry of Foreign Affairs 2007). Such a debate was an eye opener because the main focus was on major funding mechanisms that could sustain healthcare financing in the context of both developed and developing countries. However, the weakness of the debate was that it was based on existing studies which were conducted in developed countries because of the paucity of studies conducted in developing countries. It would be interesting to explore how leadership's increased focus on specific disease programmes such as HIV and AIDS, tuberculosis, and malaria has affected the opportunity cost of addressing other urgent health matters such as the escalating epidemic of non-communicable diseases, and the need for investing in innovation and technology in changing the future of healthcare in disease high burden countries and regions.

A retrospective and prospective analysis of the 2014 West African Ebola epidemic highlights lack of budget as a limitation of WHO (Gostin and Friedman 2014). Lack of legal framework to interact with the public sector, private sector, NGOs and development agencies is highlighted as another weakness of WHO (Gostin and Friedman 2014).

According to an article by Montegut (2007), the other limitation of WHO has been the disease-focused vertical approach to global healthcare instead of a broad-based horizontal approach. Other authors argue that a combination of vertical and horizontal approaches and flexibility to suite each particular context could be the best approach.

The fundamental structural changes of the global health architecture of the twenty-first century have been characterised by the emergence of influential stakeholders in the global health leadership arena. Stakeholders such as the Bill & Melinda Gates Foundation, GAVI, and the Global Fund, have come at the back of a declining prior dominance of WHO and the World Bank.

The embracing of global health by the G8, and the emergence of the Health 8 or H8 provides a locus for discussion on global health policy and an opportunity for collaborative global health leadership efforts. However, the weakness is that the G8 has lack of capacity, and the H8 is still trying to find its role in the global health leadership milieu. It can be argued that since the G8 comprises leaders of the advanced market economies, how could the health agenda for middle- and low-income countries be decided by a few rich countries? Perhaps, this point of view calls for purposefulness, organisation and synergy between an empowered and more effective WHO at the top and sustainable, equitable national health systems at the root core (Gostin and Friedman 2014).

There is an increasing need to define, understand and manage the global health system amidst the challenges of globalisation (Johnson and Stoskopf 2010). The constantly changing global health landscape requires leaders to have joint commitment and eyes to see and act on global health challenges that are happening now, and eyes to see and act on global health challenges that will happen in the future (Fried et al. 2012). It requires global health leaders to walk the talk, to have new thinking and new ways of doing and acting to address current global health challenges and to prevent future challenges (Fried et al. 2012).

Leadership in Sub-Saharan African Health Systems

Health leadership in Sub-Saharan Africa is faced with many challenges, largely due to weak health systems and the heavy burden of disease such as HIV and AIDS, TB, malaria, and the epidemic of non-communicable diseases. Health systems in Sub-Saharan Africa are further paralysed by poverty, disasters such as drought and flooding, and political instability in some of the countries (Merson et al. 2012).

The findings of a 2007–2008 health systems review conducted in five Sub-Saharan African countries including Kenya, Malawi, Namibia, Uganda and Zambia showed that all these countries had weak health policies and inadequate health coverage (Tumusiime et al. n.d.). The weak health policies were an indication of weaknesses in health leadership and governance of the surveyed countries. Although it was a strength of this review that some of the sources of information were population-based surveys, it was a weakness that the sources of information were multiple and could not be ascertained (Tumusiime et al. n.d.).

The 2014 Ebola epidemic that ravaged multiple countries in West Africa including Liberia, Sierra Leone, Guinea, and to a less extent Mali, Nigeria, and Senegal, exposed the frailties of health systems leadership of the region (Gostin and Friedman 2014). This indicates that the health systems of many Sub-Saharan African countries do not have the capacity to deal with emergency disease outbreaks or epidemics. The 2014 Ebola epidemic in West Africa also presented an opportunity for learning and strengthening of health systems leadership in Sub-Saharan Africa.

A non-randomised quantitative study conducted in Kenya to test the effectiveness of leadership between those leaders and workers who had received leadership training and those who had not received training, showed the benefits of leadership training (Seims et al. 2012). This study revealed that strengthening leadership skills through team-based approaches resulted in significantly improved and sustained service delivery outcomes (Seims et al. 2012). The significance of the study was that it highlighted the importance of teamwork and collaborations in addition to leadership skills. As such, leadership skills should also be imparted to those who are led so that there could be synergy and sustainability of efforts. The weakness of this study was that it placed more emphasis on the technical skills and overlooked the other contextual factors that affect health systems. Since the improved health outcomes were sustained for six months, it would be interesting to see if the improved health outcomes would have been sustained for a longer period. A qualitative study would have provided a better insight pertaining to the reasons for the health outcomes as there could be other context-specific factors involved.

A qualitative study involving in-depth interviews of seventeen healthcare leaders in four African countries including Ethiopia, Ghana, Liberia and Rwanda, revealed that leadership needs to go beyond technical competency. Such a finding was important because it highlighted the recognition of a broader dimension of leadership that included non-mechanistic contextual factors. It was interesting that the motivation for conducting such a study was the fact that there was little research done to understand the context of health leadership in Africa. The fact that most of the leadership capacity building research was contextualised from a high-income country perspective was also a stimulus to conduct such research from an African context. The weakness of the study was that it only focused on leaders from the public health sector. As such, there was a need to explore the experiences of leaders from a broader angle that encompassed the public sector, private sector, NGOs, and development agencies in order to gain deeper insight as to why leadership in health is not as effective as it should.

Much as the South African national health leadership has committed to reducing inequalities in healthcare provision, there is a growing public impatience with the inability of the South African health system to deliver as well as it could. The disparities are glaring between the public health sector which largely serves the majority of the South African population who cannot afford, and the private health sector which largely serves the minority of the population which comprises those who can afford. Although the South African government contributes about 40% of all expenditure on health, the public sector is under pressure to deliver services to about 80% of the population. Despite this, most resources are concentrated in the private sector, which sees to the health needs of the remaining 20% of the population.

Understanding the factors that contribute to trends in public financing of health is a sensitive topic, particularly the role of ministries of finance. It is commendable that at least, the process of introducing a National Health Insurance (NHI) is in progress with the ultimate goal of balancing the terrain pertaining to the issue of access to quality healthcare care by all in South Africa. The question is how long will it take to fully implement the NHI, how will it be sustained amidst the growing challenges of health systems leadership, the fragmented efforts of many stakeholders, and the widening inequality gap between those who can afford and those who cannot, and the global economic challenges?

South Africa being the country with the highest burden of HIV and AIDS in the world, continues to face many challenges in effectively managing HIV and AIDS amidst the renewed government's vigour and political will. Some of the challenges have been due to the overcrowding of the HIV and AIDS arena by multiple and fragmented efforts of different stakeholders, including the public sector, private sector, non-governmental organisations (NGOs) and the development or donor agencies. The health system's competing demands of managing the HIV and ADS burden, the tuberculosis burden, the epidemic of non-communicable diseases, maternal and child mortality, and deaths through violence and accidents, also form part of the equation (Chopra et al. 2009).

Recognizing the diversity and interrelationship of urgently needed health policy areas, such as health systems leadership strengthening, equitable healthcare financing, multi-stakeholder harmonisation, and service delivery performance, is vital to understanding and addressing the gaps for improvement of health outcomes and responsiveness of the health system. Ultimately, leadership is responsible for ensuring that there is population health improvement, equitable healthcare financing, well-coordinated and high performing health service delivery that meets the expectations of the population.

A three-year participant observation study conducted in Mozambique revealed that the deluge of NGOs and their expatriate workers had fragmented the local health system, undermined local control of health programs, and contributed to growing local social inequality. Similarly, though not necessarily in sub-Saharan Africa, an exploratory qualitative study presenting the viewpoints of government, NGOs and donors in Pakistan, revealed that fragmented efforts contributed to further weakening of health systems. The study highlighted that the NGO model was ineffective, and that lack of collaboration between international aid workers and their local counterparts was a critical issue in primary health care. The recommendations were that there should be further research on these important dynamics, as they remained understudied, particularly in sub-Saharan African countries such as South Africa. As such, it would be critical to understand the impact of leadership on multi-stakeholder harmonisation in disease high burden countries and regions which are typically characterised by multi-stakeholder fragmentation.

In a presentation of case studies that focused on the improvement of health systems in Africa, there was a projected gloomy picture exacerbated by the fragmented investment in specific diseases programmes such as HIV and AIDS. Whilst international donor agencies have helped establish HIV and AIDS-specific systems and processes distinct from those of other health programmes, these HIV and AIDS-specific processes use many of the same resources as the country's broader health system. Drawing from the Joint United Nations Programme on HIV and AIDS's call for the redesigning of the AIDS response for long-term impact through leadership and collaborations, to achieve better outcomes by 2031, it would be important to explore how leadership's increased focus on specific disease programmes such as HIV and AIDS has affected healthcare service delivery performance in disease high burden countries, particularly low- and middle-income countries whose health systems are often faced with many constraints.

Collection of evidence is a prerequisite for a context-specific action. Such collection of evidence should be aligned with a clear understanding of the key functions that a health system must undertake and should be responsive to local conditions (World Health Organization (WHO) 2000). This evidence requires a common framework for monitoring and evaluation of the health systems strengthening actions so that there could be compatibility of data, transparency of methods, and accountability.

One of the advantages of the collection of evidence is that it acts as a repository or body of knowledge which is like a guide on what works and what does not, so that each country is better equipped to adopt and adapt the lessons learned from every other nation, and in this way, knowledge and action will reinforce each other, bringing the world closer to the common goals of better health for all.

There are lessons to be learned from the health systems strengthening actions of Rwanda, where health has been improving since 2000, which shows that comprehensive evidence-based interventions can create robust, responsive, and efficient health systems. It is believed that by combining implementation experience with continuous experimentation and robust impact evaluation is poised to generate replicable lessons that can improve health and health equity in Rwanda and throughout the world.

At the same time, it has to be acknowledged that health sector reforms cannot be developed from a single global or regional policy formula, as any reform will depend on the country's history, values and culture, and the population's expectations (Senkubuge et al. 2014). One of the major downfalls of some of the health systems of some countries is the misconception that things are just too complicated and can automatically be fixed by technologies and other evidence-based actions without having a better understanding of what that particular health system really requires. For example, there is such a severe shortage of health human resources in some of the SADC countries, and as such, any health systems strengthening actions that overlook this very issue are bound to fail. Could this be an issue of leadership?

The significance of a certain type of leadership to drive the health systems reforms, needs to be highlighted. In fact, leadership or stewardship is regarded as the core component of health systems strengthening because leadership is ultimately responsible for oversight of the overall health system (World Health Organization (WHO) 2000). Given the many actors in the health systems, strong leadership is needed to ensure effective coordination and communication between the many different stakeholders (Kingue et al. 2013).

3.3 Human Resources for Health

Whilst it is often acknowledged that workers are the most important asset, many governments and organisations fall short when it comes to putting effective incentives, policies and systems in place for generating and sustaining high performance among workers. This is acutely felt in resource-poor settings such as in sub-Saharan Africa where there is a growing challenge of low morale of health workers, particularly, in the public sector.

A mix of financial and non-financial incentives is important as part of a strategy to attract, retain and motivate staff, including health workers in resource-poor settings (Global Health Workforce Alliance (GHWA) 2008). The feasibility of using financial and non-financial incentives is dependent on the particular context such as the socioeconomic and cultural context of the setting (Chaix-Coturier et al. 2000).

In some of the resource-poor settings of Southern Africa, it may be feasible to use financial incentives such as rural allowance for health workers who are based in rural or remote areas as means to attract, motivate and retain health professionals in the rural areas (Ditlopo et al. 2011). In addition to salaries, bonuses for good performance, medical aid allowance, paid leave, housing allowance, transport allowance, an interesting financial incentive that has been implemented in South Africa is the occupation-specific dispensation aimed at attracting, motivating and retaining health professionals in the public sector (Ditlopo et al. 2011).

However, it is worth mentioning that some of the financial incentives become a challenge to sustain in some of the resource-poor settings. Sometimes there may just be unintended negative consequences of the financial incentives mainly due to poorly designed and poorly implemented policies such as the occupation-specific dispensation which has ended up causing friction among the health professionals in the South African public sector (Gerston 2004). As such, even if health systems are adequately financed, it is possible that poor leadership, poor planning and inappropriately implemented policies may make it difficult to sustain the financial incentives, thereby resulting in a negative impact on the staff's morale (Ditlopo et al. 2013).

Financial incentives are more important in terms of attracting staff to the organisation, whereas non-financial incentives such as recognition and rewards are more important in terms of retaining staff. Other non-financial incentives that are feasible include praise for attainment of organisational objectives, acknowledgement and recognition for performance, constructive feedback to strengthen the staff's self-worth, enrichment of tasks to enhance the staff's self-worth and self-motivation, and flexible working hours to enhance self-motivation and allow staff to tailor their work according their strengths (Jooste 2009). Further, relief from heavy workloads, opportunities for career growth and development, positive working environments and employee assistance and support could be important for improving staff morale and self-worth (Global Health Workforce Alliance (GHWA) 2008). Studies show that there is an association between leadership style, working conditions, employee morale and productivity, yet, this is often played down (Mabuza 2018c; Mabuza and Shumba 2018).

The challenge with non-financial incentives is that they require leaders to be closely connected to their staff in a transparent and meaningful way so that the staff can feel valued, but, the reality is that many leaders claim not to have enough time because they are always busy (Domenico 2007). Strong leadership, proper planning and more constructive engagements between leaders and workers are vital to ensure that incentive policies are appropriately implemented and sustained (Global Health Workforce Alliance (GHWA) 2008).

The migration or exodus of health care workforce such as physicians from poorer settings is indeed an important issue that is seriously affecting many low- and middle-income countries. For example, it is reported that more than 37% of South Africa's doctors and more than 7% of its nurses have migrated to developed countries such as Australia, Britain, Canada, Finland, France, Germany, New Zealand, Portugal, and the United States of America (Nduru 2006). The loss of healthcare professionals in resource-poor settings leaves already struggling health systems in an even more dire state as loss of years of investment leaves these poor settings with a loss of hope (World Health Organization (WHO) 2006a, b).

Such a situation needs urgent international interventions and working together for health as the acute shortage of health professionals is putting sub-Saharan Africa and many other affected developing countries in other parts of the world in a quandary (Nduru 2006). However, the challenge is that the solution is not as straightforward as it may seem, because there are many factors involved, as the migration of health care professionals is not only taking place from developing countries but also within developing countries of the same region or continent (World Health Organization (WHO) 2006a, b).

For example, whilst sub-Saharan countries such as Eswatini and South Africa are lamenting about a shortage of health care professionals due to the massive exodus of their health care professionals to developed countries, the irony is that both Eswatini and South Africa are themselves receiving many health professionals who migrate from other African countries. The existence of a policy not to recruit health professionals from fellow developing countries in the African continent has to a little extent assisted the South African Department of Health in stemming the internal brain drain to South Africa (Nduru 2006).

At face value, it may appear as if the main reason for migration of the health workforce is financial incentives, but on close examination of the situation, there may be deeper reasons as some authors observe this phenomenon as one of the most controversial aspects of globalisation having attracted considerable attention in the health policy discourse at both the technical and political level (Taylor et al. 2011).

It is believed that the migration of health professionals from developing countries to developed countries will continue because developing countries cannot realistically match the financial lure of the developed economies, but there are realistic strategies of proven effectiveness to limit the negative effects of the brain drain such as the following (Cometto et al. 2013):

- Placing greater emphasis on non-wage retention strategies, including improving working and living conditions;
- Diversifying the skills mix to harness the potential of non-physician clinicians and community health workers; the credentials awarded to these cadres only recognisable in their own country, making them less vulnerable to international migration;
- Circular migration; that is promoting a triangular flow of talent and skills by encouraging some migrant health workers to return to their home country (Cometto et al. 2013).

The loss of human resource capacity compounded by the emigration of experienced and qualified health professionals has had a severe impact on the health system in South Africa (George et al. 2013). It has to be acknowledged though that this challenge is not isolated in southern Africa, but other regions such as the Caribbean, south East Asia, and South America also face similar challenges. But what makes this crisis so severe and compounded in many sub-Saharan African countries including South Africa is the fact that sub-Saharan Africa has 25% of the world's diseases burden such as HIV, AIDS and TB, and yet, it possesses only 1.3% of trained human resources for health (George et al. 2013).

Seeing the rapidly increasing emigration of skilled public sector employees leading to acute shortage of human resources including human resources for health, the South Africa government introduced the Occupation-Specific Dispensation (OSD) in 2007. The main aim of the OSD was to improve the public services' ability to attract and retain employees including public sector health professionals though substantial pay hikes, thereby reducing incentives to emigrate.

However, in 2009, public sector doctor relations with their employer, soured by clumsy, inconsistent provincial implementation of the long awaited OSD pay hikes and further delayed mid-level category doctors pay talk, were on a knife edge (Bateman 2010). This friction between the doctors and the South African government led to a full-blown public sector doctors' strike that lasted for almost six months, and virtually paralysed the health system. Although this issue was subsequently addressed, in some way, it is not uncommon to come across a number of public sector health professionals who still feel betrayed by the South African government because it did not keep the initial promise. This has caused friction even amongst the medical personnel themselves, because there is a feeling that certain categories of doctors and nurses got a raw deal whilst others benefited. A recent study shows that more than 51% of doctors in the Eastern Province of South Africa view the OSD as now being a frustration for them mainly due to delayed payments.

Another aspect of the friction that ensued is that of other health professionals such as Pharmacists who perceive the implementation of the OSD as far removed from that initial promise and many pharmacists in the public sector feel betrayed (Gray and van der Merwe 2009). They feel that the employer (the national and provincial Departments of Health) has engaged in bad faith negotiation, has ignored reasoned inputs, and has little or no regard for the contribution pharmacists make to the safe and effective use of medicines (Gray and van der Merwe 2009). Pharmacy personnel as a group feel that their medical colleagues have secured a better deal, in recognition not only of their professional status and numbers, but also their perceived political power (Gray and van der Merwe 2009).

In addition to the workforce shortages, skill-mix imbalances, and maldistribution of professionals has also been a challenge that has compromised the performance of health professionals and the health system (Frenk et al. 2010). Further, the post-secondary training of health professionals is often overlooked in the context of the challenge to attract and retain the healthcare workforce.

In Southern Africa, some health professionals have emigrated because their medical school training which relies on 20th and twenty-first century models that emphasise diagnosis and treatment has not equipped them to face the real challenges facing the populations they serve (Mabuza 2018a, b; Pruitt and Epping-Jordan 2005). Much as this is a challenge, it is encouraging that educational leaders, health professional bodies, and the World Health Organisation recognise such models as inadequate for health workers caring for a growing population of patients with health problems that persist across decades or lifetimes (Pruitt and Epping-Jordan 2005).

According to The University of Sidney (2012), institutions of higher learning play a critical role in training health professionals, but the numbers trained, and the type of education provided is not necessarily well connected to the country's health needs. With rising numbers of health and medical graduates, a major issue is whether they will have opportunities to work in areas which interest them or for which their courses have prepared them (The University of Sidney 2012).

Training should be restructured to include a new set of core competencies (knowledge, skills, abilities, personal qualities, experience, or other characteristics)-new "tricks" that prepare twenty-first century health workers to manage today's most prevalent health problems (Pruitt and Epping-Jordan 2005).

The following ten recommendations provide guidance for efforts to strengthen medical education in sub-Saharan Africa (Mullan et al. 2011:

- Launch campaigns to develop capacity of medical school faculties, including recruitment, training, retention;
- Increase investment in medical education infrastructure;
- Build structures to promote inter-ministerial collaboration for medical education;
- Fund research and research training at medical schools;
- Promote community-oriented education based on principles of primary health care;
- Establish national and regional postgraduate medical education programmes to promote training, excellence, and retention;
- Establish national or regional bodies that are responsible for accreditation and quality assurance of medical education;
- Increase donor investment in medical education aligned with national health needs;
- Recognise and review the growing role of private institutions in medical education;
- Revitalise the African Medical Schools Association.

The education of health workers must seek to: strengthen the overall intellectual culture of a society; define principles for public aspiration; give life to and enlarge the best and most proven ideas of the age; refine the grounds for the private exchanges that take place in our lives; facilitate the exercise of political power; and enable professionals to detect what is important and discard what is irrelevant, accommodate oneself with others, have common ground between colleagues across societies, and ask good questions and find the means to answer them, and have the resources to adapt to national and global circumstances (Horton 2010).

3.4 Essential Health Packages

Essential medical laboratory services could provide evidence-based recommendations to support essential health packages (EHPs) (Dacombe et al. 2006). There are different interpretations of EHPs, but in general they could be defined in the context of a sector-wide approach as aspirational or short-term tools meant to apportion tailored, cost effective health services, aimed at addressing health priorities, and are sometimes considered as a safety net for the poor or vulnerable populations (Ensor et al. 2002; World Health Organization (WHO) 2008).

Implementation of essential medical laboratory services has some constraints such as in Malawi as highlighted below (Dacombe et al. 2006).

Constraints:

- Policymakers' lack of understanding of the resource requirements of a functional laboratory and how a laboratory functions, and health workers' lack of awareness of vital diagnostic approaches to EHP conditions (Dacombe et al. 2006; Mueller et al. 2011).
- Screening blood for infections can be very costly especially if the "gold standard" methods are employed such as light microscopy for detection of malaria parasites, and sputum-smear microscopy for detection of TB bacilli, as these are difficult to provide in the remote settings as such screenings require huge investments in high level technical expertise, quality monitoring and equipment maintenance which are lacking at the primary care level (Dacombe et al. 2006)
- The magnitude of the problem such as high prevalence of blood-borne infections in Malawi could overwhelm the capacity of the laboratory services (Dacombe et al. 2006).
- Patients and their relatives may have to travel far to have their blood screened in a district laboratory, and this may be an added burden not only on the sick but on households of the sick as well in terms of transport costs and poor infrastructure (Dacombe et al. 2006)
- The community's negative perception of the laboratory services could result in underutilisation of the laboratory services (Derua et al. 2011).

Possible solutions:

- It would be crucial to assess and collect locally relevant evidence about the needs of the communities and the feasibility of providing laboratory services to address those needs and to support the delivery of an essential health package (Dacombe et al. 2006)
- Effective leadership and human capacity building as well as adequate equipment and supplies could address the issue of the magnitude of the demand for laboratory testing due to the huge disease burden in certain settings (Ndihokubwayo et al. 2010).
- Improving the quality of care and standards of the laboratory services through internal quality assurance linked to external quality assurance mechanisms could improve efficiency and also address the issue of the public's negative perception of the laboratory services (Dacombe et al. 2006)
- Bringing the laboratory services into the primary care setting could be more feasible and could relieve the burden on laboratories at the secondary level of care, and could also be easily accessible to the community (Dacombe et al. 2006)
- Provision of rapid diagnostic tests such as for anaemia, HIV, antenatal syphilis, and malaria could be more feasible and less costly when provided at the primary care setting (Dacombe et al. 2006).

Effective essential medical laboratory services are crucial as part of an integrated EHP (Dacombe et al. 2006). However, greater attention needs to be given to removing the constraints of delivering effective medical laboratory services to support EHPs (Dacombe et al. 2006).

In a number of sub-Saharan African countries, lack of knowledge, understanding and awareness of laboratory functions by policymakers, health professional and patients is so pronounced that it stifles progress towards delivering cost-effective and equitable health services. There is an urgent need for policymakers, health professionals and patients that are both informed and active (Haines et al. 2004).

The starting point should be the strengthening of institutions and mechanisms that can more systematically promote interactions between researchers, policymakers and other stakeholders who can influence the process (Haines et al. 2004). Finding more effective ways of increasing knowledge and understanding about essential medical laboratory services to support health services delivery should be a priority for researchers, health professionals and policymakers (Haines et al. 2004). Even when the evidence and systematic ways of increasing knowledge and understanding are available, further work is needed to translate it into guidelines or messages that are understandable to patients and health professionals (Haines et al. 2004).

Training health professionals at institutions of higher learning should be structured in such a way that it equips them with core competencies and skills that will enable them to face the real challenges of implementing essential health packages including essential medical laboratory services (Pruitt and Epping-Jordan 2005). Promoting interdepartmental collaboration such as in the training curricula of doctors, nurses, and medical laboratory professionals will require increasing the capacity of institutions of higher learning (Mullan et al. 2011). It is encouraging that the innovative educational approach that integrates leadership and management training into the traditional medical curricula in Botswana, could enhance the employability of policymakers and health professionals that are well informed (Magowe et al. 2014).

Mitton et al. (2007) suggest the use of new technologies such as knowledge transfer and exchange (KTE) which is an interactive exchange of knowledge between research users and research producers with the primary purpose of increasing the likelihood that research evidence will be used in policy and practice decisions. Drummond et al. (2008) add that health technology assessments (HTAs) can be used to inform policymakers by using the best evidence-based information to inform best practices in health care service delivery. Such new technologies could enhance or increase policymakers' knowledge and understanding of essential medical laboratory services.

However, it is worth noting that implementing new technologies could be a challenge in low-income countries, as low-income countries face additional challenges to using research evidence due to weak health systems, lack of professional regulation and lack of access to evidence (Haines et al. 2004). Jasser highlights an important point about contextualising interventions and training to the setting (Bheekie et al. 2009). More than ever before the world needs comprehensive responses to complex problems (Frenk 2006).

Interestingly, there have been creative solutions for the implementation of medical laboratory services in low- and middle-income countries such as Uganda. The wide coverage, cost-effectiveness and consistency of the HUB specimen Transport Network System appears to be the answer to addressing the non-sustainable previously implemented specimen transport methods via the post office (Kiyaga et al. 2013).

Since low- and middle-income countries are often acutely challenged when it comes to implementing sustainable health care interventions, the specimen Transport Network System that was successfully implemented in Uganda is a model for efficiency in low- and middle-income countries (Go Molecular n.d.). The success of such an efficient laboratory services revolved around effective leadership, planning, coordination and innovation, among others.

It has been fascinating to see the Greater Sekhukhune-CAPABILITY Outreach Project that was undertaken in a rural district in Limpopo, South Africa, aimed at initiating a district clinical genetic service including a medical laboratory service to gain knowledge and experience to assist in the implementation and development of medical genetic services in South Africa. It is worth noting that this initiative was impeded by a developing staff shortage in the province and pressure on the health service from the existing HIV/AIDS and TB epidemics.

However, these impediments stimulated the pioneering of innovative ways to offer medical genetic services in these circumstances including tele-teaching of nurses and doctors, using cellular phones to enhance clinical care and adapting and assessing the clinical utility of a laboratory test, QF-PCR, for use in the local circumstances.

What this tells us is that sometimes, in the midst of a challenge or constraint there is a solution, and at the same time such a solution should be context-specific in order to ensure that there is cost-effectiveness of the intervention. Constraints during the implementation of health interventions could also be an opportunity to learn and to go back to the drawing board to be able to come up with more feasible approaches to effectively deliver health services.

Although some concerns have been raised about lack of electricity in the rural areas of many low- and middle income countries which makes it difficult to implement new health technologies, such issues can be addressed through adding applications and accessory attachments to mobile phones that turn them into diagnostic tools (Mossman et al. 2014). In the case of "Health Care at My Fingertips" in Kenya, programs are using wireless e-health tablets to take high resolution photographs and perform diagnostic evaluations (Mossman et al. 2014).

Whilst essential health packages (EHPs) have increasingly been considered as an important tool of health policy in terms of cost-effectively addressing health priorities in accordance with the local burden of disease, the mechanisms of delivery of essential health packages have often been overlooked (Mueller et al. 2011).

It is a limitation on its own to overlook the mechanisms of delivery of essential health packages as this could fail to achieve what the essential health packages are intended for, and could also incur unnecessary costs and defeat the very essence of essential health packages which is to deliver rationed health services cost-effectively and equitably (WHO 2008).

There is need for clear understanding, scope, purpose, level of delivery and the shape of the delivery of the essential health service, otherwise the implementation of the essential health package would be limited or constrained (Victora et al. 2004; WHO 2008). It is a limitation if the implemented essential health packages end up only benefiting those who can afford, whilst the poor and vulnerable have considerable barriers to accessing such services (Ensor et al. 2002). Shortage of essential medicines is another limitation that could hamper the implementation of the EHPs (Greene 2010).

Some authors consider the following practical issues as critically important (Walley and Wright 2010; WHO 2008):

- Universal solutions: since there are no universal solutions to the implementation of essential health packages, it implies that solutions to issues of essential health packages should be context-specific, and this requires a great deal of analytical capacity within that setting, and yet the unfortunate reality is that such analytical capacity is in short supply in many resource-poor settings such as in sub-Saharan Africa (Walley and Wright 2010).
- Measurement problems: whilst in theory, essential health packages are delivered and prioritised in accordance with the disease burden of that particular setting, the reality is that it is not easy to measure disease burden as there is no reliable tool, even though some quantification is required (Walley and Wright 2010).
- Resource shortfalls: since many resource-poor settings face serious challenges as they are unable to fund even the bare minimum of health services, it would be crucial to involve donors and to have a strong case and motivation to convince donors to fund such essential health packages (Walley and Wright 2010).
- Maintain current gains: it is possible that some countries may already have had some successes with certain cost-effective health intervention programmes such as immunisation coverage (Walley and Wright 2010). As such, such successful intervention programmes could not be considered as a priority in terms of the essential health packages, but the issue here is that it would be a mistake that should be guarded against to divert funds from such programmes to interventions that are part of the essential health package (Walley and Wright 2010).
- Future disease trends: it would be a mistake to merely focus on the current diseases burden and to overlook future diseases trends that may not necessarily be overtly obvious today as such a mistake could prove very costly later on (Walley and Wright 2010). Given the projection that Africa will see an unprecedented increase in tobacco use over the next few decades, the anti-tobacco legislation in South Africa could prove cost-effective in terms of proactively addressing possible future disease burden related to tobacco smoking (Baleta 2010).
- Public/political acceptability: involvement of the public and health professionals in in this approach could prove beneficial in terms of their buy-in (Walley and Wright 2010). It is also critical to bear in mind that in political terms, there has to be a good reason why funds and resources have to be diverted towards this approach to the exclusion of other services (Walley and Wright 2010). It has to be noted that EHPs can be politically unpopular especially if the argument of holding the government accountable is employed (WHO 2008). As such, lack of political buy-in could be one of the main limitations of implementing EHPs (WHO 2008).
- There has to be strong leadership, and it has to be known what service providers will be involved, what will happen if changes in budget allocations are made from other services (Greene 2010; WHO 2008).

- Monitoring and evaluation of the EHP: it has to be clear as to who will do the monitoring and how and when the monitoring will be conducted (WHO 2008).

The limitations and practical issues of implementing EHPs should be considered to ensure effectiveness of the EHP approach to delivering health services (Mueller et al. 2011). An understanding of the needs and the inherent capacity constraints can clarify the appropriate solution. As such, what is regarded as evidence-based best practice or innovation that is cost-effective in developed economies may not be applicable to the health-related technologies needed in low- and middle-income countries.

3.5 Public-Private Partnerships

Whilst it is appreciated that public-private partnerships may create a powerful mechanism for addressing difficult health service delivery problems by leveraging on the strengths of different partners, they also package complex ethical and process-related challenges (Nishtar 2004). At the level of central administration, a strong central structure, using private-sector expertise, is needed to promote and guide health policy implementation, but the benefits and the imaginative development of policy are weakened by the continuing policy drivers of ideology and off-budget finance, and there is little evidence of a political will to seek a level playing field in the choice between sources of finance (Spackman 2002).

Public-private partnerships have attracted political attention in South Africa as politicians and industry experts say that partnerships between the public and private sectors may solve the shortage of over 80,000 health professionals including highly skilled and qualified medical laboratory technicians in South Africa (Green 2013). It is believed that if South Africa wants to deliver a comprehensive and sustainable health care, there is need for resources of both the public and private sectors, as collaborations over a sustained period are likely to succeed (Green 2013).

However, while theoretically sound, at a practical level it is worth mentioning that public private partnerships can go horribly wrong and cost the state more, as what happened in Britain whereby public private partnerships in the national health system ended up enriching investors rather than benefiting the British public (Fakir 2011). In fact, such a public private partnership was such that the private sector raised the capital to build hospitals and charged the government a monthly fee which has now become an egg on face of the British government (Fakir 2011).

As such, developing countries such as the Kingdom of Eswatini and the Republic of South Africa are cautioned not to blindly implement public private partnerships if they are not needed (Fakir 2011). New ventures such as public-private partnerships should be built on need, appropriateness, and lessons on good practice learnt from experience or elsewhere (Widdus 2001). If governments go ahead or are forced to adopt the public private partnership model, they should be sure that their own capabilities are such that they are able to stand up to the lure and bullying of private sector players, and be able to cap the amount of profits private players can take (Fakir 2011). In this context, a strong public management capacity is needed to regulate the new market, since without good systems and good information transfer, fragmentation and confusion may ensue (Walley and Wright 2010).

Whilst there is enthusiasm and potential for gain in terms of efficiency in using public-private partnerships in the delivery of health services for a wider range of health problems, the success of public-private partnerships in this context appears to be mixed (Barr 2007).

3.6 Healthcare Financing

Healthcare financing is one of the critical challenges facing health systems of low- and middle-income countries, and, more recently, healthcare financing features prominently on the global health policy agenda. The challenges are largely brought about by the dilemma of fragile health systems, amid an ever-increasing disease burden, and the prevailing socioeconomic shocks. This is no simple matter, and questions are asked as to how health should be financed, as it is inevitable that the actions needed to attain desired health outcomes must be financed somehow, regardless of the prevailing health systems challenges of those countries.

For example, on 1 June 2018, on the occasion of the official opening of the Central Medical Stores in the Kingdom of Eswatini, it was interesting that the Global Fund's Head of Strategy and Policy, Harley Feldbaum, asserted that the Kingdom of Eswatini should think about innovative ways of financial sustainability for health, as donor funding had flat-lined, and that major increases were unlikely. It is a truism that unless recipient countries urgently take action and come up with mechanisms for sustainable financing for health, the health systems of such countries are in danger of major collapse.

In the context of the vision to end AIDS as a public health issue by 2030, there is some merit in terms of intensification of efforts for the same day initiation of antiretroviral therapy (ART) by international donor agencies, towards achievement of targets, in the short term. However, there is also concern about efficiency and whether the recipient low- and middle-income countries will be able to sustain such efforts beyond the international donor funding. An observation is that there is a general inadequacy of resources in the public health sector of a number of low- and middle-income countries such as in sub-Saharan Africa. In such countries, the supply of therapeutic drugs is not sustainable, which complicates the burden of disease even further, especially among the poor, as the inequities in terms of health access become more skewed in favour of those who can afford, especially in the context of an out-of-pocket payments financing modality. As such, more focus is now on the other financing modalities such as government funding (which is usually insufficient) and health insurance (of which mandatory health insurance is still non-existent or not fully implemented in many low- and middle-income countries).

With the realisation of the inefficiencies of their respective health systems and that donor funding is not going to last forever, many recipient low- and middle-income countries are beginning to seriously assess possible financing mechanisms to improve or replace the existing financing mechanisms. One such mechanism is the basket fund mechanism which involves the pooling of funds from various sources such as government, private sector, and donors to support priorities and ensure adequate resource allocation for agreed upon programme areas. While early experiences of basket funds in countries such as Nigeria, show that they enhance availability of funds, accountability and transparency, basket funds should be part of a multi-pronged approach to improve healthcare financing.

There is consensus that equity in healthcare financing should be related to an individual's ability to pay. More specifically, it is accepted that individuals (or families) with different ability to pay should make 'appropriately dissimilar payments' for healthcare with higher income individuals paying more than those with a lower income (referred to as vertical equity). At the same time, it would also be equitable for individuals (or families) with the same ability to pay to contribute the same amount towards their health care costs (referred to as horizontal equity). However, there is less agreement on what is meant by 'appropriately dissimilar payments.' When considering the equity of health care financing, one cannot simply consider who bears the burden of paying for health services; it is equally important to consider who derives the benefit from each source of financing. Thus, it is the combination of the distribution of health care payment burdens relative to ability to pay, and the distribution of health service benefits relative to need, that determine the equity of individual health care financing mechanisms (McIntyre 2007).

3.6.1 Global Aid Architecture

Many economically advanced governments regard official development aid (ODA) as an important tool for promoting economic development, and as an important part of their foreign strategy (Myers 2016). The United Nations (UN) challenged all economically advanced governments to contribute at least 0.7% of their gross national income to ODA, even though, to date, a few of such countries have met this target (Myers 2016). As of 2016, the most generous countries in terms of foreign aid were: Sweden (1.41%), United Arab Emirates (1.09%), Norway (1.05%), Luxembourg (0.93%), Denmark (0.85%), Netherlands (0.76%), United Kingdom (0.71%), Finland (0.56%), Turkey (0.54%), Switzerland (0.52%), and Germany (0.52%). The United States of America (USA) came tops in terms of total spend (over $30 billion) through bilateral organisations such as the World Bank or the United Nations (UN).

The global aid architecture which has traditionally consisted of bilateral agencies and non-governmental organisations (NGOs) has undergone major transformations over the past two decades or so. These changes have largely been influenced by increasing pressure to show results of aid; increased demands on official aid budgets, leading to the search for innovative financing mechanisms; changing global conditions such as globalisation, climate change, and persistent political instabilities or conflicts; increased public scrutiny on aid; and the proliferation of new donors, among others. Although global aid programmes have a unique and necessary contribution to make, they are fraught with challenges, such as duplication and overlap with each other, leading to inefficiencies of operation and poor accountability for results (Lele et al. 2012).

Coupled with the growing spending on development assistance for health, stimulated by the UN Millennium Development Goals (MDGs) and UN Sustainable Development Goals (SDGs), there has been an interesting transformation of the public health landscape by the emergence of a plethora of vertically funded global health initiatives (Waddington et al. 2009). Some of the major funders of vertical global health initiatives include the Global Alliance for Vaccines and Immunization (GAVI), Global Fund to Fight AIDS, Tuberculosis and Malaria (GFATM), and the United States President's Emergency Plan for AIDS Relief (PEPFAR), among others. It would be interesting to know if this plethora of vertically funded programmes in the health sector is strengthening countries' attempts to improve health or is simply the 'path of least resistance' solutions which avoid some of the difficult complexities of sustainable development.

The influx of so many players into the development assistance arena challenges the overall coordination of the global aid architecture, and, more so, the historic and current dominance of the United States of America (USA). The recent remarkable surge or evolution of China's foreign aid has implications for global aid architecture as it relies on aid principles that are divergent from those of traditional donor countries (Huang and Peiqiang 2012). In fact, there are ongoing debates about who should call the shots in the global aid architecture. Recommendations are that there should be a global coordinating body or mechanism and standards to ensure equity and fairness both within the donor countries' arena and between the donor countries and recipient countries' arena.

The USA has been a dominant player in global health efforts for more than a century, and, more so, in recent times, where such engagement is sparked by economic, health, and security concerns (Kates et al. 2009). It is reasoned that, perhaps, the main reason for the USA to assume the de facto first responder for global health crises is due to the absence of effective international institutions (Glassman and Silverman 2016). The global health engagement of the USA has developed within structure (foreign assistance structure and public health structure), programs and funding (Kates et al. 2009).

While the foreign assistance structure is predominantly development-oriented and has close links to foreign policy, the public health structure has its roots in disease control and surveillance efforts (Kates et al. 2009). Most funding and oversight of global health resides within the foreign assistance structure. The main programmatic and funding roles in the USA global health response are played by the State Department and United States Agency for International Development (USAID) play, followed by the Department of Health and Human Services (HHS), and also by a number of other agencies which carry out some global health activities (Kates et al. 2009).

The USA continues to be the main funder of the global health response, particularly in low- and middle-income countries, even though programming is concentrated in those countries with the heaviest burden of disease, those countries with fragile economies, and those countries where the USA has strategic interests (Kates et al. 2009). Such funding has significantly increased over time, mainly driven by HIV/AIDS, and, yet, it still constitutes only a small fraction of the overall USA federal budget (Kates et al. 2009). Most of the global health funding from the USA follows a vertical, disease or problem focused approach, is provided through bilateral channels, primarily through the international affairs budget and through the State Department, USAID, Department of Health and Human Services and its operating divisions (Kates et al. 2009).

It cannot be denied that initiatives such as the President's Emergency Plan for AIDS (PEPFAR) and the President's Malaria Initiative have been effective to a certain degree (Glassman and Silverman 2016). However, it is argued that the USA's global health response follows outmoded and inefficient models which fail to reflect emerging challenges, threats, and financial constraints (Glassman and Silverman 2016). The immediate quick responses in committing funds to fight emerging and remerging diseases such as Ebola is commendable, but committing funds without strengthening systems is a problem, and unsustainable. As she was speaking to USA law makers in a congressional hearing in May 2018, it was interesting to see the USA Global AIDS Coordinator Deborah Birx questioning the effectiveness of the US$3 billion spent on supply chain since 2009 and also made reference to glitches in the USAD's US$9.5 billion project (Henry J Kaiser Family Foundation 2018). As such, it is recommended that the USA should prioritise and strengthen global health leadership and accountability, health and economic impact, partnerships for sustainable health investment, and drive reforms at related multilateral organisations such as WHO, GAVI, and Global Fund (Glassman and Silverman 2016).

Much as the USA is the largest donor to global health efforts, the USA has its own domestic health policy and programme challenges. In fact, the USA is ranked as the worst performing health system out of a total of eleven richest countries, particularly in the context of measures of access, affordability, health outcomes, and equality between the rich and the poor (Khazan 2017). The USA health policy challenges include lack of cross-party political consensus, lack of stringent spending controls, poor accountability and oversight of insurance companies, and prohibition of the creation of institutes for the assessment of the cost-effectiveness of pharmaceuticals, health services and technologies in the context of the implementation of the Patient Protection and Affordable Care Act – commonly known as the Affordable Care Act (ACA) or Obamacare.

The plethora of vertically funded programmes has had some positive effects in the sense that this has brought much needed resources to help contribute towards the strengthening of health systems especially in low- and middle-income countries. Judging from what has been observed in the Southern African Development Community (SADC), those vertically funded programmes concerned with HIV/AIDS have not only increased access and uptake of HIV/AIDS services, but they have also resulted in a broader use of HIV-specific resources for the improvement of primary health care in general. Merson et al. (2012) highlight that vertically funded HIV/AIDS-specific programmes have resulted in the upgrade of health facilities and infrastructure, training and empowerment of health care workers, and an overall improved primary health care service in countries such as Haiti and Rwanda, among others.

On the other hand, the vertically funded programmes in the health sector have also had negative effects on countries' attempts to strengthen health systems. Much as the HIV/AIDS specific vertically funded programmes have increased access to health care facilities, this has also increased the pressure on the health care workforce in the public sector, to such an extent that the increased workload has somewhat demoralised the poorly paid health care workforce, especially in disease burdened countries. Such programmes have been costly in the sense that they tend to concentrate on a particular area of diseases expertise and neglect others, and that such programmes can be difficult to establish, monitor, or to even assess their effectiveness (Merson et al. 2012).

The disease-based approach takes a unilateral and narrow view to health provision in the sense that it employs systems such as planning, management and financing that are separate from other systems, while the system/sector based approach is horizontal and takes an integrative view to health provision, and uses existing health system structures. The vertical approach focuses on fighting one disease at a time whereas the horizontal or sector-wide approach (SWAp) invests sector-wide to make health systems work to administer prevention and treatment for all diseases (Easterly and Frechi 2010).

Merson et al. (2012) define a SWAp as an approach to a locally owned programme for a coherent sector in a comprehensive and coordinated manner, moving toward the use of country systems. Sector wide approaches have been perceived as being the answer to competition and duplication, as well as improving health system equity and efficiency by ensuring a more effective way of managing resources in line with national needs and priorities (McIntyre 2007).

The vertical disease-based approach has minimal impact because of the involvement of varied players and activities having competing, overlapping, and, only rarely, shared approaches (Birn et al. 2009). This results not only in fragmentation of efforts but also in competition and duplication because of poor coordination.

The UN Millennium Development Goals (MDGs) somewhat created a strong emphasis on specific disease initiatives, such as the HIV/AIDS, Malaria and Tuberculosis initiatives, with the assumption that if the goals of such specific initiatives were achieved, the health system would also be strengthened. The irony though is that such specific disease initiatives appear to overlook the fact that many low- and middle-income countries have low capacity to deliver, and therefore the specific disease initiatives may end up weakening the already weak health systems.

From the perspective of a failing disease-focused TB or Malaria programme to a sector-wide approach (SWAp), there would be a need to ensure that there is coordination, reduction of duplication of service provision and development of a single, sustainable coherent vision that is led by the recipient government with reliance on local knowledge and methodologies (Birn et al. 2009).

It is encouraging though, that there has been growing recognition of the limitations of the disease-based or vertical approach, lately. As a result, there has been a move towards an integrative sector-based approach being adopted in a number of settings in a number of low- and middle-income countries. The advantage of a system- or sector-based approach is that it is comprehensive and allows the synchronisation of planning and pooling of resources. This can enhance equitable access to health care services and the inequalities or differences in health status experienced by the local population will be addressed, but the disadvantage is that it is not that easy to monitor and measure a system-based approach.

Proponents of the disease-based approach such as the HIV/AIDS programme claim that it is advantageous because it is cost-effective, more focused and the results are measurable (Birn et al. 2009). The disadvantage is that it fails to consider the root causes or the complexities of the constraints beyond specific disease programmes such as public sector employment rules, and sustainability issues.

It is of concern that so much intensification of efforts and investment is channelled towards HIV treatment, and not so much on prevention of new infections. The opportunity cost is also an issue, as there seems to be so much focus on HIV and AIDS, and not so much on other major public health issues such as the emerging epidemic of a plethora of chronic non-communicable diseases and co-morbidities crippling the health system. It is also of concern that there is poor or lack of integration of HIV prevention interventions as well as poor or lack of continuum between HIV prevention, treatment and care at both coordination and implementation levels of the HIV and AIDS response. The vertical focus on public health issues is inefficient and unsustainable.

A disease-based approach appears to worsen health inequities and inequalities in the local population, while a system- or sector-based approach appears to address this issue. On the other hand, it is argued that SWAps are a good idea in theory but a disaster in practice, in the sense that SWAps focus on the process of coordinating aid delivery, which has become an end in itself, obscuring the need to actually increase successful treatment and decrease deaths (Easterly and Frechi 2010). For example, it is reported that only a few of the World Bank SWAp projects in sub-Saharan Africa from 2001 to 2008 have shown successful health outcomes. In fact, it was only in Tanzania where a SWAp might have been linked to an actual health outcome: higher rates of TB treatment success (Easterly and Frechi 2010).

To move from a failing disease-focused TB or Malaria programme to a SWAp, there would be a need to create incentives to focus on results, not the process, drastically increase transparency of project information and evaluation, and do independent programme evaluation (Easterly and Frechi 2010).

While the limitations of disease-focused approaches have been highlighted by a number of studies, sector-wide approaches (SWAps) have offered some promise in terms of harmonising aid and assimilating various sectors and role players with the goal of strengthening health systems, but on the other hand the overall success and sustainability of SWAps is in doubt (Walley and Wright 2010). As such, it would be crucial to re-evaluate systems and structures in healthcare provision.

An evaluation in 2010 of health SWAps in six countries (Bangladesh, Ghana, Kyrgyzstan, Malawi, Nepal, and Tanzania) produced mixed results (Merson et al. 2012). On the one hand, the SWAps had been successful in putting in place tools and processes for improved sector coordination and oversight and had made headway in improving the harmonisation and alignment of development assistance (Merson et al. 2012). On the other hand, SWAps had been only modestly successful in achieving improvements in the efficiency of resource utilisation, the ability to focus on results, and the enforcement of sector-wide accountabilities (of government and donors) (Merson et al. 2012). The majority of completed programmes of work had made only modest progress in achieving their nationally set development objectives (Merson et al. 2012).

Some authors observe that the difficulty with evaluating SWAps is that sustained reforms take time and that in SWAps there is no universal standard to determine the point at which tangible benefits to population health can be demonstrated. It is therefore suggested that accurate and comprehensive monitoring programmes tailored to specific system contexts must be set up, preferably based on demographic surveillance systems.

Walley and Wright (2010) argue that the emergence of large disease-specific global funds such as the Global Fund for AIDS, Tuberculosis and Malaria threatens to re-fragment health systems which were integrating funding and service provision. It has been observed that the Global Fund has somewhat created a dependency in a number of low- and middle-income countries, particularly, in sub-Saharan African. This appears to leave these recipient countries in a dilemma, because on the one hand, these countries have the intention to implement SWAps, but on the other hand the major donors do not want to get involved with the SWAps, and this undermines the SWAps' effectiveness.

Moving from a failing disease-focused program to a SWAp may seem attractive, but SWAps have their own inherent challenges largely because they vary in different contexts, and therefore very difficult to monitor and evaluate in terms of their population health impact. Both the disease-specific approach and the sector-wide approach (SWAp) have a role to play in reducing inequalities. However, the context of low- and middle-income countries poses many challenges, unless the more fundamental causes of poverty and inequity are addressed, as many of the poorest countries are trapped in a cycle of debt, unfair trade restrictions and undemocratic international policymaking that protects the wealthy at the expense of the poor.

These challenges are exacerbated by the tendency for international donors to react or respond to a crisis situation such as the burden of HIV/AIDS, Malaria and Tuberculosis in low- and middle-income countries such as in the sub-Saharan Africa. The reactionary tendency or crisis mentality stimulated by effective advocacy programmes puts more emphasis on the treatment of communicable diseases such as Tuberculosis and in the process inadvertently compromises or undermines the long-term view of sustainability and strengthening the health system.

It is interesting that the South African government has committed to employing a SWAp or an integrated health system. However, the dominance of international donors and global health initiatives on communicable diseases such as the Global Fund to fight AIDS, Tuberculosis and Malaria has made this look more like a disease-focused approach, as there does not seem to be an agreed-upon strategy by all role players. Despite the strong commitment to implement SWAp in Zambia, the envisaged efficiency improvements do not seem to have been attained, possibly because the SWAp has not been fully developed or that not all parties have completely embraced it. This calls for urgent evaluation of the approach. For example, the Department for International Development (DFID) agreed with the Government of Malawi to commission an impact evaluation of SWAp, and this evaluation was done in phases.

Even if there is a move from a collapsing disease-focused approach to a SWAp or an integrated approach, the bottom line is that if the fundamental causes of poverty and inequity are not addressed, such an approach is bound to fail, and particularly so if the long-term view is ignored or overlooked. Clearly, a SWAp may not be appropriate in all cases – particularly where there is no agreed-upon strategy, where demand for this approach is not initiated by the government, where opinions differ between a government and donors (Lele et al. 2012).

3.7 Technical Assistance and International Health Consultancy

There are a number of ways in which technical assistance can be defined and provided, but, technical assistance is about a one-off, or repeated short-term or a long-term provision of expertise, and tools to build individual and institutional capacity as an instrument to influence effective policy implementation and practice especially in the recipient country (Tyson and McNeil 2009). Although technical assistance remains the favoured aid tool in the health sector, there is much criticism about its effectiveness in building individual and organisational capacity for sustainable development.

Some of the criticism levelled against technical assistance is that it tends to push the agenda of the donor countries, it undermines the internal institutions and systems of the recipient country, and it distorts whatever capacity the recipient country might already have built prior to the technical assistance, it is expensive, and unsustainable because it does not enhance ownership by the recipient country. It is hardly surprising that in the Southern African Development Community (SADC), there are often complaints from some of the civil society groups because of the on-going chopping and changing of technical assistance which takes the recipient country a few steps forward and many steps backwards as this can be confusing, expensive and unsustainable.

Successful provision of technical assistance in the health sector should be based on relevance of the technical assistance to the setting or recipient country, driven and owned by the recipient setting or country to ensure effectiveness in building individual and organisational capacity for sustainable development. According to

Land et al. (2007), the two dimensions of effective technical assistance include progressively shifting the management responsibilities to the recipient country and alignment of the technical assistance with the recipient country's defined strategies and systems, as well as ensuring that technical assistance personnel support is of high quality and is systematically applied as it is an integral part of capacity development. Capacity development entails the process by which society adapts and strengthens the way in which it goes about managing its affairs over time (Land et al. 2007).

Tyson and McNeil (2009) highlight that there are lessons to be learned by those commissioning and by those receiving the technical assistance, and the authors distil the critical success conditions of technical assistance into ten parts including: clear understanding of the technical assistance assignment; clarity about what can and cannot be delivered; provision of the right technical assistance for the task; understanding of the local context in which the technical assistance will be applied; ensuring that recommendations are pragmatic and realistic; clear communication channels; acknowledging that slow progress is not always bad; strong monitoring and evaluation culture; learning from the situation at hand; and not having a predetermined agenda in mind.

If technical assistance is properly done, it can be of great benefit to the health sector in terms of building capacity for effective policy and practice, but if technical assistance is poorly done it can cause more harm than good because it can be expensive and unsustainable (Tyson and McNeil 2009). Technical assistance that is adapted, systematically applied and harmonised with the recipient country's defined strategies and systems, internally owned, and regularly monitored and evaluated, can be successful (Tyson and McNeil 2009).

Side by side with technical assistance in low- and middle-income countries, is the increasing role of international health consultants. By definition, international health consultants are individuals or groups of individuals working in the field of health, who have specialised knowledge, expertise, skills, and core competencies that qualify them to provide advice and services internationally (World Health Professions Alliance (WHPA) 2007). Given the widespread array of international health consultants, the appropriateness and role of international health consultants can sometimes be confusing to the potential clients. As such, it is not uncommon to see international health consultants being used in instances where it is not appropriate to use them.

International health consultants can be used to diagnose a problem and recommend solutions just like in the context of a doctor-patient relationship or an audit. In that context, the international health consultants have power over the clients. An example of the role of international health consultants in this instance is that of influencing the client to take a certain direction in terms of policy agendas.

International health consultants can also be used when the recipient institution or government purchases expert assistance that is not available internally so that they could diagnose the problem and utilise the expertise of the client to solve the problem. This could be regarded as expert consulting, and in that context, the client has power over the consultant. An example of the role of the consultant in this instance is as a watchdog especially when it is considered too complex and risky to manage certain aspects such as finances and resources locally. Another example of the role of international health consultants in this instance is in project management where there are specialised skills required such as to manage the complexities of the project life cycle. International health consultants can also play a role in providing support for advocacy such around health systems strengthening and poverty reduction. The role of the consultant as technical advisor also falls within this ambit because it is not just about giving recommendations, but it also involves support and assistance in dealing with particular operational challenges such as poverty alleviation.

The other circumstance where international health consultants can be used is when the client requires the know-how of the consultants to facilitate the solution of a problem which the client takes ownership, in such a way that both the consultant and the client become partners. In that circumstance the role of the consultant is merely to facilitate a solution in partnership with the client, and this implies that neither the client nor the consultant has more power over the other. This kind of involvement between the consultant and the client can be regarded as process consulting.

An example of the role of international health consultants in this instance is in capacity development whereby the consultants contribute towards the strengthening of skills, systems and policies and to ensure that there is sustainability in terms of implementation, monitoring and evaluation. The role of the consultant as technical advisor can also fall within this context in the case of weak health systems, as the consultants can contribute towards the development of efficient systems providing technical assistance at national and community level to establish strong and sustainable health care systems as long as the client takes ownership of the problem. Process consulting is the most ideal in terms of sustainability because the client takes ownership of the problem.

Before embarking on a career in international health consulting, it is a crucial skill to develop the ability to understand the challenges in the context of that particular community and to make recommendations relevant to that context to ensure efficiency and sustainability of better health care services (WHPA 2007). This requires some flexibility and pragmatism to ensure that resources are not unnecessarily wasted and inappropriately utilised on solutions that are not relevant to the context of the setting, bearing in mind that the situation may change unexpectedly during the course of the technical assistance (Land et al. 2007).

It is also important to have developed the ability to provide the service through a behaviour that is consistent with the laws and regulations governing professional practice and according to laws and regulations governing the consultant and client country (WHPA 2007).

The aspiring international healthcare consultant should have developed the ability to adapt to different situations and such adaptability is also important in terms of applying ethical principles and codes of conduct in different contexts particularly in the client's context so that the needs of the client can be met (WHPA 2007).

3.8 International Institutions' Public Health Policies Over Time

The way in which Public Health Care (PHC) is defined and applied in the high income countries may not necessarily be applicable in the context of low-income countries, bearing in mind the underlying social, political, and economic causes of poor health in the different settings (Magnussen et al. 2004). The following discussion describes two initiatives related to Primary Health Care (PHC) that aimed to reduce health inequalities. The successes and failures of these initiatives will also be highlighted, as well as the programme's impact on equity.

With the realisation that modern medicine-based health systems did not provide sustainable solutions to health problems affecting developing countries, the World Health Organization introduced the concept of health for all in the Alma Ata declaration of 1978 (Birn et al. 2009). The Alma Ata declaration underpinned primary health care as essential health care made universally accessible to all people in their own setting in the way that such health care service is acceptable and affordable to those people, through their full participation (Walley and Wright 2010).

The primary health care philosophy may include: environmental healthcare; maternal and child health care; health promotion; access to health data and health information; prevention and control of communicable diseases; access to primary curative services; rehabilitative services; and services to people in the community, including school health, workplace health services, and community development projects.

Public Health initiative 1: The multivariate malaria initiative showed that after a large-scale Phase III clinical trial in seven African countries, the most advanced malaria vaccine (RTS.S.) continued to offer protection to children and infants even 18 months after the initial vaccination (Zakus 2013).

Successes and failures: Given the malaria related high mortality of young children in low income countries, it was a huge success that this initiative gave a glimmer of hope by the 50% reduction of malaria cases in young children during the clinical trials (Zakus 2013). It is a failure and a concern that approval for this malaria vaccine will be determined by the European Medicines Agency (EMA) and yet this vaccine was tested in Africa (Zakus 2013). Are the European standards applicable to the African setting?

Impact on equity: This is seen as having an impact on equity especially if the vaccine is available in all malaria-affected areas, so that the health condition of the affected populations can be improved.

Public health initiative 2: The millennium development goals are of interest because all the eight goals directly or indirectly represent facets of the primary health care philosophy.

Successes and failures: The success of the MDGs initiative is that it has enhanced global advocacy, encouraged political consensus, and focus on monitoring of development projects. The failures of the MDGs initiative are lack of ownership, poor implementation, and the fact that they seem to lack focus on key development issues which may be because the uniqueness and inclusiveness of input from different settings were not considered when the MDGs were developed.

One sees the MDGs as having had a positive impact on equity because they addressed the socioeconomic and other issues that influence equality, even though many countries, particularly low-income countries struggled to meet the targets.

There has been some successes and failures of the GOBI-FFF initiative. GOBI-FFF is an acronym for Growth monitoring, Oral rehydration, Breast feeding, Immunization, Food supplementation, and Female literacy (Birn et al. 2009).

It is interesting that the success of the GOBI-FFF initiative was largely visible, particularly, with regard to the fast decline of child mortality where there was community-based primary health care as opposed to selective primary health care. Although a fast decline in child mortality would not necessarily have been expected in settings where there was community based primary health care, a long-term sustainable decline in child mortality would be expected in such settings because such settings are characterised by addressing the underlying causes of mortality rather than narrow targets (Walley and Wright 2010).

Subsequent to the Alma Ata Declaration of 1978, it was felt that the broad view of primary health care adopted through the Alma Ata Declaration was too ambitious and had less promise of producing results. It is rather ironic that the very same World Health Organization (WHO) and the United Nations Children's Fund (UNICEF) which were instrumental in the organisation of the 1978 Alma Ata Conference subsequently turned around and also adopted the selective primary health care approach with the hope of achieving quick results (Birn et al. 2009).

In a way, this sounds confusing, but at the same time, it is hardly surprising, because the task team of the GOB-FFF initiative that comprised the WHO, UNICEF, and the World Bank might have been obliged to show accountability and efficient use of resources (Birn et al. 2009). The unfortunate reality is that selective primary health care's premise for quick results, does not necessarily translate to sustainability of efforts. The failure of selective primary health care is that it overlooks or ignores the underlying causes of morbidity or mortality (Magnussen et al. 2004). As such, selective health care is not a lasting solution to address the issue of inequity, particularly in low- and middle-income countries.

In many low- and middle-income countries, it is not uncommon to see some of the primary health care programmes falling short because they do not consider the bigger picture. For example, with regard to the HIV and AIDS programme, there has been so much focus on changing behaviour and provision of antiretroviral treatment, instead of looking at the underlying cause of the high incidence of HIV in some of the sub-Saharan Africa countries (Schwartlander et al. 2011). The issue of poverty is central to the huge burden of HIV and AIDS in the Southern Africa region, and addressing this issue requires proper planning and a multi-sectoral approach to ensure that there is sustainability of efforts and health outcomes. Moreover, there is need to have a deeper understanding of the communities, and why programmes fail, rather than to continue pumping in money for "quick fixes" through international development agencies, which is not sustainable. Yes, the immediate results may be achieved through immediate "piece meal" changes, but, ultimately, the consequences of unsustainable programmes are much bigger and costly for the low- and middle-income countries to handle.

Consideration should be given to comprehensive primary healthcare and the unique situation of each setting in order to sustainably address the underlying cause of morbidity or mortality, instead of looking at narrow targets (Magnussen et al. 2004).

There is no doubt that the Alma Ata Declaration has been a subject of on-going debate, largely because it highlighted major changes in the direction of health care, and the fact that the goal of health for all has turned out to be a very ambitious goal. In that context, maybe it would not be unfair to liken the Alma Declaration to a ship that never really gained its bearings.

Nevertheless, the Alma Ata Declaration formed a useful foundation from which to make reference in the context of health care initiatives. Even the small steps are successes on their own, as long as there is a sustainable comprehensive plan and direction to get somewhere along the continuum of health care for the benefit of humankind. The important thing is not necessarily to take giant steps, but it is to realistically take meaningful steps and to strive towards delivering a holistic healthcare system that is sustainable.

As those meaningful small steps are taken, and striving towards comprehensive primary health care, the following key points would be particularly crucial: the need to work towards equity and health in healthcare; inter-sectoral action to respond to the determinants of health; the importance of preventive and promotive approaches to health; use of technology which is appropriate to the specific context; participation of individuals and communities in decisions about their health (Walley and Wright 2010).

The Scaling Up Nutrition (SUN) plan developed by the United Nations Children's Fund (UNICEF) is particularly noteworthy because it emphasised the importance of good nutrition, but it has to be mentioned that UNICEF depends on the generosity of donors to support child nutrition. Ethiopia has certainly taken meaningful steps by rolling out nutrition interventions with full participation of the communities and also taking into consideration the unique needs of those communities. This subscribes to the concept of primary health care as laid down in the Alma Ata Declaration because it emphasises community-based care and also places emphasis on the right of individuals to participate as members of the healthcare team. After all, nutritional concerns in low-income countries are diverse, and as such, prevention of nutritional concerns such as deprivation, hunger, and consequent deficiencies that impair health, quality of life, and survival was identified as fundamental to achieving the first Millennium Development Goal to halve the burden of hunger between 1990 and 2015 (Merson et al. 2012).

The community focus of UNICEF in some of the low-income sub-Saharan African countries, has also seen an increase in the number of vertical nutrition programmes. The sad reality is that vertical programmes are bound to fail because they do not take into consideration the unique political and socioeconomic situation of the particular setting (Birn et al. 2009).

Over the years, there have been a number of shifts in health/development policy, influenced mainly by the World Health Organisation (WHO), and International Financial and Economic Institutions (IFIs) such as the World Bank (WB), International Monetary Fund (IMF) and the World Trade Organisation (WTO) (Birn et al. 2009).

Although prior to 1980, the United Nations through the WHO was the dominant actor in shaping health/development policy, by the 1980s, the dominance of the WHO was challenged by other actors such as the WB who began to see their role on a bigger scale and scope as the perceived inefficiencies and bureaucracy of the United Nations and the practical dilemmas of providing primary health care particularly in the low-income countries became more evident (Birn et al. 2009). Through its Health, Nutrition and Population (HNP) arm, the WB began to get directly involved with financing health, nutrition and population development projects in low-income countries.

As such, the new focus of the World Bank (WB) put emphasis on efficiency with the aim of promoting healthy and equitable societies through the governing principles of cost-effectiveness, private sector competition and user fees (Birn et al. 2009). By the 1990s, and through the World Development Report of 1993, the WB became so influential in shaping health/development policy as the WB assumed the role of being the preeminent financier of health and development projects throughout the world, particularly in low-income countries (Birn et al. 2009).

The recent emergence of new players and initiatives such as the Global Fund, the Bill and Melinda Gates Foundation somewhat reduced the dominance of the WB as the preeminent international health financier (Birn et al. 2009). As time progressed, the WB was criticised for following a market-orientated stance which subscribed to the ideologies of capitalism which exacerbated and deteriorated the circumstances of the poor in the low-income countries rather than genuinely uplifting them (Birn et al. 2009). Although the WB subsequently prioritised health systems strengthening, it still received criticism because its financial muscle seemed to give it a grip and control over low-income countries' health/development affairs (Hunter 2007).

Through its International Development Association (IDA) the WB has successfully assisted in Senegal with the implementation of community nutrition health programme through collaborative efforts of all stakeholders (World Bank 2014a). In Lao PDR and Indonesia, the WB has assisted with financing knowledge exchange of policy makers between these two countries to enhance nutrition interventions (World Bank 2014b).

The WB's involvement in coordination and partnerships with other actors with regard to infrastructure and structural adjustments has been an important aspect of influencing health/development policy that had a major impact upon public health in low-income countries. It remains to be seen what the impact of the recently announced WB/WHO joint framework for monitoring progress towards universal health coverage will be (World Bank 2014a). It has to be acknowledged that partnerships or joint efforts may not always work out because actors may have different interests or agendas (Merson et al. 2012).

The shift in health/development policy since 1980 through to the current day has been largely influenced by the individual and/or collaborative role of the WHO, and

IFIs such as the WB, and lately by the emergence of new players and initiatives such as the Global Fund.

Some quarters in the low- and middle-income countries have raised their concerns about the World Bank's non-philanthropic posture. Since the World Bank's official goal is to reduce poverty, does its lending arm inadvertently induce more poverty in the low-income countries that it purports to help?

An observation is that the challenges facing countries of the Southern African Development Community (SADC) such as Angola, Botswana, Eswatini, Lesotho, Malawi, Mozambique Namibia, South Africa, Zambia, and Zimbabwe, are very complex and exacerbated by the triple burden of chronic high unemployment, poverty and inequality amid a slow and volatile domestic and global economic environment. When one looks at the complexity of the multiple challenges facing these countries, it is unlikely that lending money to them is going to be a lasting solution, as issues of poor governance and poor implementation have been reported in some of the low- and middle-income countries, even in other parts of the world, such as Asia and the Americas, among others. There needs to be much more than just the loans from the World Bank. For instance, how does the World Bank effectively address the challenge of poor implementation of programmes in the countries that it has provided loans to?

Given the growing epidemic of non-communicable diseases and chronic diseases of lifestyle in the low-income countries, in recent times, the World Bank was also criticised because of the $4.25 billion allocated to loans for health between 1997 and 2002, only 2.5% was explicitly devoted to chronic disease control programmes (Merson et al. 2012).

It seems as if the harsh criticism against the World Bank started in the 1980s following its new ideological focus which put emphasis on lending to service low-income countries' debt, and structural adjustment policies designed to streamline the economies of developing nations. For example, some of the heavy criticism levelled against the World Bank in the 1980s came from the United Nations Children's Fund (UNICEF) which reported that the World Bank's structural adjustment policies had resulted in deterioration of health, nutritional and educational levels of millions of children in Africa, Asia, and Latin America (Jolly and Stewart 1987).

Interestingly, the World Bank tried to respond to this heavy or harsh criticism in a number of ways. For example, the World Bank began to include non-governmental organisations and environmental groups in its loans in order to try and address the past effects of its development policies that had prompted the criticism (Goldman 2005).

Dr. Jim Yong Kim, the 12th President of the World Bank, conceded that there had been so much criticism levelled against the World Bank, but he believed that the World Bank was also learning from its mistakes and from its successes in different parts of the world, and that this search for global knowledge to solve local problems will be an integral part of the World Bank's everyday work (World Bank 2014c).

Perhaps, one of the main reasons the World Bank is criticised for advancing Western ideals such as globalisation, is because of the United States of America's monopoly as the president of the World Bank has always been nominated by the

United States of America, except, of course, in 2012, where for the first time, two non-United States citizens were nominated (Indo-Asian News Service 2012).

When the incumbent president of the World Bank visited South Africa, recently, one of the comments made by both the then incumbent South African State President and the South African Minister of Finance was that they would really like to see the World Bank transform, as they felt that its leadership picture was unacceptable because it had always excluded representation of the low-income countries. Their argument was that it was totally unfair for a large organisation such as the World Bank which claims to be committed to reducing poverty and addressing inequalities in low-income countries, and yet these low-income countries did not have any voice in the decision-making echelons of the World Bank.

Many people share the same sentiments not only about the World Bank, but about other non-democratic but very globally influential international organisations such as the International Monetary Fund (IMF) and the United Nations (UN) as well. In fact, a number of economic and developmental experts believe that the World Bank's influence of health policy is dominated by a market-led paradigm that fosters privatisation and overlooks the underlying determinants of disease, and as such, it is not trying to alleviate poverty but it is helping rich nations and individuals get richer, and making it impossible for poor nations ever to pay off their debts (Birn et al. 2009).

In such circumstances, there is no doubt that the inequality gap gets wider and wider and pushing more and more people into poverty in the deeply indebted low-income countries (Merson et al. 2012). We are currently witnessing this phenomenon in many parts of Southern Africa, whereby the proponents of globalisation such as the World Bank have propagated the use of genetically modified food, only to find that the consequences are dire as the poor rural population who depend on maize cultivation for their livelihood, can no longer save their seeds, but have to buy them. What one often sees is that in the rural areas, the deepening poverty and hunger have severely complicated the whole picture of the huge disease burden such as HIV and AIDS and chronic non-communicable diseases.

While on the one hand the World Bank purports to reduce poverty in low-income countries, on the other hand, it also creates and worsens poverty through its globalisation and market-orientated ideals. After all, market-led solutions have often undermined the poorest and most vulnerable communities (Oxfam International and WaterAid 2006).

3.9 Quality Improvement in Health

Whilst quality assurance in health care aims to ensure that the needs of the client are met and even exceeded in terms of the improvement of health through the provision of health services, this also encompasses the clinical element where quality is just as important (Teare 1998). In fact, it is of little value to have a health system structure that purports to be responsive to the client's needs if the clinical aspect of health care and the client's inputs are overlooked. It is also of little value to solely focus on the clinical aspect of quality if the overall health service is not responsive to the client's needs.

Health services should not simply purport to be responsive to the client's needs, but the client should play a key role in determining if such services are indeed responsive to his/her needs, and this also encompasses the clinical quality of care. After all, quality service delivery in healthcare includes acceptability of the services to the client; relevance and appropriateness of the health service to the client; continuity of care whereby the care provided is coordinated between the policymakers and authorities (upstream) and the health care practitioners or clinicians (downstream); client's perspective in terms of his/her involvement in decision-making processes in matters pertaining to his/her health; safety of the care environment; timelines of care; and effectiveness and efficiency (Muller et al. 2006).

In some low- and middle-income countries, it has reached a stage where the general public is increasingly becoming disillusioned with the poor clinical quality of care in many public health sector clinics and hospitals (Palitza 2014). When one digs deeper as to what the real cause of the poor quality of care is, some of the reasons that come up are indicative of deficiencies upstream, such as poorly organised health services, lack of competent leadership, and lack of resources, among others. Given the increasing number of complaints by the public or the client, the authorities have somewhat shifted the blame to the clinicians. As such, there has been a number of initiatives aimed at improving the practice and behaviour of clinical staff as part of the healthcare human resources development programme. Whilst human resources development aimed at improving the clinical quality of care is welcome, the argument is that the deficiencies upstream such as poorly organised health services appear to be overlooked.

In that sense, well organised health services and high clinical quality of care are equally important in the context of ensuring health care quality assurance. Focusing only on providing health services that are considered to be responsive to the needs of the client, makes one wonder how the health care services are responsive to the needs of the client in the first place if the clinical quality of care is overlooked. In theory, it may be easy for policymakers or the authorities to presume that they have implemented health care services that are responsive to the needs of the client, but in practice such services may not meet the client's expectations.

Responsiveness is more of a social goal that should take the expectations of the client into account in terms of how he/she is treated (World Health Organization (WHO) 2000). If the client is not treated well by the health care practitioner or clinician, the client may end up having a negative perception about the health care service and may end up not willing to use the service (World Health Organization (WHO) 2000). On the other hand, if the client is treated well by the health care practitioner or clinician, the client may have a positive perception about the quality of the health care service (World Health Organization (WHO) 2000). As such, it seems as if clinical care is almost like a window to the health service.

Responsiveness of health care services is as important as the clinical quality of care, but there is need for political commitment to provide legal and institutional framework to support quality assurance in health care services. The Policy on Quality in Health Care for South Africa gives some hope, even though it is still a challenge putting it into practice. The delivery of quality health care should be considered as a whole encompassing a connection or synergy between the upstream and the downstream of the river of health care (Walley and Wright 2010).

The issue of powerlessness of the client is worrying, particularly in the public health sector of a number of low- and middle-income countries. Perhaps, the powerlessness of the client is magnified by the inferiority complex and the perception that clients are at the mercy of clinicians who ‘know-all’. In fact, doctors are somewhat trusted and ‘worshipped’ in many parts of the low- and middle-income countries. This kind of ‘doctor-worshipping’ is a bit dangerous because it opens room for clinical or medical malpractice, and the client would just have to live or die with it as he/she is powerless to challenge the doctor or nurse. Some clients have disclosed that they were scared of challenging the doctor or nurse because if they did, they feared being victimised by the clinicians.

This is a concern because medical malpractice puts the safety of patients at risk, as it compromises quality of care. It is interesting to see that that there is a sharp increase in medical malpractice litigation in countries such as South Africa as patients are increasingly becoming aware of their rights (Pepper and Slabbert 2011). Many of these are related to claims of misdiagnosis, practising outside the scope of practice, and refusal to treat patients both in the public and private sector (Malherbe 2013). In this regard, there is an urgent need to improve quality and patient safety.

The client has an important influence within the framework of health care quality assurance, specifically, the dimensions of accessibility, efficiency, effectiveness, equity, and safety (Walley and Wright 2010). Three key roles can be assigned to the client, as follows:

Client as contributor to health care quality assurance:

- Definer of health care quality: through his/her prior experience of health care it is appropriate for the client in joint partnership with the health care provider to be able to define what is good quality healthcare and what is not. This may be realistic in the urban areas of some of the low- and middle-income countries where the majority of the population is empowered and there is the added influence of civil groups and worker representatives. It may be unrealistic in the rural areas of such low- and middle-income countries where the majority of the population’s main priority is other burning issues that affect them, such as poverty.
- Evaluator of health care quality: it is appropriate for the client to express his/her satisfaction or dissatisfaction with the quality of health care, but realistically, the rural population of many parts of the sub-Saharan African countries may find it uncomfortable to express their dissatisfaction as compared to the urban population.
- Informant of health care quality: it is appropriate to assess the quality of health care through information obtained from the client pertaining to his/her experience during the health care process and the outcome of this process. This would be realistic and appropriate in many low- and middle-income countries as there

is already a realisation of the importance of a holistic health systems approach, at least, in theory.

Client as target of health care quality assurance:

- Co-producer of health care quality: whilst it is appropriate to monitor the responsibilities of both the provider and the client, the reality is that it is such a challenge to monitor the client's responsibility such as adherence to antiretroviral therapy in a number of low- and middle-income countries (Kober and van Damme 2006).
- Controller of health practitioner behaviour: whilst it is appropriate that the client actively participates in health care decisions, the reality is that the client has very little influence in controlling the practitioner behaviour particularly in the public health sector of developing countries.

Client as reformer of health care:

- Direct participation in health care system: this is appropriate, but it cannot be denied that the practitioner-client exchange in many of the sub-Saharan African countries tends to be skewed in favour of the practitioner rather than being balanced.
- Administrative support in health care: it is appropriate that the quality enterprise in low- and middle-income countries does encourage participation of the client such as through surveys, but realistically there is a challenge when it comes to direct involvement of the client in quality assurance policy formulation.
- Through markets: this is appropriate and realistic in the private health sector of a low- or middle-income country where the client can choose from a wide range of providers, unlike in the public health sector.
- Political action: political action would not be appropriate in low- and middle-income countries where there is already significant political commitment, but there is still room for improvement in terms of recognition of the important role of the client in health care quality assurance (IntraHealth International 2010).

Policymakers and health providers need to realise the important role of the client to influence sustainable health care quality assurance for better health outcomes. There is need for policymakers to ensure that clients are informed and involved in the decision-making process, particularly in low-income countries where the clients generally feel they have no power to influence the quality of health care. Walley and Wright (2010) suggest the following ways of improving quality and patient safety:

- Keeping up to date: evidence-based practice
  - Lifelong learning: this encourages healthcare practitioners to keep up to date in a rapidly changing world, and it also encourages them to admit when they do not know rather than try and bluff their way through ignorance

- Health informatics: easily accessible computerised health information in hospitals and clinic keeps health workers up to date and enhances the efficiency of performing their jobs, and this also includes the use of cell phones for urgent referrals.

- Guidelines or protocols: can provide an effective method of research evidence which could act as a reminder on how to treat certain illnesses.
- Knowledge into practice: knowledge should be accompanied by training in skills and practical competence (Walley and Wright 2010).

Whilst the client should reclaim his/her power to influence quality of care, policymakers, leadership and health care practitioners should also play a part to improve quality and patient safety at the clinical care level. While it facilitates an emphasis on respect for patient autonomy, viewing patients as consumers may be detrimental to the doctor-patient relationship as it inadvertently results in the commodification of health care (Rowe and Moodley 2013).

Imagine the possibility of policymakers and doctors or healthcare providers being patients. Such an analogy is crucial because it puts the policymaker and healthcare provider in a 'vulnerable' position which could perhaps make them see things from the perspective of the client. In southern Africa, generally, policymakers and doctors access better quality care in the private sector, because they can afford, whilst the majority of the population can only afford poor quality care in the public sector, which underlies the health inequity in southern Africa (Ruff et al. 2011).

According to Kay et al. (2008) health care professionals also face the same challenges faced by the general public when they access health care. Interestingly, many doctors tend to portray a 'macho' medical culture image and hide or minimise their vulnerabilities, combined with widespread compulsion to work hard (Jones 2006).

The question is would health practitioners be happy to receive the same kind of care that they deliver to their clients? One of the published and much discussed studies showed that doctors might recommend different treatments for their patients than they would for themselves (Manheimer 2011). In fact, this study showed that doctors were far more likely to prescribe for patients a potentially life-saving treatment with severe side effects than they were to pick that treatment for themselves (Manheimer 2011). More interesting in that study was the doctor-patient who realised how vulnerable he was as he went through the whole treatment regimen for squamous cell carcinoma of the throat, and later pointed out that, if anything, it was the recognition of vulnerability that has made him a better doctor today who delivers the best quality of care to patients (Manheimer 2011).

If all policymakers and health care professionals recognised the vulnerability of being a patient, could this make them deliver better quality of care? It is of concern that in many parts of southern Africa, especially in the rural areas, the client is so vulnerable, largely because of the paternalism or 'doctor knows best'. As such, the client suffers in silence and cannot hold the health practitioner accountable. It is hardly surprising that the majority of people in the rural areas of these countries confide in traditional medicine practitioners whom they believe give them quality care and enough time to listen (Peltzer 2009).

The health practitioner should at least be aware of the client's vulnerability in order to establish rapport and optimise communication with the client, and the health practitioner-client relationship should have a form of shared care with patient empowerment to take a major degree of responsibility for his/her care (Pulia 2011). If the client is informed and empowered to know his/her rights to quality health care, and recognition that health professionals are also human beings, there is a realistic chance for the client to play a key role to influence health care quality assurance.

Realistically, clients may find it difficult to freely express their dissatisfaction with the quality of the physician's or healthcare provider's care. This difficulty to express dissatisfaction seems to be more pronounced in the rural areas of many low- and middle-income countries. A counter argument could be, is there really a significant difference between the rural and the urban population of low- and middle-income countries, in this regard?

To answer this question, it is important to begin by highlighting the context of a certain middle-income sub-Saharan African country, steeped in culture, generally characterised by respect, peace and politeness of the population which values collectivism and closeness of relationships. There is a tendency for the rural population to view themselves as being of low socio-economic status, whilst the urban population is perceived to be of a high socio-economic status, even though this may not necessarily be true. Perhaps, this underlines the psychology of social status (Waytz 2009).

These characteristics of the population affect doctor-patient communication in the sense that they reinforce social distance between the doctor and the patient, mainly because in that particular country's culture there is an embedded tendency for hierarchical respect towards elders or people of higher social status. Since physicians are generally perceived to be of a very high social status, perhaps, also reinforced by the physicians' or nurse's paternalistic communication style, the clients have a tendency to show hesitant and diffident behaviour, the importance of maintaining harmony and therefore difficulty to freely express their dissatisfaction with the physician's or nurse's quality of care.

The abovementioned middle-income sub-Saharan African country scenario can almost be paralleled to the findings of a study conducted in South East Asia which showed that physicians unintentionally adhere to behaviour that underlines social distance, while clients seem dissatisfied with that type of behaviour. Clients by contrast, seem to have developed a tendency to prefer a closer relationship, which physicians unintentionally fail to acknowledge or notice.

Whilst physicians may have enjoyed dominance in the physician-client communication, such dominance seems to be waning especially in the burgeoning private health sector of parts of low- and middle-income countries. Added to this is the rising consumerism that has required health practitioners to attend more to clients' wants rather than their medically defined needs, and the picture of professional decline looks persuasive.

The change in contract between physicians and clients suggests that physicians are changing from being authorities to being partners with clients, and to some physicians this transition is unsettling. But perhaps the change is deeper still as physicians today are confronted with increasing demand to ensure and improve care of their clients, and wealthy clients demand more control because they feel the physician is inadequate.

The new emancipation of the client may raise new problems in the relationship between healthcare practitioner and client, as there is now increasing concern about unrealistic client autonomy and increased consumerism and the expectation that this may foster laissez-faire attitudes and loss of morale among healthcare practitioners (Grol 2001).

3.10 Monitoring Performance

It is a painful reality that most countries have an inability to generate the data needed to monitor performance in health care delivery (AbouZahr and Boerma 2005).

Given the increasing importance of performance indicators in health policy, the availability of quality data is crucial, but bearing in mind the potential problems associated with obtaining and utilising the data. Some of the major problems include the potential to undermine the conditions required for quality improvement, perverse incentives and the difficulty of using data to promote change. AbouZahr and Boerma (2005) observe that international donors in health are largely responsible for the problems, having prioritised urgent needs for data over longer-term country capacity-building.

There is a lot that is happening to try and make quality data available in many low- and middle-income countries, and there are many different actors involved at different levels of the health care system, and so many different sources of data and the use of different indicators, thus creating more confusion for decision-makers (Mate et al. 2009). As such, there is an urgent need for a framework for integrating, validating, analysing, and disseminating the fragmentary and at times contradictory information that is available (Lopez et al. 2006).

Health surveillance and information systems have also been implemented to generate, analyse and disseminate such data (Mate et al. 2009). The reality is that health information systems rarely function systematically as they are products of historical, social and economic forces, and they are complex, fragmented and unresponsive to needs (AbouZahr and Boerma 2005).

Some policymakers may think that investing more money will solve the problem, however the reality is that money alone is likely to be insufficient unless accompanied by sustained support to country systems development coupled with greater donor accountability and allocation of resources AbouZahr and Boerma (2005).

According to Murray et al. (2004), the availability of valid, reliable, and comparable health information to inform local, regional, national, and global decisions can be furthered through four interconnected efforts:

- Improving the technology and methods for population health measurement, strengthening national capacity and motivating governments to collect and analyse useful health data;
- Establishing global norms and standards for what are the core health related measurements and how to measure them; and
- Reporting to the globe valid, reliable, and comparable assessments of inputs, service delivery, and achievements for health.

The monitoring of performance indicators in health performance management systems has heavily influenced debate over their value. Whilst the importance of the availability of quality data cannot be denied, the main challenge is the capacity to apply it, and this creates more confusion, as policy-makers end up taking the data at face value and taking decisions that are not applicable or appropriate to the particular context of the setting.

Given the uniqueness of different settings, should different countries have their own set of indicators to monitor performance of health care delivery? In contrast, Lewis and Pettersson (2005) propose performance indicators that offer the potential for comparable measures as useful tools for cross-country comparisons and for tracking relative health performance.

Whether cross-cutting or country-specific indicators are used, the crucial thing is to ensure that there is good governance, since good governance is central to enhancing performance in health care delivery (Lewis and Pettersson 2005). Crucial to high performance are standards, information, incentives and accountability (Lewis and Pettersson 2005).

However, it has to be borne in mind that ensuring good governance is not always easy especially where there is rapid transformation of jurisdictions such as in post-apartheid South Africa (Coovadia et al. 2009). Given the restructuring of jurisdictions in South Africa, the public health system has also been transformed, but failures in leadership and stewardship and weak management have led to inadequate implementation of what are often good policies (Coovadia et al. 2009). As such, inadequate implementation of good policies appears to compromise efforts towards good governance such as in health care service delivery, thereby making it seem as if good governance is done in a vacuum (Taylor 2000).

Much as the importance of a context-specific approach in terms of each country having its own set of indicators is valid, good governance should also be approached from a deeper angle as it is not that obviously clear in different settings. In fact, some authors observe that the good governance agenda is unrealistically long and growing longer over time, because there is little guidance about what is essential and what is not, what should come first and what should follow, what can be achieved in the short term and what can only be achieved over the long term, what is feasible and what is not (Grindle 2004). If more attention is given to sorting out these questions, "good enough governance" may become a more realistic goal for many countries faced with the goal of reducing poverty. Working toward good enough governance means accepting a more nuanced understanding of the evolution of institutions and government capabilities; being explicit about trade-offs and priorities in a world in which all good things cannot be pursued at once; learning about what is working rather than focusing solely on governance gaps; taking the role of government in poverty alleviation seriously; and grounding action in the contextual realities of each country (Grindle 2004).

The distinctive good governance issues and challenges that must be faced in health care delivery are often neither fully recognised nor addressed, yet, governance can serve as a critical facilitator of, or a barrier to, achieving high performance in health care delivery (Alexander et al. 1995).

Good governance and indicators to monitor performance are crucial and can also be a guide in healthcare service delivery (Lewis and Pettersson 2009).

Budget and resource management:

- It is feasible to monitor indicators of budget processes that track how credible, transparent and comprehensive the budget is, even though there could be a challenge in monitoring sector-specific indicators because of overlaps between sectors (Savedoff 2011). These indicators reflect good governance because they enable accountability, standards and information (Savedoff 2011).
- Monitoring indicators of budget leakages could be a challenge especially because it is not easy to pinpoint where the budget leakages occur at many different areas of the health system (Lewis and Pettersson 2009). These indicators reflect good governance because they enable incentives, accountability and corruption reduction.
- It is feasible to monitor indicators of payroll irregularities as long as the human resources payroll systems are updated (Lewis and Pettersson 2009). These indicators reflect good governance because they enable incentives, accountability and corruption reduction (Lewis and Pettersson 2009).
- It is a challenge to monitor indicators of in-kind supply leakages especially in countries with weak institutions and procurement systems (Lewis and Pettersson 2009). These indicators reflect good governance because they enable incentives, accountability and corruption reduction (Lewis and Pettersson 2009).

Individual providers:

- It is a challenge to monitor indicators of job purchasing including side payments, bribes, nepotism and favouritism, because measuring perception is prone to high probability of error (Lewis and Pettersson 2009). These indicators reflect good governance because they enable incentives, accountability and reduction of corruption (Lewis and Pettersson 2009).
- It is feasible to monitor indicators of physician credentials because the enforcement of licencing requirements is usually in place, even though there are still loop-holes in some countries (Forster et al. 2011). These indicators reflect good governance because they enable incentives and accountability (Lewis and Pettersson 2009).

- Indicators of health worker absenteeism are feasible to monitor because absenteeism is easy to measure as long as time and attendance human resource systems are up to date (Lewis and Pettersson 2009). These indicators reflect good governance because they enable incentives, accountability and reduction of corruption (Lewis and Pettersson 2009).

Health facilities:

- It is feasible to monitor indicators of health worker performance, even though patient satisfaction surveys may not necessarily give a true picture (Hickson et al. 2002). These indicators reflect good governance because they enable incentives and accountability (Lewis and Pettersson 2009).
- It is feasible to monitor indicators of facility performance as long as facility reporting systems and surveillance are in place (Chan et al. 2010). These indicators reflect good governance because they encourage accountability and standards (Lewis and Pettersson 2009).

Informal payments:

- It is challenging to monitor indicators of under-the-table payments to individuals due to difficulty getting reliable information. These indicators reflect good governance because they enable incentives, accountability and corruption reduction (Lewis and Pettersson 2009).

Corruption perceptions:

- It is challenging to monitor indicators of the perceptions of corruption, because measuring perceptions is prone to high probability of error (Lewis and Pettersson 2009). These indicators reflect good governance because they enable incentives, accountability and corruption reduction (Lewis and Pettersson 2009).
- It is feasible to monitor indicators of institutional quality, if healthcare quality systems are implemented (Lewis and Pettersson 2009). These indicators reflect good governance because they enable standards and accountability (Lewis and Pettersson 2009).

References

AbouZahr, C., & Boerma, T. (2005). Health information systems: The foundations of public health. *Bulletin of the World Health Organization, 83*, 578–583.

Ahuja, R. (2017). National Health Policy 2017: Addressing the "fragmentation" challenge. *Health Express*, April 07, 2017. Available from https://www.orfonline.org/expert-speak/national-health-policy-2017-addressing-fragmentation-challenge/. Accessed 29 May 2018.

Alexander, J. A., Zuckerman, H. S., & Pointer, D. (1995). The challenges of governing integrated health care systems. *Health Care Management Review, 20*(4), 69–81.

Alva, S., Kleinau, E., Pomeroy, A. & Rowan, K. (2009). *Measuring the impact of health systems strengthening: A review of the literature*. US Agency for International Development.

Baleta, A. (2010). Africa's struggle to be smoke free. *The Lancet, 375*(9709), 107–108.
Barr, D. A. (2007). A research protocol to evaluate the effectiveness of public-private partnerships as a means to improve health and welfare systems worldwide. *American Journal of Public Health, 97*(1), 19–25.
Bateman, C. (2010). Occupation specific dispensation – A hapless tale. *The South African Medical Journal, 100*(5), 268–272.
Bheekie, A., Adonis, T., & Daniels, P. (2009). Contextualising undergraduate pharmacy training in service-learning at the university of the Western Cape. *Education as Change, 11*(3), 157–167.
Birn, A., & Richter, J. (2017). *U.S. Philanthrocapitalism and the global health agenda: The Rockefeller and Gates Foundations, past and present*. New York: Global Policy Forum.
Birn, A., Pillay, Y., & Holtz, T. H. (2009). *Textbook of international health: Global health in a dynamic world*. Oxford: New York.
Canadian Institute for Health Information. (2018). *How Canada compares: Results from the Commonwealth Fund's 2017 international health policy survey of seniors*. Ottawa, ON: CIHI.
Chaix-Coturier, C., Durand-Zaleski, I., Jolly, D., & Durieux, P. (2000). Effects of financial incentives on medical practice: Results from a systematic review of the literature and methodological issues. *International Journal for Quality in Health Care, 12*(2), 133–142.
Chan, M., Kazatchkine, M., Lob-Levyt, J., Obaid, T., Schweizer, J., Sidibe, M., Veneman, A., & Yamada, T. (2010). Meeting the demand for results and accountability: A call for action on health data from eight global health agencies. *PLoS Medicine, 7*(1), e1000223.
Chopra, M., Lawn, J. E., Sanders, D., Barron, P., Abdool-Karim, S. S., Bradshaw, D., Jewkes, R., Abdool-Karim, Q., Flisher, A., Mayosi, B. M., Tollman, S. M., Churchyard, G. J., & Coovadia, H. (2009). Achieving the health millennium development goals for South Africa: Challenges and priorities. *The Lancet, 474*(9694), 1023–1031. Retrieved May 11, 2015, from http://www.thelancet.com/journals/lancet/article/PIIS0140-6736(09)61122-3/fulltext.
Cometto, G., Tulenko, K., Muula, A. S., & Krech, R. (2013). Health workforce brain drain: From denouncing the challenge to solving the problem. *PLoS Medicine, 10*(9), e1001514.
Coovadia, H., Jeukes, R., Baron, P., Sanders, D., & McIntyre, D. (2009). The health and health system of South Africa: Historical roots of current public health challenges. *Lancet, 374*, 817–834.
Dacombe, R. E., Squire, S. B., Ramsay, A. R. C., Banda, H. T., & Bates, I. (2006). Essential medical laboratory services: Their role in delivering equitable health care in Malawi. *Malawi Medical Journal, 18*(2), 77–79.
Danish Ministry of Foreign Affairs. (2007). *Controversies in health care financing: perspectives and debate*. Special Session at the 6th Congress of iHEA.
Department for International Development (DFID). (2006). *How to note: How to provide technical cooperation personnel*, June. Available from http://www.jica.go.jp/cdstudy/library/pdf/20071101_13.pdf. Accessed 15 Jan 2016.
Derua, Y., Ishengoma, D. R. S., Rwegoshora, R. T., Tenu, F., Massaga, J. J., Mboera, L. E. G., & Magesa, S. M. (2011). Users' and health service providers' perception on quality of laboratory malaria diagnosis in Tanzania. *Malaria Journal, 10*, 78.
Ditlopo, P., Blaauw, D., Bidwell, P., & Thomas, S. (2011). Analysing the implementation of the rural allowance in hospitals in North West Province, South Africa. *Public Health Policy, 32*(Suppl).
Ditlopo, P., Blaauw, D., Rispel, L. C., Thomas, S., & Bidwell, P. (2013). Policy implementation and financial incentives for nurses in South Africa: A case study on the occupation-specific dispensation. *Global Health Action, 6*(10), 19289.
Domenico, F. D. (2007). Staff your most valuable asset. *The American Chiropractor*, 4 March.
Drummond, M. F., Schwartz, J. S., Johnsson, B., Luce, B. R., Neumann, P. J., Siebert, U., & Sullivan, S. D. (2008). Key principles for the improved conduct of health technology assessments for resource allocation decisions. *International Journal of Technology Assessment in Health Care, 24*(3), 244–258.
Dwyer, J. & Wilhelmsen, S. (n.d.). *Leadership and management*. Retrieved May 10, 2016, from http://www.globalhealthmagazine.com/cover_stories/leadership_and_management

Easterly, W. & Frechi, L. (2010). *The World Bank's "horizontal" approach to health falls horizontal*. Available from www.aidwatchers.com/2010/06/the-world-bank

Eghan, K. (2018). Strong pharmaceutical systems are crucial to attaining UHC. *Health systems strengthening,* May 24, 2018. Available from https://www.msh.org/blog-categories/health-systems-strengthening. Accessed 28 May 2018.

Ensor, T., Dave-Sen, P., Ali, L., Hossain, A., Begum, S. A., & Moral, H. (2002). Do essential service packages benefit the poor? Preliminary evidence from Bangladesh. *Health Policy and Planning, 17*(3), 247–256.

Evans, T. G. (2018). Canada and global health: Accelerate leadership now. *Lancet, 391*, 1648–1649.

Fakir, S. (2011). Lessons for South Africa from England's messy public-private partnerships, *The South African Civil Society Information Service*, 10 February.

Feiring, B. (2003). *Indigenous peoples and poverty: The cases of Bolivia, Guatemala*. Minority Rights Group International: Honduras and Nicaragua.

Forster, A. J., Turnbull, J., McGuire, S., Ho, M. L., & Worthington, J. R. (2011). Improving patient safety and physician accountability using the hospital credentialing process. *Open Medicine, 5*(2).

Frenk, J. (2006). Bridging the divide: Global lessons from evidence-based health policy in Mexico. *Lancet, 368*, 954–961.

Frenk, J., Chen, L., Bhutta, Z. A., Cohen, J., Crisp, N., Evans, T., Fineberg, H., Garcia, P., Ke, Y., Kelley, P., Kistnasamy, B., Meleis, A., Naylor, D., Pablos-Mendez, A., Reddy, S., Scrimshaw, S., Sepulveda, J., Serwadda, D., & Zurayk, H. (2010). Health professionals for a new century: Transforming education to strengthen health systems in an interdependent world. *The Lancet, 376*, 1923–1958.

Fried, L. P., Piot, P., Frenk, J. J., Flahault, A., & Parker, R. (2012). Global public health leadership for the twenty-first century: Towards improved health of all populations. *Global Public Health, 7*(S1), S5–S15.

Fryatt, R., Mills, A., & Nordstrom, A. (2010). Financing of health systems to achieve the health millennium development goals in low-income countries. *The Lancet, 375*(9712), 419–426.

George, G., Atajuna, M., & Gow, J. (2013). Migration of south African health workers: The extent to which financial considerations influence internal flows and external movements. *BMC Health Services Research, 13*, 297.

Gerston, L. N. (2004). *Public policy making: Process and principles*. New York: ME Sharpe.

Gilson, L., & Agyepong, I. A. (2018). Strengthening health system leadership for better governance: What does it take? *Health Policy and Planning, 33*(Suppl_2), ii1–ii4. https://doi.org/10.1093/heapol/czy052.

Glassman, A. & Silverman, R. (2016). Restructuring US global health programs to respond to new challenges and missed opportunities. The white house and the world. Available from https://www.cgdev.org/publication/ft/restructuring-us-global-health-programs-respond-new-challenges-and-missed-opportunities. Accessed 28 May 2018.

Global Health Workforce Alliance (GHWA). (2008). *Guidelines: incentives for health professionals* [Online]. Geneva: Global Health Workforce Alliance.

Go Molecular. (n.d.). *Sample transport in Uganda: a network for efficiency*. Available from http://www.gomolecular.com/thrive/sta

Goldman, M. (2005). *Imperial nature: The World Bank and struggles for social justice in the age of globalisation*. New Haven: Yale University Press.

Gostin, L., & Friedman, E. A. (2014). Ebola: A crisis in global health leadership. *The Lancet, 384*, 1323–1325. Retrieved May 10, 2015 from http://www.thelencet.com.

Gray, A. & van der Merwe, L. (2009). Occupation-specific dispensation – An exercise in bad faith negotiations or promise for the future, *South African Pharmaceutical Journal*, November/December, 52–56.

Green, A. (2013). Public private partnerships may answer doctor shortage, *Mail & Guardian*, 19 August.

Greene, J. A. (2010). When did medicines become essential? *Bulletin of the World Health Organization, 88*(7), 483.
Grindle, M. S. (2004). Good governance: Poverty reduction and reform in developing countries. *Governance, 17*(4), 525–548.
Grol, R. (2001). Improving the quality of medical care. *The Journal of the American Medical Association, 28*(20), 2578–2585.
Haines, A., Kuruvilla, S., & Borchert, M. (2004). Bridging the implementation gap between knowledge and action for health. *Bulletin of the World Health Organization, 82*, 724–732.
Ham, L. (2001). *Consulting on health policy in Canada*. Citizens as partners: Information, consultation and public participation in policy-making. OECD.
Heading, G. (2009). *Strategic leadership, culture and change in health services*. Alexandria: Cancer Institute NSW.
Health Policy Project. (2015). *Health insurance feasibility study in Afghanistan: Phase one summary findings*. Washington, DC: Futures Group, Health Policy Project.
Henry J Kaiser Family Foundation. (2018). Kaiser daily Global Health policy report, May 21, 2018. Available from https://www.kff.org/daily-news/may-21-2018/. Accessed 28 May 2018.
Hickson, G. B., Federspiel, C. F., Pichert, J. W., Miller, C. S., Gauld-Jaeger, J., & Bost, P. (2002). Patients complaints and malpractice risk. *Journal of the American Medical Association, 287*(22), 2951–2957.
Hodzic, S. I. (2017). *Healthcare systems, patients' rights and patient Organisations' involvement in healthcare policy and Programme development: A situational analysis of the Western Balkans*. European Patients Forum.
Horton, R. (2010). A new epoch for health professionals' education. *The Lancet, 376*, 1875–1877.
Huang, M. & Peiqiang, R. (2012). *China's foreign aid and its role in the international aid architecture*. Emerging economies and global policies, pp. 75–78.
Hunter, J. (2007). *Managing for health*. New York: Routledge.
Indo-Asian News Service. (2012). US monopoly on World Bank presidency challenged. Available from www.dnaindia.com
IntraHealth International. (2010). *New health care system planned for Swaziland*. Available from http://www.intrahealth.org/page/new-health-. Accessed 19 Apr 2014.
Johnson, J. A., & Stoskopf, C. (2010). *Comparative health systems: Global perspectives*. New York: Jones & Bartlett. Retrieved April 11, 2015, from http://www.jblearning.com/catalog/97814496.
Jolly, R., & Stewart, F. (1987). *Adjustment with a human face: Protecting the vulnerable and promoting growth*. New York: Oxford University Press.
Jones, P. (2006). *Doctors as patients*. Twickenham: Radcliffe Publishing.
Jooste, K. (2009). *Leadership in health services management*. Lansdowne: Juta.
Kates, J., Fischer, J. & Lief, E. (2009). The U.S. government's global health policy architecture: Structure, programs, and funding. The Henry J. Kaiser Family Foundation. *U.S. Global health Policy*. Available from www.kff.org. Accessed 28 May 2018.
Kay, M., Mitchell, G., Clavarino, A., & Doust, J. (2008). Doctors as patients: A systematic review of doctors' health access and the barriers they experience. *The British Journal of General Practice, 58*(552), 501–508.
Kelley, E. T., Arispe, I. & Holmes, J. (2006). Beyond the initial indicators: Lessons from the OECD health care quality indicators project and the US national healthcare quality report. *International Journal for Quality in Health Care*, 45–51. Retrieved April 11, 2015, from http://inqhc.oxfordjournals.org
Khazan, O. (2017). What's actually wrong with the U.S. health system. *The Atlantic*. Available from https://www.theatlantic.com/health/archive/2017/07/us-worst-health-care-commonwealth-2017-report/533634/. Accessed 28 May 2018.
Kingue, S., Rosskam, E., Bela, A. C., Adjidja, A., & Codjia, L. (2013). Strengthening human resources for health through multisectoral approaches and leadership: The case of Cameroon. *Bulletin of the World Health Organization, 91*, 864–867.

Kiyaga, C., Sendagire, H., Joseph, E., MConnll, I., Grosz, J., Narayan, V., Esiru, G., Elyanu, P., Akol, Z., Kirungi, W., Musingizi, & Opio, A. (2013). Uganda's new national laboratory sample transport system: A successful model for improving access to diagnostic services for early infant HIV diagnosis and other programs. *PLoS One, 8*(11), e78609.

Kober, K., & van Damme, W. (2006). Public sector nurses in Swaziland: Can the downturn be reversed? *Human Resources for Health, 4*, 13.

Kumar, A., & Ozdamar, L. (2004). International comparison of health care systems. *International Journal of the Computer, The Internet and Management, 12*(3), 81–95.

Kumar, S., Kumar, N., & Vivekadhish, S. (2016). Millennium Development Goals (MDGs) to Sustainable Development Goals (SDGs): Addressing unfinished agenda and strengthening sustainable development and partnership. *Indian Journal of Community Medicine, 41*(1), 1–4. Available from https://www.ncbi.nlm.nih.gov/pmc/articles/PMC4746946/. Accessed 29 May 2018.

Land, T., Hauck, V. & Baser, H. (2007). Aid effectiveness and the provision of TA personnel: Improving practice, *Policy Management Brief*, 20, November.

Lele, U., Sadik, N., & Simmons, A. (2012). *Changing Aid Architecture: can global initiatives eradicate poverty?* [Online].

Lewis, M., & Pettersson, G. (2005). *Governance in health care delivery: Raising performance.* World Health Workforce Alliance, Geneva: World Health Organization.

Lewis, M. & Pettersson, G. (2009). Governance in health care delivery: Raising performance, *Policy Research Working Paper*, 5074. Washington, DC: World Bank.

Lopez, A., Mathers, C., Ezzati, M., Jamison, D. T., & Murray, C. J. L. (2006). Global and regional burden of disease and risk factors, 2001: Systematic analysis of population health data. *The Lancet, 367*(9524), 1747–1757.

Mabuza, M. P. (2018a). *Health and society: Critical and contemporary perspectives.* Beau Bassin: Lambert Academic Publishing.

Mabuza, M. P. (2018b). *Management of health systems: Critical perspectives.* Beau Bassin: Lambert Academic Publishing.

Mabuza, M. (2018c). Impact of an onsite occupational health clinic on organisational performance and employee wellbeing at a southern African maritime port. *Eurasian Journal of Medicine and Oncology, 2*(3), 152–164. https://doi.org/10.14744/ejmo.2017.24008.

Mabuza, M. P., & Shumba, C. (2018). A qualitative exploration of doctors and nurses' experiences on the management of TB and HIV coinfection in a TB-HIV high burden community in northern KwaZulu-Natal, South Africa. *Journal of Public Health in Africa, 9*, 770. https://doi.org/10.4081/jphia.2018.770.

Magnussen, L., Ehiri, J., & Jolly, P. (2004). Comprehensive versus selective primary health care: Lessons for global health policy. *Health Affairs, 23*(3), 167–176.

Magowe, M. K., Lediwe, J. H., Kasvosve, I., Martin, R., Thankane, K., & Semo, B. (2014). An innovative educational approach to professional development of medical laboratory scientists in Botswana. *Advances in Medical Education and Practice, 4*(5), 73–81.

Malherbe, J. (2013). Counting the costs: The consequences of increased medical malpractice litigation in South Africa. *The South African Medical Journal, 13*(2), 83–84.

Manheimer, E. D. (2011). When doctors become patients, *The New York Times*, 2 September [Online]. Available from http://www.nytimes.com/2011/09/03/opinion

Mate, K. S., Bennett, B., Mphatswe, W., Parker, P., & Rollins, N. (2009). Challenges for routine health system data management in a large public programme to prevent mother-to-child transmission in South Africa. *PLoS One, 4*(5), e5483.

McGuire, J.W. (2013). *Conditional cash transfers in Bolivia: origins, impact, and universality.* Annual meeting of the international studies association, San Francisco, April 3-6.

McIntyre, D. (2007). *Learning from experience: Health care financing in low- and middle-income countries.* Geneva: Global Forum for Health Research.

Merson, M. H., Black, R. E., & Mills, A. J. (2012). *Global health: Diseases, programs, systems, and policies.* London: Jones & Bartlett.

Ministry of Foreign Affairs of Denmark. (2013). Denmark-Bolivia Country Policy Paper 2013–2018. Copenhagen. www.danida-publikationer.dk
Mishra, P. & Agarwal, A. (2017). *Public health in India: gaps in intent, policy, and practice.* Available from https://www.thehinducentre.com/the-arena/current-issues/article9917871.ece. Accessed 28 May 2018.
Mitton, C., Adair, C. E., McKenzie, E., Patten, S. B., & Perry, B. W. (2007). Knowledge transfer and exchange: Review and synthesis of the literature. *The Milbank Quarterly, 85*(4), 729–768.
Montegut, A. J. (2007). To achieve "health for all" we must shift the world's paradigm to "primary care access for all". *Journal of the American Board of Family Medicine, 20, 514–517.*
Mossman, K., McGahan, A., Mitchell, W. & Bhattacharyya, O. (2014). Evaluating high-tech health approaches in low-income countries, *Stanford Social Innovation Review*, 11 February.
Mueller, D. H., Lungu, D., Acharya, A. & Palmer, N. (2011). Constraints to implementing the essential health package in Malawi, *Public Library of Sciences*, e20741.
Mullan, F., Frehywat, S., Omaswa, F., Buch, E., Chen, C., Greysen, S. R., Wassermann, T., Abubakr, D. E. E., Awases, M., Boelen, C., Isidore, M. J., Dovlo, D., Ferro, J., Hailleamlak, A., Iputo, J., Jacobs, M., Koumare, A. K., Mipando, M., Monekosso, G. L., Olapade-Olaopa, E. O., Rugarabamu, P., Sewankambo, N. K., Ross, H., Ayas, H., Chale, S. B., Cyprien, S., Cohen, J., Haile-Mariam, T., Hamburger, E., Jolley, L., Kalars, J. C., & Neusy, A. (2011). Medical schools in sub-Saharan Africa. *The Lancet, 377*, 1113–1121.
Muller, M., Bezuidenhout, M., & Jooste, K. (2006). *Healthcare service management.* Cape Town: Juta.
Murray, C. J., Lopez, A. D., & Wibulplprasert, S. (2004). Monitoring global health: Time for solutions. *The British Medical Journal, 329*, 1096–1000.
Myers, J. (2016). *Foreign aid: These countries are the most generous.* World Economic Forum. Available from https://www.weforum.org/agenda/2016/08/foreign-aid-these-countries-are-the-most-generous/. Accessed 22 Nov 2018.
Ndihokubwayo, J. B., Kasolo, F., Yahaya, A. M. & Mwenda, J. (2010). Strengthening public health laboratories in the WHO Africa region: A critical need for disease control, *The African Health Monitor*, (12), April-June.
Nduru, M. (2006). World health day: Medical brain drain puts southern Africa in a quandary, *Inter Press Service*, 7 April.
Nishtar, S. (2004). Public-private 'partnerships' in health – A global call to action. *Health Research Policy and Systems, 2*, 5.
Nishtar, S., Niinisto, S., Vazquez, T., et al. (2018). Time to deliver: Report of the WHO independent high-level commission on NCDs. *Lancet, 6736*(18), 31258–31253.
Opio, A., Wafula, W., Amone, J., Kajumbula, H., & Nkengasong, J. N. (2010). Country leadership and policy are critical factors for implementing laboratory accreditation in developing countries. *American Journal of Clinical Pathology, 134*, 381–387.
Osborn, R. (2017). *2017 Commonwealth Fund International Health Policy Survey of Older Adults in 11 Countries.* The Commonwealth Fund.
Oxfam International and WaterAid. (2006). *In the public interest: health, education, and water and sanitation for all* [Online]. Available from http://www.oxfam.ca/sites/default/files/in-the-public-interest-health-education-and-water-and-sanitation-for-all.pdf
Palitza, K. (2014). South Africa: Lack of quality health care causes rises in orphans, *Inter Press Service,* 20 April.
Peltzer, K. (2009). Traditional health practitioners in South Africa. *The Lancet, 374*(9694), 956–957.
Pepper, M. S., & Slabbert, M. N. (2011). Is South Africa on the verge of a medical malpractice storm? *The South African Journal of Bioethics & Law, 4*(1), 29–35.
Porter, M. E., & Lee, T. H. (2013). *The strategy that will fix health care.* October: Harvard Business Review.
Pruitt, S. D., & Epping-Jordan, J. (2005). Preparing the 21st century global healthcare workforce. *The Lancet, 330*, 637–639.

Pulia, M. (2011). Simple tips to improve patient satisfaction. *American Academy of Emergency Medicine, 18*(1), 18–19.
Quick, J. D. (2011). *Strong leadership, management, and governance practices improve health impact*. Available from https://www.msh.org/blog/2011/03/29/strong-leadership-management-and-governance-practices-improve-health-impact. Accessed 28 May 2018.
Rowe, K., & Moodley, K. (2013). Debate: Patients as consumers of health care in South Africa: The ethical and legal implications. *BMC Medical Ethics, 14*, 15.
Ruff, B., Mzimba, M., Hendrie, S., & Broomberg, J. (2011). Reflections on health-care reforms in South Africa. *Journal of Public Health Policy, 32*, s184–s192.
Sahoo, M.K. (2018). India's new National Health Protection Scheme: How feasible is it? *The Critical Mirror*, March 23, 2018. Available from http://thecriticalmirror.com/analysis/indias-new-national-health-protection-scheme-how-feasible-is-it/2018/03/23/. Accessed 29 May 2018.
Savedoff, W. D. (2011). Governance in the health sector: A strategy for measuring determinants and performance, *Policy Research Working Paper*, 5655. Washington, DC: World Bank.
Schwartlander, B., Stover, J., Hallett, T., Atum, R., Avila, C., Gouws, E., Bartos, M., Ghys, P. D., Opuni, M., Barr, D., Alsallaq, R., Bollinger, L., de Ftreitas, M., Garnett, G., Holmes, C., Legins, K., Pillay, Y., Stanciole, A. E., McClure, C., Hirnschall, G., Laga, M., & Padian, N. (2011). Towards an improved investment approach for an effective response to HIV/AIDS. *The Lancet, 377*(9782), 2031–2041.
Seims, L. R., Alegre, J. C., Murei, L., Bragar, J., Thatte, N., Kibunga, P., & Cheburet, S. (2012). Strengthening management and leadership practices to increase health-service delivery in Kenya: An evidence-based approach. *Human Resources for Health, 10*(25). Retrieved May 10, 2015 from https://human-resources-health.biomedcentral.com/articles/10.1186/1478-4491-10-25.
Senkubuge, F., Modisenyane, M., & Bishaw, T. (2014). Strengthening health systems by health sector reforms. *Global Health Action, 7*, 1–7.
Serrate, P. C., Lausanne, R. C., Jean-Calude, M. M., Espinosa, C. S. & Gonzalez, T. C. (2007). *Study on intersector practices in health in Cuba: report to the Pan American Health Organization*. National School of public health. Escuela Nacional de Salud Publica de la Republica de Cuba (ENCAMP). Havana.
Smith, P. C., & Papanicolas, I. (2012). *Health system performance comparison: An agenda for policy, information and research*. Copenhagen: World Health Organization.
Spackman, M. (2002). Public-private partnerships: Lessons from the British approach. *Economic Systems, 26*, 283–301.
Sullivan, T. M., Limaye, R. J., Mitchell, V., D'Adamo, M., & Baquef, Z. (2015). Levaraging the power of knowledge management to transform global health and development. *Global Health: Science and Practice, 3*(2), 150–162.
Suy, R., Yen, Y., Chatterjee, R., et al. (2017). Cambodian health policy: Challenge and development. *International Journal of Humanities and Applied Social Science, 2*(2), 23–32.
Swiss Agency for Development and Cooperation (CDC). (2016). *Swiss cooperation strategy Kosovo 2017–2020*. Directorate of Political Affairs: Bern.
Taylor, D. W. (2000). Facts, myths and monsters: Understanding the principles of good governance. *The International Journal of Public Sector Management, 13*(2), 108–124.
Taylor, A. L., Hwenda, L., Larsen, B. I., & Daulaire, N. (2011). Stemming the brain drain – A WHO global code of practice on international recruitment of health personnel. *New England Journal of Medicine, 365*, 2348–2351.
Teare, R. E. (1998). Interpreting and responding to customer needs. *Journal of Workplace Learning, 10*(2), 76–94.
The University of Sidney. (2012). The challenges of preparing the health workforce of the future, *News*, 15 August.
Tumusiime, P., Gonani, A., Walker, O., Asbu, E. Z., Awases, M. & Kariyo, P. C. (n.d.). Health systems in sub-Saharan Africa: What is their status and role in meeting the health millennium development goals? *Health Systems and Reproductive Health*, Special Issue 14.

Tyson, S., & McNeil, M. (2009). How to… provide effective technical assistance. *BJOG, 116*(s1), 93–95.
USAID. (2012). *The intersection of knowledge management and health systems strengthening: implications from the Malawi Knowledge for Health Demonstration Project* [online].
Van de Pas, R. (2017). Global health in the Anthropocene: Moving beyond resilience and capitalism. *International Journal of Health Policy and Management, 6*(8), 481–486.
Victora, C. G., Hanson, K., Bryce, J., & Vaughan, J. P. (2004). Achieving universal coverage with health interventions. *Lancet, 364*, 1541–1548.
Waddington, C., Hadi, Y., Pearson, M., Alebachew, A., Eldon, J., James, J., Khan, M. S., & Varghese, B. (2009). *Global aid architecture and the health millennium development goals*. Oslo: Norwegian Agency for Development Cooperation.
Walley, J., & Wright, J. (2010). *Public health: An action guide to improving health*. Oxford: New York.
Waytz, A. (2009). The psychology of social status, *Scientific American*, 8 December.
Widdus, R. (2001). Public-private partnerships for health: Their main targets, their diversity, and their future directions. *Bulletin of the World Health Organization, 79*, 713–720.
Woltring, C., Constantine, W., & Schwarte, L. (2003). Does leadership training make a difference? The CDC/UC public health leadership institute. *Journal of Public Health Management & Practice, 9*(2), 103–122.
World Bank. (2014a). *Health overview*. Available from http://www.worldbank.org/en/topic/health/overview
World Bank. (2014b). *Nutrition at a glance*. Available from http://www-wds.worldbank.org/external/default/WDSContentServer/WDSP/IB/2014/01/23/000442464_20140123124540/Rendered/PDF/841040BRI0Lao00Box0382094B00PUBLIC0.pdf
World Bank. (2014c). *Speech by World Bank Group president Jim Yong Kim on universal health coverage in emerging economies*. Available from https://www.worldbank.org/en/news/speech/2014/01/14/speech-world-bank-group-president-jim-yong-kim-healthemerging-economies
World Health Organization (WHO). (2000). *Health systems: Improving performance*. Geneva: World Health Organization.
World Health Organization (WHO). (2006a). *Bridging the "know-do" gap meeting on knowledge translation in global health*.
World Health Organization (WHO). (2006b). *World health report 2006: Working together for health*. Geneva: World Health Organization.
World Health Organization (WHO). (2007a). *Building leadership and management capacity in health*. Geneva: World Health Organization.
World Health Organization (WHO). (2007b). *Everybody's business: Strengthening health systems to improve health outcomes: WHO's framework for action*. Geneva: World Health Organization.
World Health Organization (WHO). (2007c). *Towards better leadership and management in health: Report on an international consultation on strengthening leadership and management in low-income countries*. Making Health Systems Work: Working Paper No. 10. Retrieved May 10, 2015, from http://www.who.int/management/ghana/en/index.html
World Health Organization (WHO). (2008). *Essential health packages: What are they for? What do they change?*, WHO Service Delivery Seminar Series, DRAFT Technical Brief No. 2, July.
World Health Professions Alliance (WHPA). (2007). *A core competency framework for international health consultants*. Geneva: World Health Professions Alliance.
Zakus, D. (2013). Global health rounds. *Global Health Weekly, 2*(37), 1–7.

Chapter 4
The UN Millennium Development Goals (MDGs) and Sustainable Development Goals (SDGs)

Abstract Almost like the United Nations Sustainable Development Goals (SDGs), it was envisaged that the United Nations Millennium Development Goals (MDGs) would lead to commitment by governments and actors to increase their efforts towards improving public health. When one reviews the MDGs, it is notable that some of the goals were directly related to health while the others were lateral but had a great influence on health. As such, it is important that the MDGs should not be viewed in isolation because they were interlinked in some way, and therefore successful implementation would have required concerted effort from a multi-sectoral perspective. It is worth highlighting that due to a number of factors, there were variations across countries/regions in their success in meeting the targets of the MDGs. While it was good that the MDGs created impetus for commitment towards improving public health, blanket targets for the MDGs as well as vertical programmes aimed at achieving the MDGs were not helpful because they ignored the unique underlying challenges of each setting and issues of sustainability and ownership. The MDGs were not an end in themselves, as the work continues in the new developmental era of the Sustainable Development Goals (SDGs).

Keywords Clean water and sanitation · Climate action · Decent work · Economic growth · Education and literacy · Equality · Health and wellbeing · Innovation and infrastructure · Millennium development goals · Partnerships · Poverty and hunger · Sustainable development goals · Sustainable environment

4.1 Overview and Progress of the MDGs

The Millennium Development Goals (MDGs) were a set of eight time-bound and measurable goals adopted by world leaders including United Nations member states at the beginning of this millennium, with the aim of fighting poverty in its many dimensions. The MDGs remained as the overarching developmental framework between 2000 and 2015, even though the baseline for the targets was set at 1990 (Fig. 4.1).

M. P. Mabuza, *Evaluating International Public Health Issues*,
https://doi.org/10.1007/978-981-13-9787-5_4

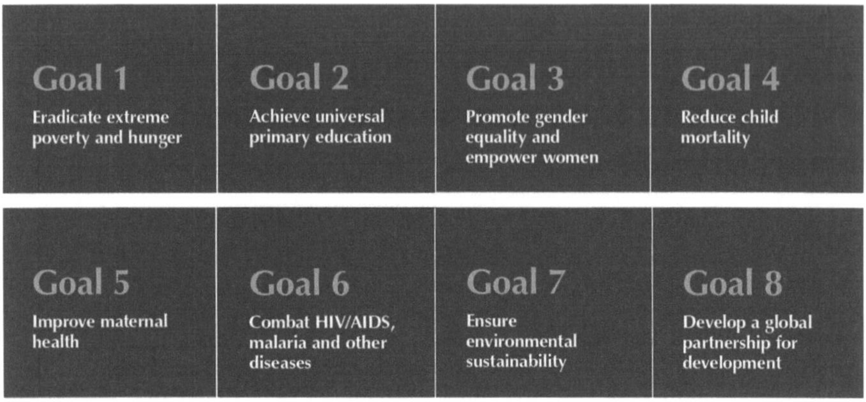

Fig. 4.1 United Nations Millennium Development Goals

While it is worth highlighting that the world community had reason to celebrate at the end of the MDG period, as the concerted global, regional and local efforts resulted in saving millions of lives and improving the conditions of many more, it also has to be acknowledged that implementation of the MDGs had shortfalls in many areas. As such, the MDGs were not an end in themselves, as the work continues in the new developmental era of the Sustainable Development Goals (SDGs) (Tables 4.1, 4.2, 4.3, 4.4, 4.5, 4.6, 4.7 and 4.8).

4.2 Critical Review of the MDGs

It is important to assess the situation so that it could be known how to go about with the implementation strategy relevant for that particular setting. Having blanket targets as reflected by the MDGs is problematic, because it fails to consider the uniqueness of each setting (Birn et al. 2009). In some cases, the inflexible nature of the MDG framework, and the focus on targets rather than broader goals, has contributed to countries distancing themselves from a global agenda that is seen as irrelevant to their particular development situation (Waage et al. 2010).

Merson et al. (2012) report that progress has been made from a global perspective as under-five child mortality (MDG 4) declined to approximately 8.1 million deaths in 2009, down from 12.4 million deaths in 1990, but it is of concern that a number of low-income countries still recorded significant increases in under-five child mortality during the same period. After all, regional differences are often pronounced, with Sub-Saharan Africa faring worse than other regions.

Table 4.1 Millennium Development Goal 1

MDG 1: Eradicate extreme poverty and hunger	
Target 1. A	Halve, between 1990 and 2015, the proportion of people whose income is less than $1 a day
Target 1. B	Achieve full and productive employment and decent work for all, including women and young people
Target 1. C	Halve, between 1990 and 2015, the proportion of people who suffer from hunger
Overall Performance as at July 2015	Extreme poverty rate:
	1990 = 47%
	2015 = 14%
	Global number of extremely poor people:
	1990 = 1926 million
	1999 = 1751 million
	2015 = 836 million
	Number of people in working middle class living on more than $4 a day, almost tripled between 1991 and 2015, and this group makes up half the workforce in the developing regions, up from just 18% in 1991.
	Proportion of undernourished people in the developing regions:
	1990–1992 = 23.3%
	2014–2016 = 12.9%

Source: United Nations (2015)

Table 4.2 Millennium Development Goal 2

MDG 2: Achieve universal primary education	
Target 2. A	Ensure that, by 2015, children everywhere, boys and girls alike, will be able to complete a full course of primary schooling
Overall Performance as at July 2015	Global out-of-school children of primary school age:
	2000 = 100 million
	2015 = 57 million
	Primary school net enrolment rate in sub-Saharan Africa:
	1990 = 52%
	2000 = 60%
	2015 = 80%
	Sub-Saharan Africa had the best record of improvement in primary education of any region since MDGs were established, with a 20%-point increase in the net enrolment rate from 2000 to 2015.
	Primary school net enrolment rate in the developing regions:
	2000 = 83%
	2015 = 91%
	Literacy rate among youth aged 15–24, globally:
	1990 = 83%
	2015 = 91%

Source: United Nations (2015)

Table 4.3 Millennium Development Goal 3

MDG 3: Promote gender equality and empower women	
Target 3. A	Eliminate gender disparity in primary and secondary education, preferably by 2005, and in all levels of education no later than 2015
Overall Performance as at July 2015	Primary school enrolment ratio in southern Asia:
	1990 = 74 girls for every 100 boys
	2015 = 103 girls for every 100 boys
	The developing regions as a whole achieved the target to eliminate gender disparity in primary, secondary and tertiary education.
	90% of countries have more women in parliament since 1995
	Women paid workers outside the agricultural sector:
	1990 = 31%
	2015 = 41%
	Proportion of women in vulnerable employment as a share of total female employment declined by 13 percentage points, between 1991 and 2015. In contrast, vulnerable employment among men fell by 9 percentage points.
	Women have gained ground in parliament in nearly 90% of the 174 countries with data between 1985 and 2015. Although the average proportion of women in parliament has nearly doubled during the same period, only one in five members are women.

Source: United Nations (2015)

Table 4.4 Millennium Development Goal 4

MDG 4: Reduce child mortality	
Target 4. A	Reduce by two thirds, between 1990 and 2015, the under-five mortality rate
Overall Performance as at July 2015	Global number of deaths of children under five:
	1990 = 12.7 million
	2013 = six million
	Global under five mortality rate:
	1990 = 90 deaths per 1000 live births
	2015 = 43 deaths per 1000 live births
	Global measles vaccine coverage:
	2000 = 73%
	2013 = 84%
	Measles vaccination helped prevent nearly 15.6 million deaths between 2000 and 2013. The number of globally reported measles cases declined by 67% for the same period.

Source: United Nations (2015)

For example, the issue of increasing child mortality in South Africa, sparked questions about what South Africa was not doing right despite the visible involvement of international organisations such as the World Health Organization (WHO), the World Bank (WB) and other donor organisations in the country? It is reported that vertical intervention programmes are an issue because they fail to involve the communities to ensure sustainability of such programmes, and it is also reported

Table 4.5 Millennium Development Goal 5

MDG 5: Improve maternal HEALTH	
Target 5. A	Reduce by three quarters, between 1990 and 2015, the maternal mortality ratio
Target 5. B	Achieve, by 2015, universal access to reproductive health
Overall Performance as at July 2015	Global maternal mortality ratio (deaths per 100,000 live births):
	1990 = 380
	2000 = 330
	2013 = 210
	In southern Asia, the maternal mortality ratio declined by 64% between 1990 and 2013, and in sub-Saharan Africa it fell by 49%
	Global births attended by skilled health personnel:
	1990 = 59%
	2014 = 71%
	In northern Africa, the proportion of pregnant women who received four or more antenatal visits increased from 50% to 89% between 1990 and 2014
	Contraceptive prevalence among women aged 15–49, married or in a union, increased from 55% in 1990 worldwide to 64% in 2015.

Source: United Nations (2015)

Table 4.6 Millennium Development Goal 6

MDG 6: Combat HIV/AIDS, malaria and other diseases	
Target 6. A	Have halted by 2015 and begun to reverse the spread of HIV/AIDS
Target 6. B	Achieve, by 2010, universal access to treatment for HIV/AIDS for all those who need it
Target 6. C	Have halted by 2015 and begun to reverse the incidence of malaria and other major diseases
Overall Performance as at July 2015	Global antiretroviral therapy treatment:
	2003 = 0.8 million
	2014 = 13.6 million
	New HIV infections fell by approximately 40% between 2000 and 2013, from an estimated 3.5 million cases to 2.1 million.
	ART averted 7.6 million deaths from AIDS between 1995 and 2013.
	Number of insecticide-treated mosquito nets delivered in sub-Saharan Africa between 2004 and 2014:
	900 million
	Over 6.2 million malaria deaths have been averted between 2000 and 2015, primarily of children under five years of age in sub-Saharan Africa. The global malaria incidence rate has fallen by an estimated 37% and the mortality rate by 58%.
	Between 2000 and 2013, tuberculosis prevention, diagnosis and treatment interventions saved an estimated 37 million lives. The tuberculosis mortality rate fell by 45% and the prevalence rate by 41% between 1990 and 2013.

Source: United Nations (2015)

Table 4.7 Millennium Development Goal 7

MDG 7: Ensure environmental sustainability	
Target 7. A	Integrate the principles of sustainable development into country policies and programmes and reverse the loss of environmental resources
Target 7. B	Reduce biodiversity loss, achieving, by 2010, a significant reduction in the rate of loss
Target 7. C	Halve, by 2015, the proportion of the population without sustainable access to safe drinking water and basic sanitation
Target 7. D	By 2020, to have achieved a significant improvement in the lives of at least 100 million slum dwellers
Overall Performance as at July 2015	Between 1990 and 2015, 1.9 billion people gained access to piped drinking water. Therefore, over half of the global population (58%) now enjoys this higher level of service.
	1990 = 2.3 billion
	2015 = 4.2 billion
	98% of ozone-depleting substances eliminated between 1990 and 2015.
	Therefore, ozone-depleting substances have been virtually eliminated since 1990, and the ozone layer is expected to recover by the middle of this century.
	Terrestrial and marine protected areas in many regions have increased substantially since 1990. In Latin America and the Caribbean, coverage of terrestrial protected areas rose from 8.8% to 23.4% between 1990 and 2014.
	Globally, 147 countries met the drinking water target, 95 countries met the sanitation target and 77 countries met both.
	Worldwide, 2.1 billion people have gained access to improved sanitation. The proportion of people practicing open defecation has fallen almost by half since 1990
	The proportion of urban population living in slums in the developing regions fell from approximately 39.4% in 2000 to 29.7% in 2014.

Source: United Nations (2015)

that the increase in child mortality in South Africa may also be attributable to the huge burden of HIV as research studies report that South Africa bears the greatest burden of mother-to-child transmission of any country (Chopra et al. 2009a, b). It has to be realised that poverty also complicates the whole picture even further as there is proliferation of informal settlements with poor living conditions in countries such as South Africa.

Ownership was one of the challenges facing the implementation of the MDGs, including MDG 4 and MDG 1. For example, the United Nations Children's Fund (UNICEF) and World Health Organization (WHO) have had a complex relationship over involvement in, and ownership of, MDG 4, because by the time they became involved, other organisations had taken the lead in a field that was traditionally theirs (Chopra et al. 2009a, b). As such, the MDG process was largely seen as donor driven, and issues of concern to civil society were neglected from the agenda.

Blanket targets for the MDGs such as MDG 1 and MDG 4 as well as vertical programmes aimed at achieving the MDGs were not helpful because they ignore the unique underlying challenges of each setting.

Table 4.8 Millennium Development Goal 8

MDG 8: Develop a global partnership for development	
Target 8. A	Develop further an open, rule-based, predictable, non-discriminatory trading and financial system
Targets 8.B and 8. C	Address the special needs of the least developed countries, landlocked developing countries and small island developing states
Target 8. D	Deal comprehensively with the debt of developing countries
Target 8. E	In cooperation with pharmaceutical companies, provide access to affordable essential drugs in developing countries
Target 8. F	In cooperation with the private sector, make available the benefits of new technologies, especially information and communications
Overall Performance as at July 2015	Official development assistance:
	2000 = $81 billion
	2014 = $135 billion
	In 2014, Denmark, Luxembourg, Norway, Sweden and the United Kingdom continued to exceed the United Nations official development assistance target of 0.7% of gross national income.
	In 2014, 79% of imports from developing to developed countries were admitted duty free, up from 65% in 2000.
	The proportion of external debt service to export revenue in developing countries fell from 12% in 2000 to 3% in 2013.
	As of 2015, 95% of the world's population is covered by a mobile-cellular signal.
	The number of mobile-cellular subscriptions grew almost tenfold between 2000 and 2015:
	2000 = 738 million
	2015 = over 7 billion
	Global internet penetration:
	2000 = 6%
	2015 = 43%
	As a result, 3.2 billion people are linked to a global network of content and applications.

Source: United Nations (2015)

Whilst Goal 4 (Reduce child mortality), Goal 5 (Improve maternal health) and Goal 6 (Combat HIV/AIDS, malaria and other diseases) related directly to health, the others were not directly related to health, but they had health implications (Walley and Wright 2009).

Given the magnitude of HIV/AIDS, malaria and other diseases, particularly in low-income countries such as in Sub-Saharan Africa, Goal 6 is a huge challenge. As such, international aid agencies such as the World Health Organisation (WHO) and the World Bank (WB) scaled up efforts to address HIV/AIDS, malaria and other diseases such as tuberculosis. However, it is argued that the targets for this goal were too specific and narrow, and failed to take into account the non-measurable dynamics that have a huge impact on the challenge of HIV/AIDS, malaria and other diseases (Waage et al. 2010).

Eradicating extreme poverty and hunger (MDG 1) was a challenging goal because when looking at the magnitude of poverty in low-income countries, one may even think that poverty and hunger are actually directly linked to health. Poverty has long been considered a consequence and cause of poor health and development throughout life (Merson et al. 2012). Efforts directed towards reducing hunger by half between 1990 and 2015 seemed to be on course in many parts of the world, but many parts of the low-income countries still lagged far behind as the number of people who live below the poverty line is astonishing. It has to be highlighted that making efforts towards reducing poverty and hunger would also have helped in reaching Goal 4 and Goal 5 of the MDGs given the often-causal association between survival and adequate nutrition (Merson et al. 2012). As such, both Goal 6 and Goal 1 of the MDGs were very appropriate to improve public health in low income countries. However, the very nature of the specific dimension of the abovementioned MDGs left a gap because it seemed to fail to recognise the synergies that needed to be taken into account when implementing these MDGs (Waage et al. 2010).

It was expected that governments should have shown commitment and played a leadership role through coordination of multi-sectoral actions, adequate resource allocation and accountability of policy makers and all role players to ensure sustainable implementation; institutions of higher learning and researchers should have shown commitment by providing information that could reorient priorities for action, increase output of trained personnel to drive the implementation process; civil society should have shown commitment through active participation at all levels of the implementation process of the MDGs (Chopra et al. 2009a, b). The MDGs should not have been viewed in isolation because they were interlinked in some way, and, therefore, successful implementation would have required concerted effort from a multi-sectoral perspective.

There was an interesting article mentioning the importance of the need to break the Millennium Development Goals (MDGs) in accordance with the uniqueness of the specific countries. The point was vital because it is really unfair to set blanket targets as this puts the high-income countries at an unfair advantage over the low-income countries. Easterly (2009) argues that a series of arbitrary choices made in defining "success" or "failure" as achieving numerical targets for the MDGs made attainment of the MDGs less likely in Africa than in other regions even when its progress was in line with or above historical or contemporary experience of other regions. As such, the statement that "Africa will miss all the MDGs" thus has the unfortunate effect of making African successes look like failures.

It is quite encouraging that the specific targets of MDG 8 (Develop a global partnership for development) took cognisance of the unique needs of low-income countries. For example, Target 8.B. addressed the special needs of the least developed countries; Target 8. C. addressed the special needs of landlocked developing countries and small island developing States; Target 8. D. dealt comprehensively with the debt problems of developing countries through national and international measures in order to make debt more sustainable in the long term; Target 8. E. in cooperation with pharmaceutical companies, provided access to affordable essential drugs in developing countries (United Nations 2013).

However, as far as MDG 8 was concerned, it is worrying that the cost for the global partnerships for development was expected to be shared by both the developed and the developing countries (Dennill and Vasuthevan 2005). Since many of the low-income countries are already highly indebted through loans such as from the World Bank, would it be fair to expect the low-income countries to still share the cost of the global partnerships for development?

MDG 7 (Ensure environmental sustainability) was quite crucial, particularly in low-income countries, especially with regard to the issue of sanitation and slum dwellers. Poverty is becoming somewhat of a vicious cycle in many of the low-income countries, and urbanisation causes the proliferation of slum dwellings which exacerbate poverty and the spread of diseases due to poor sanitation or lack of access to clean water. There was definitely an urgent need to develop a global partnership for development (MDG 8) in order to achieve MDG 7 and of course the other six MDGs. The countries would have benefited from integrating the principles of sustainable development in order to reverse the loss of environmental resources to accomplish MDG 7. There was need to have a fresh look at the MDGs. Addressing the growing disparities within countries would have offered the best hope for achieving the MDGs (Vandemoortele 2011).

Although significant achievements was made on many of the MDG targets worldwide, progress was uneven across regions and countries, leaving significant gaps. Millions of people are being left behind, especially the poorest and those disadvantaged because of their sex, age, disability, ethnicity or geographic location.

Gender inequality persists: Women continue to face discrimination in access to work, economic assets and participation in private and public decision-making. Women are also more likely to live in poverty than men. In Latin America and the Caribbean, the ratio of women to men in poor households increased from 108 women for every 100 men in 1997 to 117 women for every 100 men in 2012, despite declining poverty rates for the whole region.

Big gaps exist between the poorest and richest households, and between rural and urban areas. In the developing regions, children from the poorest 20% of households are more than twice as likely to be stunted as those from the wealthiest 20%. Children in the poorest households are four times as likely to be out of school as those in the richest households. Under-five mortality rates are almost twice as high for children in the poorest households as for children in the richest. In rural areas, only 56% of births are attended by skilled health personnel, compared with 87% in urban areas. About 16% of the rural population do not use improved drinking water sources, compared to 4% of the urban population. About 50% of people living in rural areas lack improved sanitation facilities, compared to only 18% of people in urban areas.

Climate change and environmental degradation undermine progress achieved, and poor people suffer the most Global emissions of carbon dioxide have increased by over 50% since 1990. Addressing the unabated rise in greenhouse gas emissions and the resulting likely impacts of climate change, such as altered ecosystems, weather extremes and risks to society, remains an urgent, critical challenge for the global community.

An estimated 5.2 million hectares of forest were lost in 2010, an area about the size of Costa Rica. Overexploitation of marine fish stocks led to declines in the percentage of stocks within safe biological limits, down from 90% in 1974 to 71% in 2011. Species are declining overall in numbers and distribution. This means they are increasingly threatened with extinction. Water scarcity affects 40% of people in the world and is projected to increase. Poor people's livelihoods are more directly tied to natural resources, and as they often live in the most vulnerable areas, they suffer the most from environmental degradation.

Conflicts remain the biggest threat to human development: By the end of 2014, conflicts had forced almost 60 million people to abandon their homes—the highest level recorded since the Second World War. If these people were a nation, they would make up the twenty-fourth largest country in the world. Every day, 42,000 people on average are forcibly displaced and compelled to seek protection due to conflicts, almost four times the 2010 number of 11,000. Children accounted for half of the global refugee population under the responsibility of the United Nations High Commissioner for Refugees in 2014. In countries affected by conflict, the proportion of out-of-school children increased from 30% in 1999 to 36% in 2012. Fragile and conflict-affected countries typically have the highest poverty rates.

Millions of poor people still live in poverty and hunger, without access to basic services: Despite enormous progress, even today, about 800 million people still live in extreme poverty and suffer from hunger. Over 160 million children under age five have inadequate height for their age due to insufficient food. Currently, 57 million children of primary school age are not in school. Almost half of global workers are still working in vulnerable conditions, rarely enjoying the benefits associated with decent work. About 16,000 children die each day before celebrating their fifth birthday, mostly from preventable causes. The maternal mortality ratio in the developing regions is 14 times higher than in the developed regions. Just half of pregnant women in the developing regions receive the recommended minimum of four antenatal care visits. Only an estimated 36% of the 31.5 million people living with HIV in the developing regions were receiving ART in 2013. In 2015, one in three people (2.4 billion) still use unimproved sanitation facilities, including 946 million people who still practise open defecation. Today over 880 million people are estimated to be living in slum-like conditions in the developing world's cities.

As the MDGs came to their deadline in 2015, the world had the opportunity to build on their successes and momentum, while also embracing new ambitions for the future that all people want. A bold new agenda at the core of which is sustainable development, has emerged to transform the world to better meet human needs and the requirements of economic transformation, while protecting the environment, ensuring peace and realizing human rights. The agenda of the Sustainable Development Goals (SDGs) must become a living reality for every person on planet earth. Targeted efforts will be needed to reach the most vulnerable people. The successes of the MDG agenda prove that global action works. It is the only path to ensure that the new development agenda leaves no one behind.

In the post-2015 development agenda, strengthening data production and the use of better data in policymaking and monitoring are becoming increasingly recognized as fundamental means for development. The MDG monitoring experience has clearly demonstrated that effective use of data can help to galvanize development efforts, implement successful targeted interventions, track performance and improve accountability. Thus, sustainable development demands a data revolution to improve the availability, quality, timeliness and disaggregation of data to support the implementation of the new development agenda at all levels. Strong political commitment and significantly increased resources will be needed to meet the data demand and sustainability for the SDG agenda and beyond.

> *The experience of the MDGs offers numerous lessons, and they will serve as the springboard for our next steps. Leaders and stakeholders in every nation will work together, redoubling efforts to achieve a truly universal and transformative agenda. This is the only way to ensure a sustainable future and a dignified life for all people everywhere.* **(Wu Hongbo, Under-Secretary-General for Economic and Social Affairs)**.

> *The global mobilization behind the Millennium Development Goals (MDGs) has produced the most successful anti-poverty movement in history. The MDGs helped to lift more than one billion people out of extreme poverty, to make inroads against hunger, to enable more girls to attend school than ever before and to protect our planet. They generated new and innovative partnerships, galvanized public opinion and showed the immense value of setting ambitious goals. By putting people and their immediate needs at the forefront, the MDGs reshaped decision-making in developed and developing countries alike. Yet for all the remarkable gains, inequalities persist, and progress has been uneven.*
>
> *Experiences and evidence from the efforts to achieve the MDGs demonstrate that we know what to do. But further progress will require an unswerving political will, and collective, long-term effort. We need to tackle root causes and do more to integrate the economic, social and environmental dimensions of sustainable development.* **(Ban Ki-moon, Former Secretary-General, United Nations)**.

4.3 Overview and Progress of the SDGs

The United Nations Sustainable Development Goals (SDGs) were ratified by world leaders in 2015, and the aim was to continue the development agenda as the Millennium Development Goals' (MDGs) journey came to an end (Fig. 4.2).

The deliberately ambitious and transformational 2030 Agenda for Sustainable Development, has at its heart a foundation for ensuring lives of dignity for all in terms of freeing humanity from poverty, securing a healthy planet for future generations, building peaceful, inclusive societies, and leavening no one behind. This collective journey is guided by a set of 17 integrated Sustainable Goals and targets as a universal agenda, applicable to all countries (United Nations 2018). With just a few years of implementation since the Sustainable Goals were ratified in 2015, the clock is ticking, and the rate of progress in many areas is not as fast as it should to meet the targets by 2030. As such, there is need for injection of a sense of urgency, effective leadership and partnerships, efficiency, cohesiveness, accountability, capacity for reliable data to measure progress, sustained momentum, and a paradigm shift that goes beyond business as usual (United Nations 2018) (Tables 4.9, 4.10, 4.11, 4.12, 4.13, 4.14, 4.15, 4.16, 4.17, 4.18, 4.19, 4.20, 4.21, 4.22, 4.23, 4.24 and 4.25).

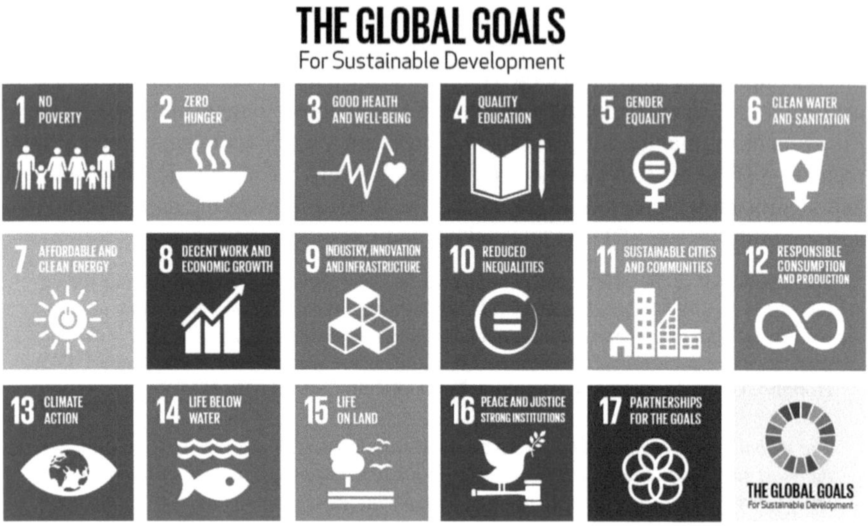
THE GLOBAL GOALS
For Sustainable Development
1 NO POVERTY
2 ZERO HUNGER
3 GOOD HEALTH AND WELL-BEING
4 QUALITY EDUCATION
5 GENDER EQUALITY
6 CLEAN WATER AND SANITATION
7 AFFORDABLE AND CLEAN ENERGY
8 DECENT WORK AND ECONOMIC GROWTH
9 INDUSTRY, INNOVATION AND INFRASTRUCTURE
10 REDUCED INEQUALITIES
11 SUSTAINABLE CITIES AND COMMUNITIES
12 RESPONSIBLE CONSUMPTION AND PRODUCTION
13 CLIMATE ACTION
14 LIFE BELOW WATER
15 LIFE ON LAND
16 PEACE AND JUSTICE STRONG INSTITUTIONS
17 PARTNERSHIPS FOR THE GOALS
THE GLOBAL GOALS
For Sustainable Development

Fig. 4.2 United Nations Sustainable Development Goals. (Source: United Nations 2018)

Table 4.9 Sustainable Development Goal 1

SDG 1: End poverty in all its forms everywhere	
Progress	While extreme poverty has eased considerably since 1990, pockets of the worst forms of poverty persist. Ending poverty requires universal social protection systems aimed at safeguarding all individuals throughout the life cycle. It also requires targeted measures to reduce vulnerability to disasters and to address specific underserved geographic areas within each country.
	Only 45% of the world's population are covered by at least one social protection cash benefit
	Economic losses attributed to disasters were **over $300 billion** in 2017
	The rate of extreme poverty has fallen rapidly: In 2013 it was a third of the 1990 value. The latest global estimate suggests that 11% of the world population, or 783 million people, lived below the extreme poverty threshold in 2013.
	The proportion of the world's workers living with their families on less than $1.90 per person a day declined significantly over the past two decades, falling from 26.9% in 2000 to 9.2% in 2017.
	Based on 2016 estimates, only 45% of the world's population were effectively covered by at least one social protection cash benefit.
	In 2017, economic losses attributed to disasters were estimated at over $300 billion. This is among the highest losses in recent years, owing to three major hurricanes affecting the United States of America and several countries across the Caribbean.

Source: United Nations (2018)

Table 4.10 Sustainable Development Goal 2

SDG 2: End hunger, achieve food security and improved nutrition and promote sustainable agriculture	
Progress	**World hunger is on the rise again:**
	815 million people were undernourished in 2016, up from 777 million in 2015.
	After a prolonged decline, world hunger appears to be on the rise again. Conflict, drought and disasters linked to climate change are among the key factors causing this reversal in progress.
	The proportion of undernourished people worldwide increased from 10.6% in 2015 to 11.0% in 2016. This translates to 815 million people worldwide in 2016, up from 777 million in 2015.
	Stunting, wasting and overweight:
	Still affected millions of children under age 5 in 2017
	In 2017, 151 million children under age 5 suffered from stunting (low height for their age), 51 million suffered from wasting (low weight for height), and 38 million were overweight.
	Aid to agriculture in developing countries totalled $12.5 billion in 2016, falling to 6% of all donors' sector-allocable aid from nearly 20% in the mid-1980s.
	Progress has been made in reducing market-distorting agricultural subsidies, which were more than halved in five years—From $491 million in 2010 to less than $200 million in 2015.
	In 2016, 26 countries experienced high or moderately high levels of general food prices, which may have negatively affected food security.

Source: United Nations (2018)

4.4 Critical Review of the SDGs

While the governments that have signed onto the ambitious 2030 Agenda for Sustainable Development exude confidence that the SDGs represent a "supremely ambitious and transformative vision, and seek to realise the human rights for all", there have been a lot of criticism from various quarters about the unrealistic nature of the SDGs. "As countries take bold steps to achieve the ambitious vision of the SDGs, they face daunting challenges such as climate change, conflict, inequality, persistent poverty and hunger, rapid urbanisation and environmental degradation" (United Nations 2018). It is observed that despite the clearly ambitiously envisaged positives of the SDGs, it is a loophole that the SDGs are not a legally binding treaty, just like their predecessors, the MDGs, and this presents a drawback as countries may skirt their commitments.

As such, the SDGs promote a false sense of achievement and make it easy for governments to go slow on their realisation of human rights. Initially, there was

Table 4.11 Sustainable Development Goal 3

SDG 3: Ensure healthy lives and promote well-being for all at all ages	
Progress	Births attended by skilled health personnel **increased** globally:
	2000–2005 = 62%
	2012–2017 = 80%
	Under-5 deaths fell between 2000 and 2016:
	2000 = 9.9 million
	2016 = 5.6 million
	HIV incidence rate for **women** of reproductive age in **sub-Saharan Africa** is **10 times higher** than the global average:
	HIV incidence per 1000 uninfected people
	Global average = 0.26
	Sub-Saharan Africa average = 2.58
	The world is **not on track** to end malaria by 2030:
	210 million cases of malaria in 2013
	216 million cases of malaria in 2016
	Many more people today are living healthier lives than in the past decade. Nevertheless, people are still suffering needlessly from preventable diseases, and too many are dying prematurely. Overcoming disease and ill health will require concerted and sustained efforts, focusing on population groups and regions that have been neglected.
	Reproductive, maternal, newborn and child health
	The maternal mortality ratio has declined by 37% since 2000. Nevertheless, in 2015, 303,000 women around the world died due to complications during pregnancy or childbirth. Over the period 2012–2017, almost 80% of live births worldwide occurred with the assistance of skilled health personnel, up from 62% in 2000–2005.
	Globally, from 2000 to 2016, the under-5 mortality rate dropped by 47%, and the neonatal mortality rate fell by 39%. Over the same period, the total number of under-5 deaths dropped from 9.9 million to 5.6 million.
	Even in the region facing the greatest health challenges, progress has been impressive. Since 2000, the maternal mortality ratio in sub-Saharan Africa has been reduced by 35%, and the under-5 mortality rate has dropped by 50%.
	In 2018, the global adolescent birth rate is 44 births per 1000 women aged 15–19, compared to 56 in 2000. The highest rate (101) is found in sub-Saharan Africa.
	Infectious diseases and non-communicable diseases
	Globally, the incidence of HIV declined from 0.40 to 0.26 per 1000 uninfected people between 2005 and 2016. For women of reproductive age in sub-Saharan Africa, however, the rate is much higher, at 2.58 per 1000 uninfected people.
	In 2016, 216 million cases of malaria were reported versus 210 million cases in 2013. There were 140 new cases of tuberculosis per 100,000 people in 2016 compared to 173 cases per 100,000 in 2000. Hepatitis B prevalence declined among children under 5—from 4.7% in the pre-vaccine era to 1.3% in 2015.
	In 2016, 1.5 billion people were reported to require mass or individual treatment and care for neglected tropical diseases, down from 1.6 billion in 2015 and 2 billion in 2010.

(continued)

Table 4.11 (continued)

SDG 3: Ensure healthy lives and promote well-being for all at all ages	
	Unsafe drinking water, unsafe sanitation and lack of hygiene continue to be major contributors to global mortality, resulting in about 870,000 deaths in 2016. These deaths were mainly caused by diarrhoeal diseases, but also from malnutrition and intestinal nematode infections.
	Globally, 32 million people died in 2016 due to cardiovascular disease, cancer, diabetes or chronic respiratory disease. The probability of dying from these causes was about 18% in 2016 for people between 30 and 70 years of age.
	In 2016, household and outdoor air pollution led to some seven million deaths worldwide
	Health systems and funding
	Globally, almost 12% of the world's population (over 800 million people) spent at least one tenth of their household budgets to pay for health services in 2010, up from 9.7% in 2000.
	Official development assistance (ODA) for basic health from all donors increased by 41% in real terms since 2010, reaching $9.4 billion in 2016.
	Available data from 2005 to 2016 indicate that close to 45% of all countries and 90% of least developed countries (LDCs) have less than one physician per 1000 people, and over 60% have fewer than three nurses or midwives per 1000 people.

Source: United Nations (2018)

Table 4.12 Sustainable Development Goal 4

SDG 4: Ensure inclusive and equitable quality education and promote lifelong learning opportunities for all	
Progress	**More than half** of children and adolescents are not achieving minimum proficiency in reading and mathematics: 58%
	More **trained teachers are needed** for quality education
	Percentage of trained teachers in primary education
	World 85%
	Southern Asia 71%
	Sub-Saharan Africa 61%
	More than half of children and adolescents worldwide are not meeting minimum proficiency standards in reading and mathematics. Refocused efforts are needed to improve the quality of education. Disparities in education along the lines of gender, urban-rural location and other dimensions still run deep, and more investments in education infrastructure are required, particularly in LDCs
	At the global level, the participation rate in early childhood and primary education was 70% in 2016, up from 63% in 2010. The lowest rates are found in sub-Saharan Africa (41%) and northern Africa and Western Asia (52%).
	An estimated 617 million children and adolescents of primary and lower secondary school age worldwide—58% of that age group—Are not achieving minimum proficiency in reading and mathematics.
	In 2016, an estimated 85% of primary school teachers worldwide were trained; the proportion was only 71% for Southern Asia and 61% for sub-Saharan Africa.
	In 2016, only 34% of primary schools in LDCs had electricity and less than 40% were equipped with basic handwashing facilities.

Source: United Nations (2018)

Table 4.13 Sustainable Development Goal 5

SDG 5: Achieve gender equality and empower all women and girls	
Progress	Child marriage in southern Asia **decreased by over 40%** between 2000 and 2017
	Women spend about **three times as many hours** in unpaid domestic and care work as men
	While some forms of discrimination against women and girls are diminishing, gender inequality continues to hold women back and deprives them of basic rights and opportunities. Empowering women requires addressing structural issues such as unfair social norms and attitudes as well as developing progressive legal frameworks that promote equality between women and men.
	Based on 2005–2016 data from 56 countries, 20% of adolescent girls aged 15–19 who have ever been in a sexual relationship experienced physical and/or sexual violence by an intimate partner in the 12 months prior to the survey.
	Globally, around 2017, an estimated 21% of women between 20 and 24 years of age reported that they were married or in an informal union before age 18. This means that an estimated 650 million girls and women today were married in childhood. Rates of child marriage have continued to decline around the world. In southern Asia, a girl's risk of marrying in childhood has dropped by over 40% since around 2000.
	Around 2017, one in three girls aged 15–19 had been subjected to female genital mutilation in the 30 countries where the practice is concentrated, compared to nearly one in two around 2000.
	Based on data between 2000 and 2016 from about 90 countries, women spend roughly three times as many hours in unpaid domestic and care work as men.
	Globally, the percentage of women in single or lower houses of national parliament has increased from 19% in 2010 to around 23% in 2018.

Source: United Nations (2018)

great hype about the SDGs, however, as time progressed the commitment about the SDGs seemed to be *ad hoc* in many countries. This go slow is grossly unacceptable as it allows for traversing the road towards realisation of human rights for all at whatever speed deemed acceptable, yet, this should be done, now, as fast as possible. The irony is that there seems to be disconnect between the language of true human rights and that of development. In true human rights terms, it is unacceptable that human beings should be deprived, suffer, or die along the way, whereas, in development language it seems 'acceptable' that human beings should be deprived, suffer or die along the way, as long as the ultimate goal is achieved no matter how long it takes. The moral failing of the present generation is that it has the greatest capacity to realise human rights for all, yet, it continues to perpetuate deprivation, suffering and dying through institutional arrangements which are skewed in favour of the affluent. It is hardly surprising that many people continue to be deprived, suffer and die through manmade phenomena such as disease, poverty, wars. In true human rights terms, this is disaster of the highest magnitude, whereas, in economic and development terms, this is a "minor" challenge, comparable to the perpetuation of slavery by the historical colonial masters, US invasion of Iraq and Viet Nam, and NATO's invasion of Libya, among others. How many human beings have continued

Table 4.14 Sustainable Development Goal 6

SDG 6: Ensure availability and sustainable management of water and sanitation for all	
Progress	**3 in 10 people** lack access to safely managed drinking water services
	6 in 10 people lack access to safely managed sanitation facilities
	Data from 79 countries show **59%** of all wastewater is safely treated
	Too many people still lack access to safely managed water supplies and sanitation facilities. Water scarcity, flooding and lack of proper wastewater management also hinder social and economic development. Increasing water efficiency and improving water management are critical to balancing the competing and growing water demands from various sectors and users.
	In 2015, 29% of the global population lacked safely managed drinking water supplies, and 61% were without safely managed sanitation services. In 2015, 892 million people continued to practise open defecation.
	In 2015, only 27% of the population in LDCs had basic handwashing facilities.
	Preliminary estimates from household data of 79 mostly high- and high-middle-income countries (excluding much of Africa and Asia) suggest that 59% of all domestic wastewater is safely treated.
	In 22 countries, mostly in the northern Africa and Western Asia region and in the central and southern Asia region, the water stress level is above 70%, indicating the strong probability of future water scarcity.
	In 2017–2018, 157 countries reported average implementation of integrated water resources management of 48%.
	Based on data from 62 out of 153 countries sharing transboundary waters, the average percentage of national transboundary basins covered by an operational arrangement was only 59% in 2017.

Source: United Nations (2018)

to be deprived, suffer and die since the SDGs were ratified, and why is this disaster allowed to prolong, yet there is capability to eradicate it as fast as possible, without further impinging on human rights? Where is the moral compass in the development discourse?

The SDGs fail to specify a clear division of labour as to what a human rights-based duty or genuine goal to eradicate severe poverty entails. The lack of clear division of labour opens room for confusion and indecisive action which jeopardises the possibilities to meet the stringent responsibilities of eradicating poverty in all its forms and achieving a better life for all people in the whole world, implied by human rights language. As such, this defers the realisation of human rights for all far into the future, thereby disrespecting the human rights of those who are in jeopardy at present.

It is a positive that the SDGs aim for a full realisation of human rights, however, it is a weakness that the SDGs fail to demand a massive roll-out to address international and intra-national inequalities in order to achieve the noble aspiration of human rights for all. This should take into consideration the non-negotiable issue of ensuring that inequalities are curtailed through increasing the income, meaningfully managing land use and energy consumption for the benefit of the poorest people in

Table 4.15 Sustainable Development Goal 7

SDG 7: Ensure access to affordable, reliable, sustainable and modern energy for all	
Progress	**55%** of renewable energy was derived from modern forms in 2015
	4 in 10 people still lack access to clean cooking fuels and technologies
	Ensuring access to affordable, reliable and modern energy for all has come one step closer due to recent progress in electrification, particularly in LDCs, and improvements in industrial energy efficiency. However, national priorities and policy ambitions still need to be strengthened to put the world on track to meet the energy targets for 2030.
	From 2000 to 2016, the proportion of the global population with access to electricity increased from 78% to 87%, with the absolute number of people living without electricity dipping to just below 1 billion.
	In the least developed countries, the proportion of the people with access to electricity more than doubled between 2000 and 2016.
	In 2016, 3 billion people (41% of the world's population) were still cooking with polluting fuel and stove combinations.
	The share of renewables in final energy consumption increased modestly, from 17.3% in 2014 to 17.5% in 2015. Yet only 55% of the renewable share was derived from modern forms of renewable energy.
	Global energy intensity decreased by 2.8% from 2014 to 2015, double the rate of improvement seen between 1990 and 2010.

Source: United Nations (2018)

the world. Unfortunately, the international development discourse focuses on global economic growth which takes a long time, thereby exacerbating poverty, homelessness, hunger, oppression, dependency, disease and premature death among those who are already in jeopardy, and in itself posing a threat to the realisation of human rights for all (McKinsey and Company 2016). Outside of SDG 10, there is scepticism about the SDGs' commitment to reducing inequalities, as inequality is not clearly articulated and not embedded in a cross-cutting manner across all 17 goals, as it should have been. Although SDG 5 does pay focus on gender equality, an observation is that there is a glaring omission of not clearly articulating ending discrimination on the basis of sexual orientation and gender identity, as many people's human rights have been violated on those grounds. The economic and political inequality is another area of concern, as the voices of the poor segments of society are broadly marginalised in both developed and developing nations. The tendency is that the economic and political institutional arrangements and rules are skewed in favour of a domination by global power elite and their associated banks, corporations and business interests, and further deepening inequalities, thereby worsening the situation of the poor majority. If such practices and tendencies are allowed to persist, how could poverty be eliminated in all its forms, and human rights for all be realised?

Table 4.16 Sustainable Development Goal 8

SDG 8: Promote sustained, inclusive and sustainable economic growth, full and productive employment and decent work for all	
Progress	**Earning inequalities** are still pervasive: Men earned **12.5% more** than women in 40 out of 45 countries with data
	Youth were **three times more likely** to be unemployed than adults in 2017:
	Adults 4.4%
	Youth 13%
	Globally, labour productivity has increased, and the unemployment rate has decreased. However, more progress is needed to increase employment opportunities, especially for young people, reduce informal employment and labour market inequality (particularly in terms of the gender pay gap), promote safe and secure working environments, and improve access to financial services to ensure sustained and inclusive economic growth.
	In 2016, real gross domestic product (GDP) per capita grew at 1.3% globally, less than the 1.7% average growth rate recorded in 2010–2016. For LDCs, the rate fell sharply from 5.7% in 2005–2009 to 2.3% in 2010–2016.
	Labour productivity at the global level, measured as output produced per employed person in constant 2005 US dollars, grew by 2.1% in 2017. This is the fastest growth registered since 2010.
	Globally, 61% of all workers were engaged in informal employment in 2016. Excluding the agricultural sector, 51% of all workers fell into this employment category.
	Data from 45 countries suggest that gender inequality in earnings is still pervasive: In 89% of these countries, the hourly wages of men are, on average, higher than those of women, with a median pay gap of 12.5%.
	The global unemployment rate in 2017 was 5.6%, down from 6.4% in 2000. The decline has slowed since 2009, when it hit 5.9%. Youth are three times more likely to be unemployed than adults, with the global youth unemployment rate at 13% in 2017.
	In high-income countries, almost every adult has an account at a bank or other financial institution, compared to only 35% of adults in low-income countries. Across all regions, women lag behind men in this regard.

Source: United Nations (2018)

Using the same metrics to measure progress towards the SDGs is rather unfair, because, wealthy countries have better capacity to realise most of the goals than poor countries. The danger is that this may perpetuate poor countries' dependency on wealthy nations, thereby court a relapse of oppression and domination, and stifle sustainable development in the poor countries. Ideally, the wealthy nations should commit to proving all the resources necessary to assist developing nations with the capacity towards realisation of the SDGs, particularly the implementation of systemic institutional reforms that will address the root causes of poverty. The responsibilities of the wealthy nations should have been clearly articulated in the targets for SDG 17, in this regard. In hindsight, even if the poor countries do not realise the SDGs by 2030, the big positive is that the SDGs would have kept government

Table 4.17 Sustainable Development Goal 9

SDG 9: Build resilient infrastructure, promote inclusive and sustainable industrialization and foster innovation	
Progress	Global carbon intensity decreased by **19%** between 2000 and 2015
	2000 = 0.38 CO2 emissions intensity (kg CO2/USD)
	2015 = 0.31 CO2 emissions intensity (kg CO2/USD)
	Proportion of population covered by a 3G mobile broadband network was **lower in the LDCs** in 2016
	LDCs = 61%
	Globally = 84%
	Steady progress has been made in the manufacturing industry. To achieve inclusive and sustainable industrialization, competitive economic forces need to be unleashed to generate employment and income, facilitate international trade and enable the efficient use of resources.
	The global share of manufacturing value added in GDP increased from 15.2% in 2005 to 16.3% in 2017, driven by the fast growth of manufacturing in Asia.
	Globally, the carbon intensity decreased by 19% from 2000 to 2015—From 0.38 to 0.31 kg of carbon dioxide per dollar of value added.
	In 2015, medium-high- and high-technology sectors accounted for 44.7% of total manufacturing value added globally. The value added reached 34.6% in developing economies, up from 21.5% in 2005.
	By 2016, the proportion of the population covered by a third generation (3G) mobile broadband network stood at 61% in the LDCs and 84% globally.

Source: United Nations (2018)

Table 4.18 Sustainable Development Goal 10

SDG 10: Reduce inequality within and among countries	
Progress	Products exported by **SIDS** facing zero tariff increased by **20%** between 2010 and 2016
	Remittances to low- and middle-income countries represented **over 75%** of total global remittances in 2017:
	$466 billion
	Efforts have been made in some countries to reduce income inequality, increase zero-tariff access for exports from LDCs and developing countries, and provide additional assistance to LDCs and small island developing states (SIDS). However, progress will need to accelerate to reduce growing disparities within and among countries.
	Between 2010 and 2016, in 60 out of 94 countries with data, the incomes of the poorest 40% of the population grew faster than those of the entire population.
	In 2016, over 64.4% of products exported by LDCs to world markets and 64.1% of those from SIDS faced zero tariffs, an increase of 20% since 2010. Developing countries overall had duty-free market access for about 50% of all products exported in 2016.
	In 2016, receipts by developing countries from member countries of the Development Assistance Committee of the OECD, multilateral agencies and other key providers totalled $315 billion; of this amount, $158 billion was ODA. In 2016, total ODA to LDCs and SIDS from all donors totalled $43.1 billion and $6.2 billion, respectively.
	Based on provisional data, among the $613 billion in total remittances recorded in 2017, $466 billion went to low- and middle-income countries. While the global average cost of sending money has gradually declined in recent years, it was estimated at 7.2% in 2017, more than double the target transaction cost of 3%.

Source: United Nations (2018)

Table 4.19 Sustainable Development Goal 11

SDG 11: Make cities and human settlements inclusive, safe, resilient and sustainable	
Progress	In 2016, **4.2 million people** died from ambient air pollution
	Damage to housing due to natural disasters showed a **statistically significant rise** between 1990 and 2013
	Many cities around the world are facing acute challenges in managing rapid urbanization—From ensuring adequate housing and infrastructure to support growing populations, to confronting the environmental impact of urban sprawl, to reducing vulnerability to disasters.
	Between 2000 and 2014, the proportion of the global urban population living in slums dropped from 28.4% to 22.8%. However, the actual number of people living in slums increased from 807 million to 883 million.
	Based on data collected for 214 cities/municipalities, about three quarters of municipal solid waste generated is collected.
	In 2016, 91% of the urban population worldwide were breathing air that did not meet the World Health Organization air quality guidelines value for particulate matter (PM 2.5); more than half were exposed to air pollution levels at least 2.5 times higher than that safety standard. In 2016, an estimated 4.2 million people died as a result of high levels of ambient air pollution.
	From 1990 to 2013, almost 90% of deaths attributed to internationally reported disasters occurred in low- and middle-income countries. Reported damage to housing attributed to disasters shows a statistically significant rise from 1990 onwards.

Source: United Nations (2018)

Table 4.20 Sustainable Development Goal 12

SDG 12: Ensure sustainable consumption and production patterns	
Progress	Globally by 2018, **108 countries** had national policies on sustainable consumption and production
	93% of the world's 250 largest companies are now reporting on sustainability
	Decoupling economic growth from resource use is one of the most critical and complex challenges facing humanity today. Doing so effectively will require policies that create a conducive environment for such change, social and physical infrastructure and markets, and a profound transformation of business practices along global value chains.
	The per capita "material footprint" of developing countries grew from 5 metric tons in 2000 to 9 metric tons in 2017, representing a significant improvement in the material standard of living. Most of the increase is attributed to a rise in the use of non-metallic minerals, pointing to growth in the areas of infrastructure and construction.
	For all types of materials, developed countries have at least double the per capita footprint of developing countries. In particular, the material footprint for fossil fuels is more than four times higher for developed than developing countries.
	By 2018, a total of 108 countries had national policies and initiatives relevant to sustainable consumption and production.
	According to a recent report from KPMG, 93% of the world's 250 largest companies (in terms of revenue) are now reporting on sustainability, as are three quarters of the top 100 companies in 49 countries.

Source: United Nations (2018)

Table 4.21 Sustainable Development Goal 13

SDG 13: Take urgent action to combat climate change and its impacts	
Progress	2017 was the **costliest** North Atlantic hurricane season on record
	The **majority of countries** have ratified the **Paris agreement** and provided nationally determined contributions (NDCs):
	Ratified Paris agreement 175
	NDCs 168
	The year 2017 was one of the three warmest on record and was 1.1 degrees Celsius above the pre-industrial period. An analysis by the World Meteorological Organization shows that the five-year average global temperature from 2013 to 2017 was also the highest on record. The world continues to experience rising sea levels, extreme weather conditions (the North Atlantic hurricane season was the costliest ever recorded) and increasing concentrations of greenhouse gases. This calls for urgent and accelerated action by countries as they implement their commitments to the Paris agreement on climate change.
	As of 9 April 2018, 175 Parties had ratified the Paris Agreement and 168 Parties (167 countries plus the European Commission) had communicated their first nationally determined contributions to the United Nations Framework Convention on Climate Change Secretariat.
	In addition, as of 9 April 2018, 10 developing countries had successfully completed and submitted the first iteration of their national adaptation plans for responding to climate change.
	Developed country parties continue to make progress towards the goal of jointly mobilizing $100 billion annually by 2020 to address the needs of developing countries in the context of meaningful mitigation actions.

Source: United Nations (2018)

leaders and global development institutions on their toes, as a stimulus for promoting accountability and better performance for the delivery of a better life and human rights for all.

> *The post-2015 development agenda, including the set of Sustainable Development Goals, strives to reflect the lessons learnt from the MDGs, and put all countries, together, firmly on track towards a more prosperous, sustainable and equitable world. However, looking ahead, there are daunting problems including climate change, conflict and wars, persistent inequalities, persistent poverty and hunger, rapid urbanisation and environmental degradation. Policymakers in every country need to reflect on how societies can be made more resilient while confronting these challenges.* (**Ban Ki-moon, Former Secretary-General, United Nations**).

Table 4.22 Sustainable Development Goal 14

SDG 14: Conserve and sustainably use the oceans, seas and marine resources for sustainable development	
Progress	Mean coverage of **marine KBAs under protection increased** between 2000 and 2018
	2000 = 30%
	2018 = 44%
	Open Ocean sites show **current levels of acidity have increased by 26%** since the start of the industrial revolution
	Advancing the sustainable use and conservation of the oceans continues to require effective strategies and management to combat the adverse effects of overfishing, growing ocean acidification and worsening coastal eutrophication. The expansion of protected areas for marine biodiversity, intensification of research capacity and increases in ocean science funding remain critically important to preserve marine resources.
	The global share of marine fish stocks that are within biologically sustainable levels declined from 90% in 1974 to 69% in 2013.
	Studies at open ocean and coastal sites around the world show that current levels of marine acidity have increased by about 26% on average since the start of the industrial revolution. Moreover, marine life is being exposed to conditions outside previously experienced natural variability.
	Global trends point to continued deterioration of coastal waters due to pollution and eutrophication. Without concerted efforts, coastal eutrophication is expected to increase in 20% of large marine ecosystems by 2050.
	As of January 2018, 16% (or over 22 million square kilometres) of marine waters under national jurisdiction—that is, 0–200 nautical miles from shore—were covered by protected areas. This is more than double the 2010 coverage level. The mean coverage of marine key biodiversity areas (KBAs) that are protected has also increased—from 30% in 2000 to 44% in 2018.

Source: United Nations (2018)

Table 4.23 Sustainable Development Goal 15

SDG 15: Protect, restore and promote sustainable use of terrestrial ecosystems, sustainably manage forests, combat desertification, and halt and reverse land degradation and halt biodiversity loss	
Progress	**Land degradation** threatens the security and development of all countries
	The red list index shows alarming trend in **biodiversity decline** for mammals, birds, amphibians, corals and cycads
	Protection of forest and terrestrial ecosystems is on the rise, and forest loss has slowed. That said, other facets of terrestrial conservation continue to demand accelerated action to protect biodiversity, land productivity and genetic resources and to curtail the loss of species.
	The Earth's forest areas continue to shrink, down from 4.1 billion hectares in 2000 (or 31.2% of total land area) to about 4 billion hectares (30.7% of total land area) in 2015. However, the rate of forest loss has been cut by 25% since 2000–2005.
	About one fifth of the Earth's land surface covered by vegetation showed persistent and declining trends in productivity from 1999 to 2013, threatening the livelihoods of over one billion people. Up to 24 million square kilometres of land were affected, including 19% of cropland, 16% of forest land, 19% of grassland and 28% of rangeland.
	Since 1993, the global Red List Index of threatened species has fallen from 0.82 to 0.74, indicating an alarming trend in the decline of mammals, birds, amphibians, corals and cycads. The primary drivers of this assault on biodiversity are habitat loss from unsustainable agriculture, deforestation, unsustainable harvest and trade, and invasive alien species.
	Illicit poaching and trafficking of wildlife continues to thwart conservation efforts, with nearly 7000 species of animals and plants reported in illegal trade involving 120 countries.
	In 2016, bilateral ODA in support of biodiversity totalled $7 billion, a decrease of 21% in real terms from 2015.

Source: United Nations (2018)

Table 4.24 Sustainable Development Goal 16

SDG 16: Promote peaceful and inclusive societies for sustainable development, provide access to justice for all and build effective, accountable and inclusive institutions at all levels	
Progress	**More than 570** different trafficking in persons flows were detected between 2012 and 2014
	Proportion of prisoners held in detention without sentencing has **remained almost constant** in the last decade
	2003–2005 = 32%
	2014–2016 = 31%
	Globally, **73%** of children under 5 have had their births registered
	Many regions of the world continue to suffer untold horrors as a result of armed conflict or other forms of violence that occur within societies and at the domestic level. Advances in promoting the rule of law and access to justice are uneven. However, progress is being made in regulations to promote public access to information, albeit slowly, and in strengthening institutions upholding human rights at the national level.
	Nearly 8 in 10 children aged 1–14 years were subjected to some form of psychological aggression and/or physical punishment on a regular basis at home in 81 countries (primarily developing), according to available data from 2005 to 2017. In all but seven of these countries, more than half of children experienced violent forms of discipline.
	More than 570 different flows involving trafficking in persons were detected between 2012 and 2014, affecting all regions; many involved movements from lower-income to higher-income countries.
	In 2014, the majority of detected trafficking victims were women and girls (71%), and about 28% were children (20% girls and 8% boys). Over 90% of victims detected were trafficked for sexual exploitation or forced labour.
	The proportion of prisoners held in detention without being sentenced for a crime remained almost constant in the last decade: From 32% in 2003–2005 to 31% in 2014–2016.
	Almost one in five firms worldwide report receiving at least one bribery payment request when engaged in regulatory or utility transactions.
	Globally, 73% of children under 5 have had their births registered; the proportion is less than half (46%) in sub-Saharan Africa.
	At least 1019 human rights defenders, journalists and trade unionists have been killed in 61 countries since 2015. This is equivalent to one person killed every day while working to inform the public and build a world free from fear and want.
	Freedom-of-information laws and policies have been adopted by 116 countries, with at least 25 countries doing so over the last five years. However, implementation remains a challenge.
	Since 1998, more than half of countries (116 of 197) have established a national human rights institution that has been peer reviewed for compliance with internationally agreed standards (the Paris Principles). However, only 75 of these countries have institutions that are fully compliant.

Source: United Nations (2018)

Table 4.25 Sustainable Development Goal 17

SDG 17: Strengthen the means of implementation and revitalize the Global Partnership for Sustainable Development	
Progress	Goal 17 seeks to strengthen global partnerships to support and achieve the ambitious targets of the 2030 agenda, bringing together national governments, the international community, civil society, the private sector and other actors. Despite advances in certain areas, more needs to be done to accelerate progress. All stakeholders will have to refocus and intensify their efforts on areas where progress has been slow.
	ODA for capacity building and national planning was **$20.4 billion** in 2016, which has been **stable since 2010**
	LDCs' share of world **merchandise exports fell** between 2013 and 2016, after a long period of increase
	2000 = 0.6
	2013 = 1.1
	2016 = 0.9
	In 2015, developing countries received only **0.3% of total ODA** to support all areas of **statistics**
	In 2017, net ODA totalled $146.6 billion in 2017, a decrease of 0.6% from 2016 in real terms. ODA as a share of donors' gross national income (GNI) remained low, at 0.31%.
	In 2016, remittances to low- and lower-middle-income countries were more than three times the amount of ODA they received.
	In LDCs, debt service as a proportion of exports of goods and services increased for five consecutive years—From a low of 3.5% in 2011 to 8.6% in 2016.
	In 2016, high-speed fixed broadband reached 6% of the population in developing countries, compared to 24% in developed countries.
	Total ODA for capacity-building and national planning amounted to $20.4 billion in 2016, representing 18% of total aid allocable by sector, a proportion that has been stable since 2010.
	The developing regions' share of world merchandise exports declined for two consecutive years: From 45.4% in 2014 to 44.2% in 2016, a sharp contrast to an average annual 1.2 percentage point increase between 2001 and 2012. For LDCs, the share of world merchandise exports decreased from 1.1% to 0.9% between 2013 and 2016, compared to the rise from 0.6% to 1.1% between 2000 and 2013.
	In 2017, 102 countries or areas were implementing national statistical plans. Sub-Saharan Africa remained in the lead, with 31 countries implementing such plans; however, only three of them were fully funded.
	In 2015, developing countries received $541 million in financial support from multilateral and bilateral donors for all areas of statistics. This amount represented only 0.3% of total ODA, short of what is needed to ensure that countries in developing regions are better equipped to implement and monitor their development agendas.
	During the decade from 2008 to 2017, 89% of countries or areas conducted at least one population and housing census.

Source: United Nations (2018)

References

Birn, A., Pillay, Y., & Holtz, T. H. (2009). *Textbook of international health: Global health in a dynamic world*. New York: Oxford.

Chopra, M., Lawn, J. E., Sanders, D., Barron, P., Abdool-Karim, S., Bradshaw, D., Jenkes, R., Abdool-Karm, Q., Flisher, A. J., Mayosi, B. M., Tollman, S. M., Churchyard, G. J., & Coovadia, H. (2009a). Achieving the health millennium development goals for South Africa: Challenges and priorities. *Lancet, 374*, 1023–1031.

Chopra, M., Daviaud, E., Pattison, R., Fonn, S., & Lawn, J. E. (2009b). Saving the lives of South Africa's mothers, babies, and children: Can the health system deliver? ' *Lancet, 374*(9692), 835–846.

Dennill, K., & Vasuthevan, S. (2005). *The health of southern Africa*. Cape Town: Juta.

Easterly, W. (2009). How the millennium development goals are unfair to Africa. *World Development, 37*(1), 26–35.

McKinsey & Company. (2016). *Can long-term economic growth be saved*? Available from www.mckinsey.com/insights/growth/can_long-term_global_growth_be_saved

Merson, M. E., Black, R. E., & Mills, A. J. (2012). *Global health: Diseases, programs, systems, and policies*. London: Jones & Bartlett.

United Nations. (2013). *The global partnership for development: The challenge we face*. Available from http://www.un.org/millenniumgoals/2013_Gap_Report/MDG%20GAP%20Task%20Force%20Report%202013_English.pdf

United Nations. (2015). *The millennium development goals report*. New York: United Nations.

United Nations. (2018). *The sustainable development goals report*. New York: United Nations.

Vandemoortele, J. (2011). A fresh look at the MDGs. *Journal of the Asia Pacific Economy, 16*(4), 520–528.

Waage, J., Banerji, R., Campbell, O., Chirwa, E., Collender, G., Dieltiens, V., Dorward, A., Godfrey-Faussett, P., Hanvoravongchai, P., Kingdom, G., Little, A., Mills, A., Mulholland, K., Mwinga, A., North, A., Patcharanarumol, W., Poulton, C., Tangcharoensathien, V., & Unterhalter, E. (2010). The millennium development goals: A cross-sectoral analysis and principles for goal setting after 2015. *Lancet, 376*(9745), 991–1023.

Walley, J., & Wright, J. (2009). *Public health: An action guide to improving health*. New York: Oxford.

Chapter 5
Disease Control and the Promotion of Public Health Equity

Abstract The surge in non-communicable diseases has almost gone unnoticed for quite a while because non-communicable diseases were not even included in the initial health development agenda, specifically the Millennium Development Goals. Given the limited capacity in many low- and middle-income countries, this surge in non-communicable diseases becomes an even huge challenge for these countries to deal with as most of them are still ill-prepared. The costly and prolonged treatment of chronic non-communicable diseases and the fact that women are the most severely affected in the context of both communicable and non-communicable diseases raises the equity problem between and within countries. Prevention of con-communicable diseases is often undermined by rapid urbanisation and globalisation.

Keywords Cancer · Cardiovascular diseases · Career management in HIV · Change management in HIV · Communicable diseases · Community mobilisation · Coordinating in HIV · Corporate social investment · Cost impact of HIV · Diabetes · Differences and behaviours in HIV · Ethics · Exposures · Genetic · Globalisation · HIV and AIDS · Lifestyle · Malaria · Multiple burden of diseases · Non-communicable diseases · Pharmaceutical · Pharmacovigilance · Prevention · Risk factors · Social behaviour change · Tuberculosis · Urbanisation · Workplace HIV policy and strategy

5.1 Tackling the Multiple Burden of Diseases

The burden of disease has become so complex in many settings largely because of fragmented interventions that focus on one aspect of the challenge and overlook the others. It is well and good to suggest that there is a need for an integrated or a simultaneous approach and to strengthen health systems in order to address this challenge. It is worth remembering that health systems encompass the institutions, organisations and resources assembled to deliver health care services that meet

M. P. Mabuza, *Evaluating International Public Health Issues*,
https://doi.org/10.1007/978-981-13-9787-5_5

population needs. The reality is that the health systems of some of the low- and middle-income countries have virtually reached a stage of paralysis, largely due to the deepening vicious cycle of poverty and the overwhelming burden of disease.

In fact, in many of the low- and middle-income countries, strengthening health systems may be easier said than done, due to a number of complexities unique to each country or sub-region. Even if there was money pumped in by the government or by international role players, the money ends up not being utilised efficiently for the purpose of strengthening health systems. For example, complex emergencies in countries such as Sudan, Central African Republic, and Somalia present serious challenges, and dismantle whatever gains might have been made in terms of strengthening health systems (Merson et al. 2012).

Poor leadership and poor service delivery in many low- and middle-income countries, present serious challenges in terms of strengthening health systems. Yet the scale of the challenge posed by the combined and growing infectious chronic illness (driven by HIV and AIDS) and non-communicable diseases in low- and middle-income countries has few parallels to other countries, and demands an extraordinary response that is within the capacity of those low- and middle-income countries to achieve.

It is high time for all, including policy makers, local and international role players to dig deeper into the root cause of this challenge than to just implement blanket strategies that will not be sustainable, bearing in mind that each context and setting is unique. Achievement of a reduction in the double burden of communicable diseases and chronic non-communicable diseases will need a new approach to health systems development. Waiting or stuttering is not an option, because the longer the wait, the more complicated and enormous the challenge will become and will even be more difficult to tackle.

Some of the challenges faced by low- and middle-income countries are lack of political will, poor governance, weakened health systems, poor access to health services, lack of or poor surveillance systems to provide reliable data for planning and prioritisation (Joubert and Ehrlich 2007). One of the major downfalls in terms of tackling the burden of disease in the most affected countries is poor coordination of efforts by the key role players.

The rapid urbanisation and the increasing globalisation of food, tobacco and alcohol industries have posed challenges to the low- and middle-income countries in the sense that this has increased exposure to the risk factors such as risky sexual behaviour associated with HIV and AIDS and also unhealthy lifestyle associated with chronic non-communicable diseases. The huge burden of both communicable diseases and non-communicable diseases puts a huge strain on the capacity of the low- and middle-income countries to deal with. low-income countries generally have lower capacity for the prevention and control of both communicable and non-communicable diseases, and, more so, in the context of globalisation.

The surge in non-communicable diseases has almost gone unnoticed for quite a while because non-communicable diseases were not even included in the health development agenda, specifically the Millennium Development Goals. Given the limited capacity in many low- and middle-income countries, this surge in non-communicable diseases becomes an even huge challenge for these countries to deal with as most of them are still ill-prepared. Whilst chronic non-communicable diseases are usually associated with aging, the unusual surge of chronic non-communicable diseases among the younger people makes it even more important and urgent to tackle both communicable diseases and chronic non-communicable diseases at the same time. There is an observation that women and the youth bear the brunt of the burden of both communicable and non-communicable diseases, particularly in low- and middle-income countries. There is therefore suggestion for sustainable and effective public health interventions and policies targeting risk reduction of communicable and non-communicable diseases among women and the youth.

It is increasingly becoming evident that the challenge posed by non-communicable diseases is no longer an issue of the high-income countries where there is a high proportion of the aging population, but this challenge is also sweeping across low- and middle-income countries, further adding to the huge burden of communicable diseases that have always affected low-income countries. The costly and prolonged treatment of chronic non-communicable diseases and the fact that women are the most severely affected in the context of both communicable and non-communicable diseases raises the equity problem between and within countries.

If this trend continues unabated, low- and middle-income countries will be more constrained to deal with the double burden of communicable and non-communicable diseases in an environment characterised by ill-health systems. Other public health issues such as climate change, political conflict, as well as natural and man-made disasters complicate the picture even more as these also overstretch the already ill-health systems. As such, this creates competing demands in terms of strategic prioritisation pertaining to tackling the double-burden of communicable and non-communicable diseases, particularly in low- and middle-income countries, and this makes it virtually impossible to address the underlying vicious cycle of poverty.

Studies show that in addition to the burden of communicable and non-communicable diseases, women are the most hardest-hit by the cycle of poverty and by the other challenges such as political conflicts and disaster, especially in the low-income countries, and this has huge implications for public health policy (Merson et al. 2012). It is hardly surprising that the World Health Organization stated in 2002 that "in many regions, some of the most formidable enemies of health are joining forces with the allies of poverty to impose a double-burden of disease, disability and premature death in many millions of people". Exposure to some of the low- and middle-income countries where the majority of the population live below the poverty line and have limited access to health care, makes one realise that this challenge is very real, and is huge.

Whereas, life expectancy in high-income countries remains relatively high, life expectancy in many of the low- and middle-income countries that carry the burden of HIV and AIDS has significantly decreased (Merson et al. 2012). However, it is anticipated that with effective antiretroviral therapy, more people living with HIV will live longer, and this suggests that both communicable and chronic non-communicable diseases should be tackled at the same time before the situation gets out of control. However, treatment of disease alone is not sustainable. There is urgent need to scale up on disease prevention efforts.

It has to be commended that in 2000, world leaders committed to the UN Millennium Development Goals (MDGs) which were a set of health-specific and non-health-specific targets to be reached by 2015 (Walley and Wright 2010). The MDGs stimulated more focus on the health and development profile and influenced policymakers to ensure that policies and strategies are implemented to ensure that targets for the MDGs are achieved by each country. As the MDGs reached their deadline in 2015, the world leaders ushered in a new development agenda known as the UN Sustainable Development Goals (SDGs), with the aim of freeing humanity from poverty, securing a healthy planet for future generations, and building peaceful, inclusive societies as a foundation for ensuring lives of dignity for all.

There is no doubt that communicable diseases such as HIV/AIDS, tuberculosis and malaria have been a huge burden in the low-income and middle-income countries for quite some time. However, it is detrimental for policy makers to channel so much attention on such communicable diseases and neglect chronic non-communicable diseases, emerging and re-emerging communicable diseases, and other public health concerns.

> *The Ebola crisis of 2013 to 2015, in West Africa, showed the vulnerability of countries that lack basic health services and the capacity for early detection, comprehensive reporting and a rapid response system for public health outbreaks. For countries without these basic health provisions, shocks created by emerging or re-emerging diseases or other events, such as climate change, can lead to even bigger crises. As the outbreak demonstrated, effective future responses will require country and global preparedness to avoid the reversal of gains in many aspects of development.*

The conspicuous omission of a specific focus on non-communicable diseases from the health development agenda or MDGs has turned out to be very costly omission, as the global burden of non-communicable diseases has now spiralled out of proportion and a huge challenge to control in many middle- and low-income countries. Myths such as the idea that there should be waiting until communicable diseases are controlled before tackling non-communicable diseases and other public health concerns, create a policy-making environment in which it is all too easy to justify neglect (Merson et al. 2012). Such neglect and in some instances the patchwork of responses against non-communicable diseases and other public health concerns by key stakeholders including policy makers is a recipe for disaster because it complicates and perpetuates the challenge, and this has serious implications on the socio-economic and cultural spheres. Low- and middle-income countries are currently faced with serious challenges such as globalisation, urbanisation, and economic development, which are powerful factors affecting chronic non-communicable diseases.

It has been observed that the rapid urbanisation in middle- and low-income countries, comes with many risk factors such as unhealthy lifestyle, of which the younger people are the most vulnerable. As such, it is hardly surprising that there is now an increase in the prevalence and incidence of chronic non-communicable diseases among the young, in such countries. Sometimes, urbanisation comes with better healthcare, and this may imply that more and more people have a chance of living longer, which increases the risk of chronic non-communicable diseases (Merson et al. 2012).

The mental health issues affecting people who live with chronic illnesses as well as the psychological trauma that affects people taking care of those who are chronically ill and dying from disease, as well as the orphans and widows and widowers or even close relatives and friends is often overlooked as a priority public health concern. While it is reported that mental illness is a growing public health concern, the challenge though is how to obtain accurate statistics and information about the real burden of mental illness.

In terms of unintentional injuries and violence, studies show that the overwhelming majority of unintentional injuries and violence occurs in low-income countries. Victims of unintentional injuries and violence may suffer long term psychological trauma (Merson et al. 2012). It is a pity that unintentional injuries and violence were not considered as a global public health priority until recently. Given the fact that approximately 90% of the world's population lives in low- and middle-income countries, it is estimated that the burden of unintentional injuries and violence will increase in these countries (Merson et al. 2012). As such, policymakers and international key actors are expected to take this challenge seriously and put strategies and policies into action to ensure that the burden of such challenges is effectively addressed.

Tackling both communicable and non-communicable disease burdens requires the highest level of political will and concerted efforts of all key role players such as the government, community, non-governmental organisations, and global actors. To some degree, now, politicians and health policy makers are timidly recognising that investing in people's health is a necessary condition for economic development, but energetic decisions are needed for the adoption of urgent and consequent strategies that must take into account the growing trend of risk factors correlated to both communicable and chronic non-communicable diseases.

At the same time there is also an urgent need for public health strategies and policies that will hear the voices of the vulnerable groups who bear the brunt of the double-burden of communicable and non-communicable diseases. Policymakers in developing countries need to be encouraged to give more prominence to the management of chronic non-communicable diseases, mental health and other issues of public health concern (unintentional injuries, violence, nutrition and environmental health) in order to reduce the global burden of disease.

The dominant vertical and mainly curatively-focused medical model (largely driven by the big pharmaceutical industry) needs to be challenged, to ensure that it embraces a holistic and integrative approach, for better and sustainable health outcomes, particularly in resource-poor settings such as low- and middle-income countries (Mabuza 2018d). Equal and genuine partnerships between mainstream modern medicine and traditional, complementary, and alternative medicine (TCAM), present great opportunities for a paradigm shift, discovery, innovation, effective and sustainable disease control, not only in low- and middle-income countries, but also in high-income countries (Mabuza 2018b; Mabuza and Shumba 2018). For example, with the widespread emergence of drug resistance in communicable and non-communicable disease control, such partnerships could create spaces for cross-pollination and evaluation of alternative agents to provide lasting solutions to the burgeoning disease burden (Mabuza 2018e). While the importance of evidence is important, it is a pity that purists believe that their way is the only way, and it is a gap that the dominant evidence-based paradigm is producing health professionals and policy makers that are largely one-dimensional in their practice, and this becomes a limitation in solving complex public health challenges, beyond the scope of the established dominant paradigm (Mabuza 2018c).

> *The scientific mind, in being totally scientific, is being unscientific. We are in a phase of history where the scientific pole is dominant; but where there is pole there is counterpole. The scientist atomises, someone must synthesise. The scientist withdraws, someone must draw together. The scientist particularises, someone must universalise. The scientist dehumanises, someone must humanise. The scientist turns his back on the as yet, and perhaps eternally, unverifiable; someone must face it.* (**John Fowles: from The Aristos**)

Policymakers with the support of the World Health Organization are in a better position to influence change and to ensure that coherent and effective strategies and policies are implemented to reduce the burden of communicable and non-communicable diseases and other issues of public health concern. Systematic action locally and internationally is needed to reduce risk exposures, support healthy behaviours, alleviate the severity of chronic disabling disorders, and mitigate the effects of socioeconomic deprivation. Reliable and accurate information about the burden of disease is a sine qua non for proper management of the burden of disease.

5.2 Cancer

Today, advanced knowledge about cancer prevention, diagnosis, treatment and care, is still not enough, as almost 50% of all cancer patients still die from the disease. Drug resistance is a major barrier to cancer treatment, and the probability of cancer relapse among treated cancer clients presents serious challenges in cancer control. The coexistence or comorbidities of cancer with other diseases such as HIV presents further cancer control challenges.

The majority of people in many low- and middle-income countries are generally at a disadvantage, largely because the terrain is not level between developed countries and developing countries, as well as between those who can afford and those who cannot afford, intra-country (Brookman-May et al. 2017). Cancer often goes ‘unnoticed’ among those who are poor or marginalised. In many low- and middle-income countries, the picture is further complicated by rapid urbanisation where there is now a growing combination of cancers related to poverty and cancers related to lifestyle and occupational exposures. The fragile health systems, significant level of lack of data, non-functional cancer registries, largely absent or poor cancer screening, significant lost to follow up of cancer cases, and the almost non-existent research capacity, pose a serious challenge to cancer control efforts in developing countries. This points towards an urgent need for new approaches and tools to prevent cancer. However, prevention cannot stand alone without proper cancer surveillance and cancer control systems. In retrospect, it is argued that the most common modelling approaches to understanding incidence, prevalence and control of chronic diseases in populations, such as statistical regression models, are limited when it comes to dealing with the complexity of those problems (Carvallo et al. 2015).

Evolving risk factors for cancers in low- and middle-income countries such as in African populations include lifestyle, infection, and genetic susceptibility. While cancer control should not be viewed in isolation, there is need to explore and investigate the contribution of inherited genetic variants to the development of cancer such as breast, cervical and oesophageal cancer in low- and middle-income countries such as sub-Saharan Africa, Asia and the Americas. There is also a need to measure the effect of exposures that are common, and which may lead to cancer, such as smoking, indoor air pollution, alcohol, and hormonal factors. The contribution of infections known to cause cancer, such as Helicobacter pylori, HIV, Human Papilloma viruses, Epstein Barr viruses, Kaposi sarcoma-associated herpesviruses, Hepatitis B/C, and certain polyomaviruses, needs to be seriously investigated. There is also an urgent need to address the issue of proven and probable cancer-causing chemicals such as in certain therapeutic drugs (recently, a certain antihypertensive drug has been recalled due to new evidence indicating that it contains a cancer-causing chemical), food (including genetically modified food), and the environment. Neglect of these issues and the disparities between those who are privileged and those who are disadvantaged and marginalised, will have serious implications in the future. Successful cancer control ensures that people are as healthy as possible, regardless of age, sex, gender, ethnicity, location, affiliation, or socio-economic status.

A strategic approach to cancer control for each geographic setting or region is needed to build on what works there and what is unique to the setting or region. It should ideally be situated within strong, robust, and sustainable healthcare systems that offer quality healthcare to all people, irrespective of their social or economic standing. However, to achieve this will need new leadership, critical thinking, investment, and understanding (Morhason-Bello et al. 2013).

5.3 Diabetes

The barriers to diabetes control are multifactorial and complex in both developed and developing countries. There is substantial evidence of the existence of the gap in the level of diabetes mellitus and its complications, prevention and control measures in low- and middle-income countries (Animaw and Seoum 2017). Generally, the health systems of low- and middle-income countries that are worst affected by the increasing burden of diabetes and other chronic diseases are not well-prepared to deal with the huge burden of disease.

In countries such as Indonesia where the rapid increase in the prevalence of diabetes is coincidentally accompanied by rapid economic and demographic evolution, are faced with four key issues in diabetes control: lack of awareness about diabetes in the general public and among some healthcare personnel and policymakers; inequity of healthcare supply and demand resulting from an expanding patient population and too few diabetes specialists; lack of resources in the public healthcare system and among the Indonesian population; too few people receiving proper treatment or insulin, resulting in poor-quality care (Fountaine et al. 2016; Novo Nordisk 2013).

Another challenge in diabetes control is that diabetes causes other complications such as cardiovascular disorders (including stroke, and heart attack, among others), kidney failure, diabetic retinopathy, diabetic neuropathy and peripheral neuropathy, which are responsible for severe morbidity and mortality (Narayan 2016). Treatment of diabetes and its complications is a challenge in countries such as India owing to several issues, including sociocultural factors, lack of appropriate facilities for diabetes care, an inadequate health system, poor monitoring and follow-up of patients, and problems in implementing effective management and educational strategies (Viswanathan and Rao 2013).

Some of the measures taken by some countries from which others can learn include the following: developing a national diabetes strategy; establishing data systems and performance-management processes; upgrading primary-care networks; using innovative healthcare models to increase screening and diagnosis, particularly in remote areas; upgrading the skills of and providing incentives to healthcare-delivery professionals; empowering patients to improve adherence to therapy; increasing awareness of healthy living and encouraging lifestyle changes; developing policies to promote and enforce healthier lifestyles (Fountaine et al. 2016).

Policy goals should be: to improve disease management for people with diabetes to reduce complication rates; establish effective surveillance to identify and support those at risk of type 2 diabetes; introduce a range of interventions to create an environment focused on prevention (Colagiuri et al. 2015).

There is urgent need to shift priorities from communicable diseases such as HIV/AIDS, and to put the diabetes challenge on the public health agenda. There is a call for governments to regulate the marketing and sale of unhealthy food, and providing subsidies for fresh organic foods, particularly in low- and middle-income countries (International Federation of Medical Students' Association 2018). Interestingly, while countries such as Mexico have introduced taxation on sugar with the aim of shifting people's consumption towards healthy food, there is a knowledge gap in terms of which drinks people are shifting to, or, importantly, whether this measure is helping to reduce obesity (Narayan 2016). While evidence shows that focusing on health promotion and disease prevention could reduce the burden of diabetes and other non-communicable diseases by over 50%, the supply of affordable healthy food is a big challenge, and, there is also a gap on how to motivate people to lead healthy lifestyle, more so, in low- and middle-income countries where there are complex intrinsic and extrinsic factors (Narayan 2016; World Health Organization 2018a, b). It is a gap that adolescents and youth are often overlooked, yet they are a tremendous resource to promote healthy behaviour at a young age, so that morbidity and premature death due to diabetes and other related diseases could be prevented.

While there is good data and knowledge on how to control diabetes in high-income countries, information from high-income countries does not necessarily apply to low- and middle-income countries. As such, there is need to understand how best to subsidise the production and supply of healthy food at affordable prices in the context of specific low- and middle-income countries; need to understand how best to motivate people to engage in healthy lifestyle, and to understand other factors for diabetes apart from being overweight (Narayan 2016).

Since diabetes causes complications including cardiovascular diseases, it is crucial that diabetes control measures are integrated with cardiovascular diseases control and prevention. In fact, diseases control should be approached as a continuum including communicable and non-communicable diseases control and prevention. Opportunities are there to embed non-communicable diseases control into communicable disease control such as HIV, TB, and malaria policies, strategies and programmes.

5.4 Cardiovascular Diseases

The dramatic rise of cardiovascular diseases (such as stroke, and related heart disease, predominantly driven by increased rates of hypertension, individual health choices, and, many external factors beyond the individual's control), and, comorbidities associated with diabetes and HIV, presents serious public health challenges in disease control (Keates et al. 2017).

Control of cardiovascular diseases (CVD) in South East Asia and sub-Saharan Africa is poor, and the barriers to CVD control include: significant numbers of individuals with cardiovascular diseases in low- and middle-income countries are unaware of their condition; poor adherence due to long duration of therapy; complicated regimens; cost of drugs; side effects of medication; lack of specific appointment time; long waiting period at clinic or office; lack of consistent and continuous primary care; instructions not understood; organic brain damage (memory deficit); medicines not available; asymptomatic nature of the condition, chronic condition require constant attention; there are no immediate consequences of stopping treatment, for example one does not feel sick; social isolation; disrupted home situation; and psychiatric illnesses (Mohan et al. 2013).

Strategies designed to tackle the evolving and increasing burden of cardiovascular diseases (CVD) and related non-communicable diseases in low- and middle-income countries will be dependent upon accurate and up to date epidemiological data on the cardiovascular or non-communicable disease profile of the population groups in a particular geographic setting or region (Keates et al. 2017). Crucially, in low- and middle-income countries where communicable disease management systems are already established, there is no need to reinvent the wheel by creating separate non-communicable disease management systems. An integrated approach between the management of communicable diseases and non-communicable diseases is the most ideal, particularly in resource-poor settings, and it also presents an opportunity for efficiency, effectiveness and sustainability, for better health outcomes.

A Settings Approach to Non-communicable Disease Prevention and Management in a Southern African Maritime Port
By Dr Mbuso Precious Mabuza

Abstract:

The purpose of this report is to focus on the existing self-care and employee wellness intervention designed to improve health outcomes in relation to the epidemic of non-communicable diseases at the Southern African Maritime Port and the surrounding communities. The health promotion intervention has been largely biomedical in its approach because it focused on the presence of disease rather than the absence of disease. The health promotion intervention has not really been successful and was met with resistance because it was purely a top-down approach which overlooked the importance for a needs assessment and participation of the target population at the outset. This intervention was not culturally relevant or culturally sensitive and it also overlooked the social determinants of health. A more holistic approach that takes into consideration the living and working conditions, and the whole ecosystem could have yielded better outcomes.

Background:

The increase in the incidence and prevalence of non-communicable has been of great concern, not only in sub-Saharan Africa, because it has now become the leading cause of mortality, globally (World Health Organization 2011). Non-communicable diseases such as diabetes mellitus, cardiovascular diseases such as hypertension and heart disease have been of particular concern in sub-Saharan Africa, largely because of the changing lifestyles not only in urban areas but in rural areas as well (Mayosi et al. 2009). Obesity and sedentary lifestyle have been touted as being among the major underlying factors in the epidemic of non-communicable diseases such as diabetes mellitus and cardiovascular diseases (Plath et al. 2008). According to Noblet and Lamontagne (2006), stress due to poverty, unemployment, despair, poor work and living conditions, has also fuelled the epidemic of non-communicable diseases and the combination of all these underlying factors has deleterious effects in terms of cardiovascular diseases and diabetes mellitus in particular. It has been reported that the magnitude of the HIV and AIDS epidemic has somewhat contributed to the insidious escalation of non-communicable diseases because HIV and AIDS has shifted the focus from other pressing health issues particularly in sub-Saharan Africa where there are also issues of poorly financed and poorly managed health systems (Kirigia and Barry 2008). Unlike communicable diseases, the management and prevention of non-communicable diseases is very complex because the causes are multifactorial (Arora et al. 2011).

The purpose of this report is to focus on the existing health promotion initiative of self-care and employee wellness designed to improve health outcomes with regard to the non-communicable diseases such as diabetes mellitus, cardiovascular diseases that are prevalent in the Southern African Maritime Port and the surrounding communities. This report will concentrate on the relevance of health promotion concepts and practices aimed at addressing the abovementioned issues identified in the Southern African Maritime Port and the surrounding communities. The workplace setting is regarded as a strategic setting for health promotion interventions because such interventions do not only impact on the workplace, but on the employees' families and the communities where employees live. In that regard, the workplace setting is better positioned to influence national health and social policies for better health outcomes (Noblet 2003).

Identification of the Setting:

The setting of focus in this study is the workplace setting of the Southern African Maritime Port whose core business is freight and logistics. The Maritime Port of focus is one of the most complex ports in the home country, because of the numerous break-bulk cargo that it handles. For example, commodities such as manganese, chrome, magnetite, haematite, granite, and many other mineral commodities are handled at the Maritime Port. The Southern African Maritime Port is also among the busiest and biggest coal terminals in Africa. The staff complement is 1000 permanent employees and 2000 contract employees, and the average age of the workforce is approximately 50 years. Blue-collar employees form approximately 90% of the entire workforce at the Southern African Maritime Port. The shift system is arranged in such a way that employees have to work for three consecutive weeks before they could get a weekend off. Employees that work for the Maritime Port mainly come from various parts of Southern Africa. The Maritime Port's hometown is generally, an established industrial centre with a glaring issue of air pollution, and the area has extremely hot summer months and the winter months are very mild.

Identification of the Public Health Issues/s Targeted:

The public health issues that are targeted in this study are the non-communicable diseases such as diabetes mellitus, and cardiovascular diseases such as hypertension and heart disease. Based on the company's medical surveillance programme, non-communicable diseases have become a huge concern because more than 50% of the company's employees suffer from at least one of the abovementioned non-communicable diseases and that instead of decreasing, the trend is increasing. This shows that something needs to be urgently done because these diseases are not being well managed or prevented, and this has a negative impact on the healthcare system and the economy.

Relevance of Health Promotion Concepts in This Issue:

The company has implemented a self-care programme to ensure that all employees are educated and empowered about taking care of their own lives. In this self-care programme the company has identified behaviour aspects that have a bearing on the escalation of non-communicable diseases in the workplace. These behaviour aspects include lack of physical activity, poor weight management, smoking, alcoholism, poor diet, poor monitoring of medical condition, poor sleep patterns, lack of rest, and stress. An external service provider has been appointed to manage the medical side of the health issues and another external service provider has been appointed to manage the wellness aspect, and these services are also extended to the employees' immediate family members. For instance, there is an on-site occupational health clinic which has also incorporated a primary healthcare component to address the non-occupational diseases such as the non-communicable diseases of focus in this study. There is an appointed registered nurse, who is dedicated to the self-care programme, and this requires the nursing sister to conduct daily and weekly educational sessions to employees in the various departments of the workplace.

The concepts of health promotion applied in the workplace setting of the Port of Richards Bay is more of a Western medical approach because it focuses on the presence of disease rather than the absence of disease (Naidoo and Wills 2009). Whitehead and Dahlgren (2006), emphasize the importance of considering the social determinants of health, which were overlooked in this intervention.

According to the Republic of South Africa's health and social policy, all people living in South Africa must have equitable access to quality healthcare, and this may be achieved through strengthening of the health system. A National Health Insurance Policy is in the process of being enacted and ratified, and this is aimed at bridging the health gap in terms of accessing quality healthcare between those who can afford and those who cannot afford because of their low socioeconomic status.

Possible Evaluation Measures:

Currently, a quantitative methodology is employed through the use of anonymous questionnaires to gain feedback from the employees that use the onsite workplace clinic in order to get the employees' perception of how they feel about their treatment at the onsite clinic as part of their medical screening and about the self-care programme in general. This purely follows a quantitative methodology rather than a combined approach.

Ideally, evaluation should be done in partnership with the target group (World Health Organization 2009). It would have possibly served a better purpose to have the combination of a qualitative and quantitative approach (Green 2000). A qualitative approach through focus groups could have highlighted the real gaps and opportunities for improvement for better health outcomes. However, the challenge with health promotion interventions is that it cannot show explicit evidence (Raphael 2000). This may require that standards be set (Judd et al. (2001). Nutbeam (1998) highlights the importance of evaluating healthy behaviours, healthy environments and effectiveness of health services.

Discussion on the Issues of Cultural Relevance and Cultural Sensitivities of the Intervention:

Studies highlight the importance of considering the unique culture of the setting. It is worth mentioning that approximately 98% of the workforce of the Southern African Maritime Port is indigenous Africans and steeped in their culture, and the remaining 2% is shared among the first language English and Afrikaans speaking employees. The fact that the whole intervention was imposed on the employees and the approach was viewed as foreign by the majority of the workforce indicates that the intervention was not culturally relevant and not culturally sensitive to the majority of the employees. The importance of considering the different context of different socioeconomic groups, implies that this intervention was probably only culturally relevant and culturally sensitive to the first language English speakers who comprised a very small minority. Reflecting on some of the envisaged health behaviours of the intervention such as encouraging people to eat a balanced diet, such interventions are not culturally sensitive because the majority of the target group are of a low socioeconomic status. Talking about a balanced diet to people of low socioeconomic status is being insensitive because the majority of the people struggle to even make ends meet. The majority of the employees are bread winners and they support very large families including extended families. Another envisaged health behaviour that was culturally insensitive was that of encouraging people to lose weight. In this part of the world losing weight is often associated with HIV and AIDS, and as a result, people are afraid of losing weight because of the stigma that has been created. People would rather prefer to gain weight as this is often associated with status and subconsciously also somewhat gives them a stamp of approval that they do not have HIV and AIDS. Such a stigma becomes a challenge in health promotion terms because it encourages obesity which is a huge risk for non-communicable diseases. It was also insensitive to preach to the employees that they should get quality sleep, rest and avoid stress because the majority of them live in informal settlements which are in a very bad state, including lack of portable water, lack of sewerage system, lack of proper waste management, and generally in a very appalling hygiene condition. If the work conditions are so bad and the living conditions are even worse, it is really unfair and insensitive to expect them to lead a good quality of life. The interventions should have addressed the living conditions in the communities where the employees live and also put controls in place to address the hazardous work environment and the shift system which does not allow enough time for the employees to rest.

The ground was not properly prepared for this intervention because a health needs assessment was not done. A health needs assessment with full participation of the target group or groups could have helped so that the intervention could be tailor-made for them, rather than being imposed. When a health promotion intervention is tailor-made for a specific group or individuals, this gives it a better chance of sustainability and ownership (Harden et al. 1999).

A Critical Review of the Success or Otherwise of the Intervention in Health Promotion Terms:

The fact that this top-down approach did not take into consideration the need to improve the work environment in terms of putting controls in place to prevent exposure of employees to occupational hazards, was a major downfall. Although employees were encouraged to go for medical screening at the onsite clinic, this was not enough because the employees were still exposed to the same risky work environment in terms of exposure to chemical hazards, physical hazards, ergonomic hazards, and psychosocial hazards. Clearly, this has been a huge failure and a waste of money, and such money could have been better used in the improvement of the work environment and to put control measures in place to ensure that employees are not exposed to unacceptable risk.

A more holistic settings approach that takes into consideration the living and working conditions of the employees and the whole ecosystem could have yielded better health outcomes (Dooris 2009). The importance of a health needs assessment that involves full participation of the target group has to be more emphasised in this regard. A clear focus on the social determinants of health and the commitment to ensure sustainability of health promotion interventions is most desirable. Baum and Harris (2006) emphasise the importance of having clear policies, partnerships and a global outlook to ensure sustainability of health promotion interventions.

Social Marketing Strategies:

Although social marketing can help to influence the social and health terrain, behaviour change is very complex in social marketing terms (McDermott et al. 2005). The envisaged outcome or product of the social marketing strategy at the Southern African Maritime Port was to change behaviour of the employees to ensure that the risk of non-communicable diseases is reduced or eliminated. The anticipated behaviour aspects include physical activity, good weight management to ensure a normal body mass index, quitting smoking or not starting at all, quitting alcohol or responsible drinking, following a balanced diet, regular medical screening, having quality sleep patterns, good rest periods, and preventing stress or managing it. The value of the envisaged health behaviour was not really taken into consideration because this was a top-down approach. The onsite clinic was used as the centre for the medical screening and the sections where the employees worked were used as outreach centres. Notice boards, emails, plasma screens, pamphlets and shift change forums were used to advertise the self-care programme with the aim of changing the behaviour of the employees for better health. The positioning was very poor because the beliefs and attitudes of the employees were not really taken into account in the sense that the messages were in English and the whole approach was westernised, and yet the Southern African Maritime Port area and surrounding communities are generally steeped in their local tradition. Moreover, the approach seemed to be over the top and missed the target because the majority of the employees were illiterate. Clearly there was a great need to segment the target audience to ensure that the messages were relevant and targeted (Grier and Bryant 2005). The potential audiences were the employees of the Southern African Maritime Port and the surrounding communities where the majority of the employees lived. The partnerships were between the Southern African Maritime Port and the service provider that was operating the onsite clinic and responsible for the Self-care programme. The target audience would not be regarded as partners because this approach was a one-way flow. It was more like telling the employees what to do rather than sharing with them and getting their input on what they thought could work to change their behaviour if they had to. There was no supportive policy environment and there was no code of good practice for occupational health. The financing of the marketing of the self-care programme was sufficient, except that the whole approach was ambitious, misdirected, and over the top.

Conclusion

It can be concluded that the self-care and employee wellness health promotion intervention at the Southern African Maritime Port was largely not successful because it was a top-down approach and a health needs assessment was not done and the target group was not involved at the outset. This approach was also not culturally relevant and not culturally sensitive but was possibly successful with the small minority group which is generally of a higher socio-economic status, and this may result in further widening the health gradient as observed by Graham (2004). The importance of doing proper planning for health promotion interventions is vital (Victorian Government Department of Human Services 2008). It is crucial to have good health policies, to form partnerships and take into account the social determinants of health to ensure that the health promotion intervention is sustainable (Graham 2009). A more holistic settings approach that combines the biomedical and the salutogenic concepts and also takes the whole ecosystem into account is a more desirable approach. The importance of social marketing in health promotion interventions cannot be underestimated (Crawshaw and Newlove 2011).

5.5 Malaria

Epidemiology of malaria is the description of what is known about the distribution and determinants of malaria (Joubert and Ehrlich 2007). Transmitted to humans by the female Anopheles mosquitoes, malaria is regarded as the most important vector-transmitted disease in the world, particularly in tropical regions of middle- and low-income countries where it causes an estimated 1 to two million deaths each year (Merson et al. 2012).

It is reported that warm and humid climatic conditions are conducive for malaria transmission, and that the efficiency of the malaria vector will depend on the species of Anopheles and the environmental conditions (Walley and Wright 2010). As such, global climate change or global warming has been implicated in epidemic malaria as more and more malaria infections in previously malaria non-endemic areas such as the highland areas which were protected by their low temperatures, are now being seen (Walley and Wright 2010).

Poor socio-economic conditions and lack of resources to effectively deal with the challenge are also implicated in the epidemic of malaria, and as such, it is hardly surprising that low income countries such as in sub-Saharan Africa are the most severely affected, even though disproportionately so (Birn et al. 2009).

Dennill and Vasuthevan (2005) add that the scale of the malaria problem has increased in southern Africa due to deterioration in the environment, disasters such as flooding, conflict and the resultant movement of people in the region, and as a result of drug-resistant malaria. It is worth mentioning that in non-immune populations, malaria affects both children and adults equally, whereas in areas of stable transmission, children and pregnant women are predominantly affected resulting in considerable mortality, due to the deadly *Plasmodium falciparum* species of the malaria parasite (Walley and Wright 2010).

Some of the current trends of the epidemiology of malaria highlight that countries such as the United States of America cannot afford not to reinforce prevention and controls against malaria, as it is clear that malaria is beginning to occur in areas that were previously thought to be malaria-free. There is no doubt that climate change may increase the zones where malaria is at risk of being able to spread within the United States of America or other countries that may have been declared malaria-free.

Studies show that countries such as the United States of America and parts of Europe still have the mosquitoes that transmit malaria, but the main reason why malaria has not thrived in the United States of America and Europe in the recent past is because of economic development and better public health interventions as opposed to many low-income countries which have struggled to implement effective and sustainable public health interventions such as anti-malaria programmes (De Zulueta 1998).

However, the latest available evidence suggests that in parts of the United States of America, for example, small outbreaks of locally transmitted malaria have occurred during unseasonably hot weather conditions (Merson et al. 2012). There is growing body of evidence that the unseasonably hot weather conditions may be attributable to global climate change, particularly global warming which seems to have complicated the whole picture in a number of ways, as malaria is now prevalent in elevated regions where it did not previously exist (Merson et al. 2012).

Travellers to and from malaria endemic areas also carry the risk of bringing malaria to previously unaffected areas (Stoppacher and Adams 2003). It is encouraging to see that the Centers for Disease Control and Prevention (CDC) provides 24 hour technical assistance to health care providers to ensure that there is rapid and accurate diagnosis of malaria for appropriate treatment of affected individuals and to prevent the further spread of malaria in the community (Centers for Disease Control and Prevention 2010). The role played by the CDC is advantageous as part of the prevention and control of malaria in the United States of America.

Malaria should really be regarded as a major global public health priority and that developed countries such as the United States of America should scale up efforts even in the malaria endemic areas of low- and middle-income countries, and rather more so with the complications of climate change, as studies project that the malaria agent, will be able to spread into new areas in the near future (Merson et al. 2012). An observation is that malaria has already spread to new areas in low income countries, and this is impacting negatively on equitable public health outcomes as the poor and vulnerable are the most severely affected as they often have poor access to health care services, especially in the rural areas.

Given the magnitude of the malaria issue, it is hardly surprising that the international community has identified malaria as a global public health priority that requires international and multi-sectoral partnerships for intervention. The Rollback Malaria Partnership employs the following tools to control malaria: long-lasting insecticidal nets; indoor residual spraying; intermittent preventive treatment during pregnancy; other vector controls including larvaciding and environmental management; and prompt diagnosis and treatment (Merson et al. 2012).

There is no doubt that all the above-mentioned preventive or control measures are crucial, but the challenge today is that the malaria parasite has almost become resistant to all the available antimalarial drugs and has become so resilient to control (Birn et al. 2009). Some authors concede that even the discovery of a vaccine will not eradicate malaria, unless there is a clear understanding of the fundamental mechanisms related to poverty and the dynamism of the determinants of malaria such as human demographics, climate change, environment, land use patterns, drug and vaccine efficiency as they inevitably change over time (Ricci 2012). It is interesting that South Africa has decided to bring back DDT for indoor residual spraying of walls for malaria control, even though this chemical is banned in many parts of the world.

The epidemiology of malaria is very complex, and the complexity is even more magnified in low-income countries, largely due to multidimensional poverty. Therefore, preventive and control efforts should take this complexity as well as the determinants of malaria into account.

5.5.1 Impact of Malaria Programmes

It would be interesting to review what impact the availability of malaria vaccine would have in malaria-endemic low–income countries. The issue of malaria is a cause for concern especially because even though the Global Malaria Action Plan (GMAP) released by the Roll Back Malaria (RBM) Partnership uses key tools to control malaria, each year, there are up to three million deaths due to malaria and close to five billion episodes of clinical illness occur throughout the world, with Africa having more than 90% of this burden.

This suggests that the key tools to control malaria have not been effective. Even if such tools were effective at some stage; they were not sustainable, particularly in the malaria-endemic areas of low-income countries such as in sub-Saharan Africa. Innovations such as the development of an effective malaria vaccine do bring a modicum of hope, especially given the worrisome spread of drug-resistant malaria. Based on the historical success of certain programmes mounted to control and then eradicate certain infectious diseases such as smallpox and polio in many parts of the world, it is anticipated that an effective malaria vaccine would decrease and ultimately eliminate malaria in the malaria-endemic areas.

It is commendable that the World Health Organisation (WHO) together with other partners, have been working together on the Expanded Program on Immunization (EPI) with the goal of universal coverage in the context of primary health care or maternal and child health programs (Birn et al. 2009). Further, the Global Alliance for Vaccines and Immunization (GAVI) together with the Bill and Melinda Gates Foundation and other partners, is working to ensure the earliest possible incorporation of other vaccines into the EPI (Merson et al. 2012). As it is believed that the RTS.S malaria vaccine will soon be licenced, models of impact of the malaria vaccine have mainly considered deployment via the WHO's EPI in areas of stable endemic transmission of malaria, and have been calibrated for such settings.

However, looking at the complex situation in many low-income countries; even if an effective malaria vaccine were to be innovated, a malaria vaccine on its own is not going to eliminate malaria if additional efforts to address access barriers, lack of resources, political and socio-cultural implications of malaria and their relationships with multi-dimensional poverty are not considered (Ricci 2012).

In that sense, the better way to win the battle against malaria is to improve the economic level of populations living in many countries of malaria-endemic areas together with the synthesis of a good vaccine (Ricci 2012). Unless additional efforts are directed towards addressing access barriers among the poor and vulnerable, malaria will remain a major cause of morbidity and mortality in sub-Saharan Africa and many regions of Asia where malaria is endemic (Ricci 2012).

5.6 Tuberculosis

Tuberculosis (TB) is an infectious, chronic or acute or sub-acute notifiable disease, characterised by lesion formation in tissues and organs in the body, by far the most frequent being the lungs, which type is the only source of communal spread. Tuberculosis, in people is mainly caused by a species of mycobacteria known as *Mycobacterium tuberculosis* (Merson et al. 2012).

Tuberculosis and infection with *Mycobacterium tuberculosis* are by far among the most important public health problems in the world, as it is estimated that approximately one third of the world's population is infected with Mycobacterium tuberculosis, but the only determinant of illness is a suppressed immune system (Merson et al. 2012). As such, the HIV pandemic has had disastrous consequences for the control of tuberculosis, particularly in the low- and middle-income countries, especially the most affected regions such as the Southern Africa Development Community (SADC) which bears the highest burden of HIV/AIDS and tuberculosis in the whole world. The emergence of multi-drug resistant tuberculosis (MDR-TB) and extensively drug resistant tuberculosis (XDR-TB) has complicated the whole picture, thereby creating more challenges regarding interventions to deal with tuberculosis, particularly in low-income countries.

While globalisation (the increased interconnectedness of countries such that there is open sharing of ideas, information flow, trade and markets, as well as technology and development) has contributed positively towards advancement in health care including tuberculosis care; globalisation has also exacerbated the poverty situation in low- and middle-income countries (Walley and Wright 2010). Climate change has also worsened the poverty situation in the sense that extreme weather conditions such as extreme drought have made it difficult for rural people to have a livelihood through subsistence farming, thereby increasing their vulnerability. Globalisation and climate change have inadvertently forced people to flock to the urban centres to seek employment, thereby exacerbating the creation of mega cities, proliferation of informal settlements, overcrowding, and poor living conditions in general which accelerates the spread of communicable diseases such as tuberculosis.

There is evidence that the poor have increased vulnerability to tuberculosis, and as such, it is hardly surprising that tuberculosis has now been regarded as the disease of the poor. The irony is that tuberculosis was brought to the low- and middle-income countries by Europeans, and yet it is the populations of the low- and middle-income countries that bear the highest burden of tuberculosis.

Although international organisations such as the World Bank have made efforts towards financing and supporting global public health interventions including efforts towards the achievement of the Millennium Development Goals (MDGs) including MDG 6 which aimed at combating AIDS, Malaria and other diseases such as Tuberculosis. Such efforts have been unsustainable, and at best they seem to foster the economic notions of globalisation to the detriment of the public health situation of low- and middle-income countries.

Given the magnitude of the local and global challenges posed by tuberculosis, and the inequalities and inequities that go with it, it is imperative that a global response to this challenge be urgent, effective and sustainable. As such, it would be important to describe how one would design a strategy to deal with tuberculosis as a public health problem.

The main approach to dealing with tuberculosis in low- and middle-income countries is based on the strategy of rapid detection of and provision of effective multi-drug therapy to all infectious persons or patients with pulmonary tuberculosis, particularly smear-positive patients (Merson et al. 2012). The mainstay to the effective multi-drug therapy is the World Health Organization's recommended directly observed treatment short course (DOTS) which involves the use of a standardised multi-drug short-course regimen, with direct observation of drug ingestion for at least the first two months of treatment (Merson et al. 2012).

In South Africa, the strategy of rapid detection and provision of multi-drug therapy to all infectious persons is the main strategy that is still widely employed across the country. However, this strategy has not been without challenges especially with the emergence of multi-drug resistant tuberculosis (MDR-TB) and extensively drug resistant tuberculosis (XDR-TB), and of course the coexistence of tuberculosis and HIV/AIDS which complicates the whole picture, and requires a different approach to dealing with tuberculosis.

Since 2006, the main strategy to deal with the burden of tuberculosis adopted by the World Health Organization is the Stop TB Strategy, and this strategy has six components which include the following: pursue high quality DOTS expansion and enhancement; address TB-HIV, MDR-TB, and the needs of poor and vulnerable populations; contribute to health system strengthening based on primary health care; engage all care providers; empower people with TB, and communities through partnership; and enable and promote research.

1. *Pursue high quality DOTS expansion and enhancement:*

Under the component of 'pursue high quality DOTS expansion and enhancement' mentioned above, there are five elements, which are: political commitment with increased and sustained financing; ensuring early case detection, and diagnosis through quality-assured bacteriology; provision of standardized treatment with supervision, and patient support; ensuring effective drug supply and management; monitoring and evaluation of performance and impact.

Firstly, there is emphasis on political commitment with increased and sustained financing. Political commitment is the most important aspect of the whole tuberculosis strategy because it bolsters and fosters national and international partnerships and ensures that there is sustainability of the programme. Political commitment is also crucial in terms of financing because it ensures that there is mobilisation of resources, and in fact, with political commitment the global financing such as the Global Fund to Fight AIDS, Tuberculosis and Malaria offers new opportunities for dealing with the burden of tuberculosis not only at local level but at global level as well (Birn et al. 2009). Political commitment can go a long way towards making a meaningful difference and success of the overall strategy to deal with tuberculosis. Without political commitment from the very onset, the strategy is bound to fall flat.

Secondly, there is emphasis on ensuring early case detection, and diagnosis through quality-assured bacteriology. This requires technical expertise and well-equipped facilities or laboratories where the diagnosis or case detection of tuberculosis can be performed such as through sputum smear microscopy and then culture and drug susceptibility testing. It is recommended that laboratory networks meet certain requirements and principles such as the adoption of national standards that are in line with international guidelines; high proficiency levels should be maintained in the decentralised diagnostic services; communication should be maintained across all levels of the laboratory networks; supervision, internal and external quality management should be maintained. Such facilities should also be used for occasional surveillance and monitoring of prevalence of tuberculosis including MDR-TB, XDR-TB, and the coexistence of TB and HIV not only in adults but in children as well. As such, this suggests that the laboratory staff should be well motivated and well trained and developed about new trends regarding the epidemiology of tuberculosis on an on-going basis to ensure that they carry out their work with excellence and high standards of quality and accuracy in terms of case detection and diagnosis.

Thirdly, there is emphasis on standardised treatment, with supervision and patient support. This is regarded as the mainstay of the strategy to deal with tuberculosis in the sense that it takes into account the importance of providing the right tuberculosis treatment services for all paediatric and adult patients, putting more emphasis on adherence to treatment guidelines according to the different categories of patients. It is particularly important that this element of the strategy to deal with tuberculosis takes cognisance of the fact that supervision and patient support should be context-specific and be carried out in a patient-sensitive manner. What is good about this element is that it does put importance on implementing locally appropriate measures to deal with physical, financial, cultural and health system barriers to accessing tuberculosis treatment. For example, in South Africa, the poorest of the poor are somewhat marginalised because there is poor access to health services particularly in the rural areas. As such, the poor people have to travel very long distances to access the nearest health services, and most of the time, transport is a big issue. Because of this challenge, many of the poor people who have been infected with tuberculosis do not have access to tuberculosis treatment, and most of the time, even if they do, there is poor adherence largely because of the barriers mentioned above and also because they do not have anything to eat. In that sense, it would be important to ensure that tuberculosis treatment outlets are expanded in the poorest settings, ensuring that patients do not have to pay or travel long distances, that the health service staff providing such services are also motivated to deal with the challenge, and more importantly to ensure that there is equitable access to healthcare services, particularly with regard to tuberculosis treatment.

Fourthly, there is emphasis on an effective drug supply and management system. One of the biggest challenges facing many low- and middle-income countries is lack of a reliable system that will ensure adequate and sustained drug supplies not only with regard to tuberculosis but with regard to ARVs as well. As such, it is very crucial to ensure that there is a reliable procurement system that will guarantee adequate and uninterrupted tuberculosis drug supplies to all relevant health services to ensure that all patients who are supposed to get the drugs get the correct drugs and at the right time. Otherwise, unavailability of quality-assured tuberculosis drugs will interrupt treatment and result in drug resistance. It is encouraging though that the Stop TB Partnership's Global Drug Facility and the Green Light Committee provide support to countries with lack of capacity to ensure that quality-assured tuberculosis drugs are available at low cost and that the healthcare staff or those responsible for the drug supply and management system are adequately trained on tuberculosis drug management.

Fifthly, there is emphasis on monitoring and evaluation of performance and impact. This requires an effective monitoring and evaluation system, and impact assessment measurement to be in place. For this to be possible there should be a standardised recording and reporting system about individual patient data and reporting and monitoring of treatment outcomes at the health facility level, identification of problems as they arise at the district level, ensuring consistently high quality tuberculosis controls at national level, and to evaluate the performance of each country at international level. There is no doubt that the recording, analysis and reporting of data may require that tuberculosis programme managers and relevant personnel undergo specific training to ensure that they are acquainted with the latest trends and requirements in this regard, and also pertaining to the use of electronic software as this may greatly facilitate this data recording, analysis and reporting that incorporates tuberculosis data from the public and private health sectors, to ensure that data reflected by the World Health Organization's report on Global TB Control is complete and accurate for that particular country. Tuberculosis impact measurement may be measured in terms of the major impact indicators such as incidence, prevalence, and mortality which are very useful in terms of gauging progress towards the Millennium Development Goals (MDGs). Tuberculosis impact measurement may also be done through impact evaluation which is the extent to which tuberculosis control interventions are responsible for changes in the abovementioned three major indicators.

2. *Address TB-HIV, MDR-TB, and the needs of poor and vulnerable populations:*

   The three elements here include: scaling up of collaborative TB/HIV activities; scaling up prevention and management of multidrug resistant TB (MDR-TB); addressing the needs of TB contacts, and of poor and vulnerable populations.

3. *Contribute to health system strengthening based on primary health care:*

   The four elements under this component of the strategy include: helping improve health policies, human resource development, financing, supplies, service delivery and information; strengthening infection control in health services, other congregate settings and households; upgrading of laboratory networks, and implementation of the Practical Approach to Lung Health; adaptation of successful approaches from other fields and sectors, and fostering action on the social determinants of health.

4. *Engage all care providers:*

   The two elements under this component of the strategy include: involvement of all public, voluntary, corporate and private providers through PUBLIC-Private Mix approaches; promote use of the International Standards for Tuberculosis Care.

5. *Empower people with TB, and communication through partnership:*

   The three elements under this component of the strategy include: pursue advocacy, communication and social mobilisation; fostering community participation in

TB care, prevention and health promotion; promote use of the Patients' Charter for Tuberculosis Care.

6. *Enable and promote research:*

There are two elements under this component of the strategy, and they are: conduct programme-based operational research; and advocacy for and participation in research to develop new diagnostics, drugs and vaccines.

Further research is needed in multiple areas of control of TB is to be achieved and sustained. Development of new drugs that are effective against Mycobacterium tuberculosis, affordable and safe, and able to clear the infection with a shorter duration of treatment is a high priority, and also development of effective vaccine against Mycobacterium tuberculosis is another high priority, but this is currently not within view. As such, in the meantime, operational research into how to enhance case detection and ensure dispensing of and adherence to proper treatment is needed (Merson et al. 2012).

The strategy to deal with TB should be as comprehensive as possible but given the fact that settings differ, and they have unique challenges, it is imperative to implement the tuberculosis strategy in a context-specific and patient-sensitive manner to ensure sustainability and effectiveness. Ideally, the comprehensive tuberculosis strategy should encompass the following aspects: pursue high quality DOTS expansion and enhancement; address TB-HIV, MDR-TB, and the needs of poor and vulnerable populations; contribute to health system strengthening based on primary health care; engage all care providers; empower people with TB, and communities through partnership; and enable and promote research.

At the same time, the barriers to prevention and control of tuberculosis should be borne in mind. It has to be acknowledged that the rapid growth of MDR-TB and XDR-TB, and the coexistence of TB and HIV/AIDS have complicated tuberculosis control efforts (Merson et al. 2012). At present, the principal obstacles to reducing TB-related morbidity and mortality in low- and middle-income countries are economic and operational in nature. As such, increased financial and technical assistance will be needed in many countries to ensure that currently available strategies for controlling TB are fully implemented (Merson et al. 2012).

Identifying priority areas for high impact to address health improvement and health inequalities, such as in the context of tuberculosis as a public health problem will have much greater effect if tackled in a structured programmatic approach. This approach should not be viewed in isolation, but it should be encompassed into an integrated health system. More importantly the involvement of the target population at all levels of the strategy, such as the planning, implementation, monitoring and evaluation is very crucial to ensure sustainability.

5.7 HIV and AIDS

The human immunodeficiency virus (HIV) is one of the viruses that can infect humans, and it progressively weakens the immune system. Acquired immunodeficiency syndrome (AIDS) and death can be the ultimate result if treatment such as antiretroviral medication is not available.

There are many theories surrounding the origin of HIV. Medical Virologists indicate that the most widely held hypothesis is that HIV-1 and HIV-2 are the result of cross-species transfer of simian immunodeficiency viruses from the chimpanzee and sooty mangabey, respectively. Some have suggested that this transfer occurred because of hunting primates, for food, but several other theories exist.

Although the first reported AIDS cases were among men who had sex with other men in the United States of America in the early 1980s, earlier serological evidence of HIV suggests that HIV may have originated in the former Belgian Congo, where the earliest known case of infection was found in a specimen from 1959. Some researchers assume that HIV-1 was probably first transmitted to humans in the late 1940s.

There is indication that today, HIV-1 is found in all parts of the globe, but HIV-2 is mainly confined in West Africa, and it is thought to be less deadly than HIV-1. As of 2018, the global number of people living with HIV was approximately 40 million, and the majority lived in Sub-Saharan Africa.

One of the biggest challenges in the fight against HIV and AIDS is complacency, particularly the perception that HIV and AIDS is no longer an emergency. The sobering reality is that the fight against HIV and AIDS is far from over. At this day and age, the following are five of the main challenges in the fight against HIV and AIDS:

- Adolescents and young people are left behind, evidenced by still rising infection rates, particularly in sub-Saharan Africa;
- Prevention has not received the importance and investment that has been given to treatment, yet, so much focus on treatment is not sustainable without scaling up efforts on prevention of new infections. Such a situation is potentially due to the influence of evidence-base and measurability of impact of treatment interventions as opposed to the complexity of measuring the impact of prevention. As such, the issue of evidence-base has had a huge bearing on funding of programmes where impact can be measured (Mabuza 2018a).
- Stigma, discrimination and criminalisation are becoming the main drivers of the spread of HIV particularly in Eastern Europe and Central Asia;
- Financing is not sustainable in low- and middle-income countries, particularly where there has been a dependency on donor funding;
- Coexistence of HIV with other diseases, such as with other communicable diseases and/or the dramatically increasing burden of non-communicable diseases, particularly in low- and middle-income countries. Some of the coinfections, such as TB-HIV coinfections, are deadly combinations as they potentiate each other through processes that are still not well understood, result in diagnostic and treatment challenges, more so, in children (Mabuza and Shumba 2018).

It is emphasised that proper leadership is paramount in the fight against HIV and AIDS, and that it is vital to have an expanded and innovative response to HIV and AIDS, and ensuring that the overall action plan incorporates the following key elements: Prevention and education; access to testing and therapy; respect of human rights; international cooperation; and increased research. Successfully winning the battle against HIV and AIDS would also require strengthening the social security systems and health systems of the developing nations, particularly those that are severely affected. For instance, the antiretroviral roll-out programmes must be sustainable to ensure that people who need therapy take the right tablets at the right time. It worth highlighting though that that the battle against HIV and AIDS is not only a medical but a global political, economic and social battle. It can be won if governments, private/public organisations, and individuals come forward and show active commitment in the true sense.

A South African Case Study on HIV and AIDS

South Africa has the most number of people living with HIV in the world, and, within this context, cohort survey data (collected in KwaZulu-Natal) by the Africa Health Research Institute revealed an "HIV hotspot" where an estimated 40.8% of adults (aged 15 years and older) were living with HIV. Such a high HIV prevalence rate in KwaZulu-Natal placed the province at the centre of the epidemic. The fact that the HIV/AIDS epidemic started later in South Africa also indicates that the major demographic impact of the epidemic came later.

It is important to mention that there is no comprehensive historical data from which to extract reliable information about trends in the epidemiology of HIV/AIDS in the community or South African company of focus in this discussion. However, for the purpose of this discussion, a profile and outcome of the Voluntary Counselling and Testing (VCT) project for the period November 2016 to December 2017 shall be the point of focus. It is noteworthy that the company's ten worksites or business units were spread across three provinces, which were Eastern Cape, KwaZulu-Natal, and the Western Cape. The bulk (65%) of the company's workforce was located in KwaZulu-Natal, and approximately 70% of the workforce were male. The average age of the workforce was 45 years.

The tables below entail the HIV positive test results for the Voluntary Counselling and Testing (VCT) project. Sixty-seven (4.5%) out of 1411 employees tested HIV positive. Tables 5.1, 5.2, 5.3, 5.4 and 5.5 illustrate the HIV positive profile as per age group, gender, work site or geographical location, and regional or provincial loca-

Table 5.1 HIV positive rate per age group

Age Group	Number of employees (HIV positive)	Number of employees tested	% HIV positive employees
20–30	7	153	4.6%
31–35	6	146	4.1%
36–40	3	106	4.1%
40+	51	985	4.8%
TOTAL	67	1411	4.5%

Table 5.2 HIV positive rate by gender

Gender	Number of employees	Number of employees tested	% HIV positive employees
Male	56	1130	4.96%
Female	11	280	3.97%
TOTAL	67	1411	4.5%

Table 5.3 HIV positive rate by employee type

Employee type	Number of employees (HIV positive)	Number of employees tested	% HIV positive employees
Permanent	60	1330	4.5%
Non-permanent	7	81	8.6%
TOTAL	67	1411	4.5%

Table 5.4 HIV positive rate by Worksite (Geographical location)

Worksite	Number of employees (HIV positive)	Number of employees tested	% HIV positive employees
Cape Town A	1	175	0.60%
Cape Town B	7	143	4.90%
Saldanha	1	121	0.80%
East London	2	48	4.20%
Port Elizabeth	8	271	3.00%
Durban A	10	225	4.44%
Durban B	3	48	6.25%
Durban C	16	163	9.80%
Durban D	7	76	9.21%
Richards Bay	12	141	8.50%
TOTAL	67	1411	4.5%

Table 5.5 HIV positive rate per province

Province	Number of employees (HIV positive)	Number of employees tested	% HIV positive employees
Eastern cape	10	315	3.2%
KwaZulu-natal	27	653	7.2%
Western cape	9	443	2.0%
TOTAL	67	1411	4.5%

tion. The majority of employees who tested HIV positive were married men, who were older than 40 years of age. This was similar to findings in other industries with similar workforce population.

The November 2016 – December 2017 VCT campaign confirmed a 28.0% (1411) participation rate out of 5034 permanent employees. Sixty-six employees (4.54%) tested HIV positive during the above period and 26 HIV positive employees were successfully enrolled for disease management.

The 28% uptake rate was a relatively small sample which limited precision with regard to HIV prevalence and trends in the company of focus. Nevertheless, the results of this study suggested that the KwaZulu-Natal province had the highest HIV prevalence. The geographical locations or worksites that had the highest HIV prevalence, that is, Durban and Richards Bay were also located in the KwaZulu-Natal province. This correlates with the country's latest HIV statistics, which showed the highest HIV prevalence in KwaZulu-Natal, compared to the other eight provinces.

Despite the low HIV prevalence in the Western Cape, there was a sign of varying degrees of the impact of HIV in different worksites within the same province, as indicated in Table 5.5. For example, there should be some concern about the HIV prevalence of 4.9% in Cape Town B compared to the much lower HIV prevalence in the other Western Cape worksites. Contrary to the country's Department of Health study and other studies, there was a higher HIV prevalence among male employees as shown in Table 5.2. It has to be pointed out though, that an overwhelming two thirds of the company's workforce comprised males. Therefore, the much smaller sample size for female employees did not project a truly representative picture.

There is need to obtain absolute commitment from top management to implement a sustainable and comprehensive HIV and AIDS programme. It is important to bear in mind the impact many employees who suffer from HIV related illnesses may have on the business in years to come, as well as the impact of employees not able to work and having to apply for disability benefits.

Impact of HIV and AIDS on the Health Sector

Increased demand for health services is particularly problematic. Health sectors already have difficulty in meeting basic medical care needs. Moreover, health facility assessments suggest that the epidemic is crowding out patients with conditions which are seemingly less severe than HIV/AIDS, thus denying them their right to care. As the demand increases, the human and financial resources decrease. HIV and AIDS compromises capacity for health care through its direct and indirect impacts on employees. Increased absenteeism among affected nurses, low morale, increased workloads, stress and burnout could be exacerbated.

Impact of HIV and AIDS on the Education Sector

The effect of HIV and AIDS weakens the capacity of the education sector through increased teacher morbidity and mortality. Increased absenteeism among teachers and a larger number of vacancies in teacher positions would imply that a constant pupil-teacher ratio would actually signify a decline in the quality of education. Moreover, HIV and AIDS will affect the supply of education services because of the costs it imposes on the system. The direct costs of HIV and AIDS to education include employee benefits, the hiring of temporary staff, recruitment and training. The indirect costs include the loss of productivity due to absenteeism, the loss of skills, declining morale and low performance among ill employees.

Impact of HIV and AIDS on the Welfare Sector

The impact of HIV and AIDS on the welfare of children has a number of dimensions ranging from orphan-hood, depletion of family assets, families splitting, child abuse, drugs and the lack of proper homes. The increasing number of orphans stretches resources and capacity to the limit, and the majority of those providing care are often already elderly, impoverished and might themselves have depended on the person who has died for physical and financial support, and are facing the same problems as child-headed households. The scourge of HIV and AIDS has eroded family values and sentiments.

There is a wide range of implications of HIV/AIDS, including the impact on the health sector, education sector and welfare sector. The impact of HIV/AIDS has been especially devastating in the health, education and welfare sectors of low to medium economies. Research shows that responses to date have been positive, but also piecemeal, and a comprehensive and enabling policy environment is required to adequately address the problem.

Strategies to Minimise the Impact of HIV and AIDS on the Health, Education and Welfare Sectors

As HIV/AIDS has far-reaching effects on sustainable development, it is critical to move beyond the immediate effects of the epidemic and review how social sector plans for health, education and welfare integrate HIV/AIDS. Therefore, the purpose of this section is to discuss the collaborative role that the health, education and welfare sectors can play in developing strategies to minimise the impact of HIV/AIDS.

The response to the HIV/AIDS pandemic should be practical and multifaceted, and the management structures in place within the health, education and welfare sectors should be adequate to handle this crisis. There should be full time managers with sufficient skills and executive power to take decisive action to counteract the threat of the pandemic.

Building partnerships based on supportive policy frameworks – across sectors and between civil society and government – is essential for effective national responses that benefit all members of the society. There is clearly a need for an expanded response to HIV/AIDS through formation of partnerships and collaborations between the government, non-governmental organisations and the private sector. Non-governmental organisations may include institutions that operate at the local level, community-based organisations and international agencies. Private industry can be an important and effective partner in advocacy, prevention and care. Businesses can contribute to vulnerability and can also be the answer. This might reverse the vulnerability if local community or social structure formulate constructive proposals to them, especially with regard to their social responsibility policies. Proposals can also be coupled with incentives, which the government might give to business to act to reduce vulnerability.

Enhancing communication channels can be a good platform for the health, education and welfare services in creating a supportive environment for people affected by HIV/AIDS.

The health care system falls within the first level of preventing HIV infection through health education and health promotion, the management of sexually transmitted infections, blood safety measures, as well as prenatal and perinatal care. Health services also play an important role of supporting welfare services, with essential care and support of infected people and their families.

Education can greatly reduce the vulnerability to HIV. People with more education have more access to information on which to base their decisions. They have more opportunities for employment and income generation. They may be more easily able to adopt safe behaviours and tolerate attitudes that reduce the impact of the epidemic on others. Therefore, the extent to which schools and other education institutions are able to continue functioning as part of the essential infrastructure of societies and communities will influence how well societies eventually recover from the epidemic.

Stronger sectoral systems could help in bridging top-down and bottom-up approaches and in formulating and implementing policies and programs. The sectors play a role in providing stronger support to households to meet their needs (health services, education services, and welfare such as orphan care) adequately; improving contributions to national output as a result of increased efficiency through better management of sectoral resources; adopting policies that may bring about behaviour change (for example improvement in girls' education, women's empowerment, and the provision of housing for families posted away from home).

The foregoing discussion underscores the need for a concerted strategy to stem the rise of HIV/AIDS, not simply from a health point of view but also from an education and welfare and development perspective. The concerted strategy should encompass aspects of good governance, care, communication, partnerships, monitoring and evaluation. Certainly, the ability of each sector to deliver results increases exponentially if related sectors coordinate their activities intersectorally and agree to prioritise objectives for development in general and/or HIV/AIDS mitigation, prevention, and care in particular.

HIV and AIDS and its Impact on the Macroeconomic Performance of a National Economy

Based on the available literature, it would perhaps be worth mentioning in passing that there are four categories of studies that attempt to evaluate the economic impact of HIV/AIDS. These include the following: Econometric modelling (where the impact of HIV/AIDS is factored into a growth model with estimated parameters); Equilibrium modelling (which attempts to identify and quantify the different channels of HIV/AIDS impact through simulations); Qualitative studies (sometimes, based on case studies of particular communities or areas); and the human capital approach (where the cost of AIDS is calculated through the foregone earnings or production of AIDS victims).

Since the early 1990s there has been a flurry of econometric and equilibrium modelling studies to attempt to model the impact of HIV/AIDS. While it is encouraging to see that leaders from certain nations such as Botswana have taken the initiative to prevent and mitigate the negative economic impact of HIV and AIDS. From a macro-economic perspective, a lot of work still needs to be done to win this battle against the HIV and AIDS pandemic. This will require more work of quantitative nature than researchers have attempted in the past.

The HIV/AIDS epidemic may affect the economy of a nation in a number of different ways, fuelled by the increase in mortality (death) and morbidity (illness). The following discussion attempts to explain some of the manifold macroeconomic consequences of the increased mortality and morbidity associated with HIV/AIDS.

The direct economic impact of HIV can be observed due to a reduction in labour force as a result of AIDS. Apart from such labour force reduction, the medication cost and the related opportunity costs and switching of expenditure to meet a higher medication cost also entail another adverse impact to the economy. This will, in turn, affect the saving and the steady state path of the economy.

Researchers such as Cuddington have identified some of the mechanisms through which the AIDS epidemics affect the macro economy. Cuddington tried to establish the link between growth, saving and investment and also tried to show the loop through which a one-time effect would produce a dynamic outcome. He posits that savings would be reduced not only as a result of a higher medical cost but also through the loop channel that reduces labour force and hence growth which is positively related with savings. In addition, the increase in the dependency ratio as a result of HIV related death also reduces savings. Such a decline in the gross domestic savings will, in turn, reduce capital formation and long-term growth.

From the demand side, the demand for education may also be reduced as children are forced to leave school earlier to support ill parents. In addition, households may switch their expenditure from education and other welfare enhancing expenditure to the financing of funeral services. This, in effect, reduces the human capital accumulation in the long run, which is associated with efficiency loss. The efficiency loss would be aggravated as AIDS shifts the composition of the labour force towards young and less-experienced workers. In the same vein, there could be a concomitant increase in the use of child labour, as a result of the increase in the numbers of orphans. A shortage of skilled workers leads to higher production costs and a loss of international competitiveness (ILO 2000:12).

The impact of HIV/AIDS would be transmitted from the micro units to the macro economy through different channels. A decline in the labour supply of the micro units due to the infection leads to a lower labour force in the economy which in effect contributes for a low level of output through a direct relationship between labour force and the level of output (ILO 2000: 12). In addition to this, output would also decline due to a lower productivity of the workers as a result of illness. This may increase strain on life insurance and pension funds, as more and more employees may require early pension due to permanent ill health or may even die prematurely. This increase in pressure on the social security system creates a huge dent in the national economy, since life insurance and pension funds are important sources of capital for both the government and the private sector (ILO 2000: 12).

Clearly, decline in output would affect the level of consumption, private investment, government revenue, and export while the latter also leads to a decline in consumer goods and intermediate goods imports (ILO 2006:15). Moreover, the general price level might also be affected as a result of the fall in output given that the fall in supply dominates the fall in demand (ILO 2006:15). The slow-down of the economy may also be accompanied by the shortage of imported raw materials that would make the fall in output worse. Apart from the output and the resultant effect of HIV, it also leads to lower labour income, increase in demand for health services and a squeezed level of domestic savings which could set a potential vicious spiral circle (Quattek 2000).

Tandon (2005:5) observes that in addition to rising health expenditure and lower income-generating potential and savings among households, private firms and businesses may also suffer from lower productivity on account of higher personnel costs due to health-related expenses on absenteeism, sickness, death, and recruitment, as well as organisational disruptions. These constitute an additional burden and deterrent both to expanding domestic investment (Tandon 2005:5) in the public sector, where significant pressure on the budget is created by a decline in the revenue from rapid and monumental increases in health and welfare costs.

The state may be required to redistribute other scarce development resources in order to enhance spending on health and social services. Possible broader effects of higher HIV incidence include repercussions for future political stability caused by dissatisfaction with the government and with widening inequality (Barnett and Whiteside 2002:159).

From the foregoing discussion it can be discerned that the prevalence of HIV/AIDS poses a very serious threat to the overall economy of a nation. This threat of a progressive collapse of the economy is particularly insidious because the effects may not be felt immediately. Clearly, rapid increase in mortality and morbidity due to the disease could set a potential vicious spiral circle, creating a negative impact on the very core of the fabric of a nation's economy.

Therefore, it is vital for policymakers to understand the macroeconomic impact of HIV/AIDS so that they could be in a position to commit resources to prevention and mitigation of the disease.

The Ready Availability of Antiretroviral Therapy as a Way of Reducing the Negative Effects of HIV and AIDS in the Economy

It has already been highlighted that the impact of HIV and AIDS has been very devastating in the sub-Saharan region, and that the increase in mortality and morbidity causes a huge negative impact on the economy. Studies reveal that the current projected declines in productivity in sub-Saharan Africa underline the pressing need to intervene with effective treatments, including antiretroviral therapy.

The primary goal of antiretroviral therapy is to decrease HIV related morbidity and mortality. At the population level, the goals of antiretroviral therapy include refurbishing the workforce, reducing the number of HIV orphans, reducing hospitalisations, providing cost efficient care, establishing priorities based on assessment of competing healthcare needs, and preventing HIV resistance (Global AIDS Learning & Evaluation Network 2002: 13). However, various studies show that antiretroviral therapy may have meaningful impact only when resources are used widely and equitably within a generally committed healthcare system.

Therefore, the purpose of this paper is to argue in favour of the ready availability of antiretroviral therapy as a way of reducing the negative effects of HIV and AIDS on the economy. At the same time concerns would also be highlighted, during the course of the discussion.

A number of reports indicate that there has been positive complementary improvement and upgrading of national healthcare infrastructure in resource poor countries that have had increased access to antiretroviral drugs. Such infrastructure includes laboratory facilities, the training of professionals, and the capacity to conduct research.

There is ample evidence from literature that indicates that the easy availability of Antiretroviral Therapy (ART) decreases the viral load and therefore the probability of sexual transmission of HIV in the case of unprotected sexual intercourse. ART also decreases the maternal viral load which then decreases the risk of perinatal transmission.

In this regard, the increase in the life expectancy of treated patients will reduce the number of AIDS orphans, decrease absenteeism that was as a result of HIV-related illnesses, decrease AIDS-related deaths, and minimise the strain on life insurances and pension funds. In the long run, the economy may recover, or at least the negative impact of HIV and AIDS may be reduced.

It is worth mentioning though that there are disturbing reports that indicate that the increased life expectancy of HIV positive people may predictably translate into an increased probability of sexual encounters between sero-discordant partners, as ART has become widely available. However, the overall impact on HIV incidence will further depend on the extent to which risk behaviours are affected by the availability of treatment.

The increased focus on HIV and AIDS and the subsidisation of antiretroviral drugs could be of some danger as other health challenges that have a huge bearing on the economy could be overlooked in terms of government spending or allocation of funds. Thus, indirectly creating another negative repercussion on the economy.

However, once indirect costs (that is, productivity losses associated with morbidity in HIV-infected individuals) are taken into account, ART is clearly cost-saving in developed societies. Without interventions to provide treatment, the negative impact of the AIDS pandemic on life expectancy, as well as on macroeconomic, demographic, and social development, will become increasingly more devastating for developing countries in the coming years. In this regard, the savings in indirect costs obtained through antiretroviral treatment are likely to be proportionally higher in developing countries than in the developed world.

Regulated government and private efforts to improve access to antiretroviral treatment should reduce inequality with regard to access to care in developing countries. Obviously, constraints on government expenditures will prevent the public and private sector from establishing strict egalitarian access to antiretroviral in many developing countries. However, a national consensus should be reached, in each country, for defining the population groups that can benefit from public support for expanded access to treatment. There is no doubt that leaving access to antiretroviral drugs to pure market forces will restrict their availability to the most privileged and maximise the risk of their diversion to "black market" sales.

In all developing countries, capacity building is a crucial step in speeding the implementation of integrated prevention, care, and treatment programs for HIV/AIDS as well as other health programs.

From the above discussion it can be concluded that antiretroviral therapy on its own is not enough as a way of reducing the negative effects of HIV and AIDS on the economy. Furthermore, it has been highlighted that a comparison cannot be drawn between the rich and the poor countries in terms of the roll-out of antiretroviral drugs and the management of the HIV and AIDS pandemic. The dichotomy between the rich and the poor nations is apparent. The cost-effectiveness of antiretroviral drugs can be rather compromised in resource-poor settings, due to a number of factors such as poor infrastructure, inadequate personnel capacity, poverty, inadequate education, and leadership. Be as it may, the availability of antiretroviral drugs can make a difference in terms of improving the quality of life, improvement in productivity, and the economy in general, as long as there are proper systems in place.

An integrated approach that recognises that prevention and treatment reinforce each other, could be of vital importance in helping to reduce the negative effects of HIV and AIDS on the economy.

HIV and AIDS Workplace Strategy

The organisation of focus is in the transport sector. This particular organisation or company is still going through a great deal of transformation as part of its four-point turnaround strategy. The company has just unveiled its new brand. The re-branding is aimed at communicating that it is now a focused and integrated freight transport company. As it completes the organisational transformation, this company will no longer be a diversified Group. Instead, it will be a freight transport Company which owns and operates rail freight, ports and pipeline assets.

Obviously, change comes with a lot of challenges. One of our challenges is to align our wellness strategy, including the HIV/AIDS strategy, with the core business strategy of this re-branded organisation. In this regard, it is imperative that good practice HIV/AIDS strategies in other industries, especially in the transport sector, be explored.

A report from the International Labour Office (ILO) (2000) upholds the view that urgent consideration should be given to the development of an ILO Code of practice on addressing the threat of HIV/AIDS in the world of work. This encompasses the following areas of focus as reflected through the World Economic Forum

(2006): Assessment of the threat and to have a clear idea of the extent and nature of the impact of HIV on the organisation; Development of a policy; Prioritising the protection of staff through workplace activities; Networking or forming partnerships with other stakeholders; Properly addressing the issue of stigma by implementing non-discrimination policies; Ensuring that employees have access to treatment, care and support; Monitoring and evaluation of the programme, since the impacts of HIV/AIDS on firms are likely to change over time.

Below is a detailed project plan to ensure implementation and sustainability of an organisation's HIV/AIDS programme. The programme elements would include: Risk and gap analysis; HIV/AIDS integration with workplace wellness programme strategy; Management and coordination; Prevention; Treatment; Care; Partnership with external stakeholders and communication strategy; Monitoring and evaluation.

Risk and Gap Analysis

Conduct a gap analysis, review the findings and ensure synergy amongst internal role players with regard to: Workplace wellness policy and strategy to ensure input from all stakeholders.

HIV/AIDS integration with a workplace wellness programme strategy.

Define the core elements of the workplace wellness programme and take a strategic decision with regard to the integration of HIV/AIDS programmes and/or structures to move towards integrated workplace wellness.

Management and Coordination

Review the current representation of the business units' HIV/AIDS/Wellness committee members, ensuring a realistic and sustainable approach with sufficient internal role players such as management, human resources, communications department, health and safety, service providers, employees/peer educators, unions.

Prevention

Develop a behaviour change communication strategy: Review the current HIV/AIDS (Wellness) communication strategy and ensure a risk-based approach towards general and ongoing awareness programmes.

Training for target groups: Based on the gap analysis feedback and current best practice, finalise the project plan and implement training for management and peer educators.

Voluntary counselling and testing/HIV testing services: Ongoing availability of on-site VCT/HTS at all business units. Consider the inclusion of off-site option for the employees. Review current VCT/HTS communication strategy.

Sexually transmitted infections (STIs): Ongoing awareness and access to treatment for employees diagnosed with STIs. VCT/HTS should be offered routinely to employees with STIs.

Workplace condom distribution programme: Ensure ongoing access and availability of condoms for employees. Decide who is primarily responsible for condom distribution at business unit level.

Directly Observed Treatment Short Course (DOTS): Inclusion of Tuberculosis DOTS programme as part of the internal clinic services.

Post Exposure Prophylaxis (PEP)/Workplace safety procedure: Ensure ongoing awareness on access to PEP, as well as workplace safety procedure.

Events based awareness campaigns: Set up a small, representative work team to draft the project plan, obtain approval and ensure implementation of the awareness campaigns.

Treatment and Care

Ensure continuation of care for employees already on disease management programme. Ensure facilitation of disease management programme enrolment for all employees testing HIV positive during VCT/HTS. Clinical staging, monitoring and ensuring that employees who are HIV+ and qualify for treatment, adhere to it. More recently, it has been decided at global health level that all persons who test HIV+ should start antiretroviral therapy (ART) as early as possible, regardless of the clinical staging. Establish fully functional structures for psychological support and counselling. Adherence counselling and monitoring for employees on the disease management programme.

Monitoring and Evaluation

Identify key process and outcome indicators to ensure ongoing monitoring and evaluation of programme uptake and effectiveness, such as: VCT/HTS participation and HIV+ profile; HIV risk assessment information; STIs treated and referred for VCT/HTS; TB DOTS participants; HIV and AIDS disease management report, that is, uptake, clinical staging, adherence and referrals for counselling; Training/awareness records and provide attendance registers; Lifestyle health risk questionnaire when introduced as part of employee wellness campaigns. Monthly reporting requirements need to be agreed to; Annual trend analysis based on the VCT/HTS risk assessment and HIV+ profile.

Partnership with External Stakeholders and Communication Strategy

Conduct a stakeholder analysis with regard to the inclusion of contractors, supply chain networks regarding HIV and AIDS awareness requirements and/or programme inclusion. Conduct a partnership analysis and decisions with regard to strengthening community partnerships or programmes. Conduct an external communication strategy with regard to the company's HIV and AIDS strategy. Encourage participation in business, industry or workplace wellness programmes to continuously benchmark and ensure best practices are implemented to mitigate the HIV risk for our employees.

From the forgoing discussion, it can be concluded that an effective, efficient, multi-sectoral and sustainable HIV and AIDS strategy is of paramount importance in the world of work. In this regard, the success or failure of the strategy is dependent on the depth and quality of the following critical elements: risk analysis; management and coordination; prevention, treatment and care; monitoring and evaluation; a multi-faceted approach; partnership with external stakeholders and a communication strategy. It is imperative that workplace policies be in place, and these must be reviewed regularly.

5.7.1 The Role of Culture in the HIV/AIDS Epidemic, and Stigma, Denial, Fear and Discrimination Related to HIV/AIDS

Not Being Able to Make Healthy Choices about Sexual Behaviour

Although various studies indicate a high prevalence of HIV among black Africans, increasing incidences of HIV have recently been reported in Eastern Europe and Asia. Research shows that certain cultural traditions could fuel the spread of HIV/AIDS. To illustrate this point, in the Luo community in western Kenya, customs like wife inheritance and widow cleansing have been cited as contributing factors to the high HIV/AIDS prevalence rate in the province. Luo custom dictates that a widow is obliged to undergo a cleansing ritual immediately after the death of her husband. In this regard, if this woman refuses to have sex with another man, she is thought to be unlucky or cursed and is usually ostracised by the community.

In the Luo community, many of life's milestones, like moving to a newly constructed home, are preceded by sex. Sex is also a ritual that has to take place at every stage of the farming process. Clearly, in the Luo community, sex seems to be more rooted in tradition.

The lower status of women in certain communities could also fuel the spread of HIV/AIDS. The cultural hold is so strong on a woman, even if she knows that she might be infected, she is unable to say no if the man wants to have sexual intercourse with her. In a polygamous scenario, the man might have several sexual partners who are not his wives, something that could fuel the spread of HIV/AIDS.

Studies in South Africa show that the low status accorded to a woman without a male partner may put pressure on the woman to end up engaging in risky sexual behaviour. Abstinence and monogamy are often seen as unnatural for men, who try to prove themselves, mainly by frequent sexual encounters, and often the aggressive initiation of these. Men are socialised to believe that women are inferior and should be under their control, and women are socialised to over-respect men and act submissively to them. The resulting unequal power relation between the sexes, particularly when negotiating sexual encounters, increases women's vulnerability to HIV infection and accelerates the epidemic.

Other studies show that men in Southern Africa generally have a negative attitude towards condoms, because of beliefs that "flesh to flesh" sex is equated with masculinity for male health. Certain sexual practices, such as dry sex (where the vagina is expected to be small and dry), and unprotected anal sex, carry a high risk of HIV because they cause abrasions to the lining of the vagina or anus. In cultures where virginity is a condition for marriage, girls may protect their virginity by engaging in unprotected anal sex. The importance of fertility in African communities may hinder the practice of safer sex. Young women under pressure to prove their fertility prior to marriage may try to fall pregnant, and therefore do not use condoms or abstain from sex. Fathering many children is also seen as a sign of virile masculinity. Urbanisation and migrant labour expose people to a variety of new cultural influences, with the result that traditional and modern values often co-exist. Certain traditional values that could serve to protect people from HIV infection, such as abstinence from sex before marriage, are being eroded by cultural modernisation (Health24.com 2008).

Extreme poverty has also been documented as one of the factors that could result in people not making healthy choices about their sexual behaviour. In poverty-stricken areas, women start having sex much earlier. They do not have good education. The poorer are also more likely to engage in sex as a source of income. Studies also show that some of the women that have been widowed as a result of HIV/AIDS generally give young boys money and keep them as sex partners.

According to studies, the newly homeless youth are likelier to engage in risky sexual behaviour if they stay in nonfamily settings – such as friend's home, abandoned buildings or the streets – because they lack supervision and social support.

Drug use also factors into the behaviour, according to the study, published in Journal of Adolescent Health. The researchers examined how individual factors, such as socio-demographics, depression and substance abuse, and structural factors, such as living situations, can influence sexual behaviour.

"While gender and some racial differences on predictors of sexual risk were found in this study, living with nonfamily members and drug use appear to be the most salient in explaining sexual risk," the researchers wrote.

There is literature evidence to prove that violence is another risk factor for HIV infection. Women in violent relationships are less able to enforce HIV preventive behaviours; women who have experienced physical and sexual abuse engage in more HIV risk behaviours; biological trauma from forced sex may facilitate HIV transmission.

Women in violent relationships cannot enforce preventive measures. Cannot discuss the terms of when and how a sexual encounter will occur. For example, cannot turn her back in bed while with partner; where did she learn of the new technologies, does she not trust the man or is she having other partnerships (perceptions of infidelity often associated with violence).

Young women and girls face special risks because of the erroneous but widespread belief that sex with a virgin can cleanse a man of infection. AIDS orphans who are often forced to fend for themselves, are also easy prey for sexual abuse and violence. The trafficking of women and girls into prostitution and sexual slavery is another deeply entrenched form of violence against young women fuelled by widespread poverty, international tourism and the forces of globalisation. Recent research shows that young men too, express their fear of the potential for violence within themselves, the threat of violence from other men and of the violence inflicted on them.

Women who were subject to violence engage in more lifetime HIV risk behaviours. This is a known fact for many years in mental health literature. They involve themselves in situations putting them at risk of HIV. For example, involved in multiple partnerships often with unprotected sexual encounters; have substance misuse including alcohol use and put themselves in environments that may subject them to gender based violence; get into situations of intimate partner violence themselves.

Lack of knowledge and misconceptions about HIV/AIDS has been reported. For instance, research shows that China's gays know little about HIV/AIDS. Meanwhile some of the gays also have female partners and some are married, which implies that this could increase the likelihood for the virus to spread to heterosexual female partners and their offspring. On the other hand, studies show that even if people know about HIV/AIDS, they still engage in risky sexual behaviour. Researchers speculate that, some people (regardless of their ethnic origin) may be lulled into complacency by the more effective HIV drugs available, hence the increase in risky sexual behaviour.

Studies in South Africa show that lack of open discussion and guidance about sexuality is often lacking in the home, and many young people pick up misinformation from their peers instead. In South Africa, dangerous myths and misconceptions about HIV/AIDS abound, even among adults.

War and other armed conflicts which often increase local and regional insecurity, worsen poverty, encourage violence against women and frequently lead to the breakdown of social services, infrastructure and a lack of food, shelter, medicines and health care professionals. These factors also increase the vulnerability of entire populations and threaten national security and stability.

In South Africa, the political transition and the legacy of apartheid have also been reported to have resulted in some people not making healthy choices regarding their sexual behaviour. Elements of the apartheid regime – such as migrant labour, the homeland system, the Group Areas Act and forced removals – contributed to the widespread poverty, gender inequality, social instability and unsafe sexual practices that now continue to influence the spread of HIV/AIDS in South Africa. This includes the incidences of rape of children, women, and the same gender rape in prisons.

Intervention for Risky Sexual Behaviour

Acknowledging that access to HIV/AIDS information does not necessarily lead to behaviour change, the following measures should be utilised to facilitate behaviour modification: interactive drama (life skills, behaviour change, and forum theatre), sports and recreation, personal development, voluntary counselling and testing.

Partnerships: An inter-sectoral approach is critical in dealing with the issues. Partnerships must be formed with other organisations/groups, namely: provincial HIV/AIDS Action Unit, Department of health, Traditional leadership, and Local authorities.

Various community interventions in rural communities led by the local Amakhosi and Indunas. The most significant of these interventions is aimed at recruiting leadership support for the promotion of responsible sexual behaviour.

Training programs for the Amakhosi and Indunas on HIV/AIDS issues. Premarital abstinence is the cultural method of choice that is promoted in these sessions. Debates around the controversial issue of virginity inspection must be facilitated. The issue is to ensure good health practices.

Researchers have found that interventions aimed at reducing sexual risk behaviours, and thereby reducing HIV among newly homeless youth, need to help youth find housing associated with supervision and social support (family and institutional settings) as well as aim to reduce drug use.

There needs to be community-based efforts to change norms of male sexual behaviour and conflict resolution. Improve women's access to HIV prevention tools which they can control, such as female condoms (femidoms). Promotion and quality assurance of VCT/HTS for individuals and couples. Partner notification policies: client-referral system with more counselling on disclosure. Increase post-test support services to increase disclosure and psychosocial support. Research needed to look at cause and effect between gender-based violence and HIV. Multiple stakeholders needed to intervene in the dual epidemics to curb the raging HIV epidemic this should be on-going and should have strong targeted program evaluation or monitoring and evaluation.

Causes that Prevent People from Discussing HIV in the Community

Fear of violence is a main barrier to HIV testing even when women's perception of HIV risk is high. Fear of violence interferes with a woman knowing her status and if she does disclose it to a significant other, this is especially so when there was no form of communication prior to testing. When testing occurs in situations outside of HTS clinics, disclosure becomes even more difficult. Disclosure is critical for adherence of all prevention care and treatment protocols.

Male youth who were violent toward female partners frequently described forced sex and sexual infidelity in these partnerships. Male youth with multiple concurrent sexual partners reported becoming violent when their female partners questioned their fidelity and reported forcing regular partners to have sex when these partners resisted their sexual advances.

Most people living with HIV and AIDS suffer or fear stigmatisation. Studies from Africa suggest that AIDS stigma is linked to people's sense of sexual morality and their fear of breaking taboos. It is thought that the fear of stigma adversely influences women's health –seeking practices. A "conspiracy of silence" exists in which HIV/AIDS is seldom openly discussed, even in heavily affected areas. People do not want to admit that a fatal disease spread by behaviour branded as "immoral" could be rampaging through their community or their country. Unfortunately, in places where denial flourishes, people are most vulnerable to the silent spread of HIV. Discussions of sexual practices or use of illicit drugs are often taboo and associated with embarrassment, shame, guilt and rejection.

Cultural norms of silence regarding sexual practices, preferences and desires can be problematic. Rarely are people open about their HIV status and many people go untested for fear of the result. It is still common for women to be blamed for spreading sexually transmitted infections (STIs), including HIV, despite the fact that women are often infected by their husbands or partners, to whom they are entirely faithful. Interventions to reduce HIV infection in mother to child transmission

(MTCT), particularly the administration of antiretroviral (ARV) prophylaxis and avoidance of breastfeeding, make it virtually impossible for HIV-infected women to keep their infection a secret from their families and people in the wider community. Many women fear discrimination, violence and even murder if they are identified as HIV infected, and thus are reluctant or completely unable to take advantage of interventions offered to protect their infants from infection.

The consequences of stigma and discrimination for HIV-infected people are profound. It has been suggested that people are more concerned about the social consequences of HIV – including issues of death, sex, misbehaviour (sin), blame, shame, rejection and stigma – than with the technical facts about HIV/AIDS.

Consequences of Disclosing one's HIV Status to Family, Workplace and the Community

As already highlighted under risks of sexual behaviour, violence is a major barrier to disclosure for HIV+ women. Violence against women and girls is defined in the Declaration on Elimination of Violence against Women as occurring in three domains: the family, the community, and perpetrated or condoned by the state. In its broader form gender based violence is act that results in, or is likely to result in physical, sexual or psychological harm or suffering to women, including threats of such acts, coercion or arbitrary deprivation of liberty, including battering, sexual abuse of female children in the household, dowry related violence, marital rape, female genital mutilation and other traditional practices harmful to women.

Combating Stigma, Fear, Denial and Discrimination in the Workplace and Community

While it may be unrealistic to think that stigma can be eliminated altogether, the studies reviewed show that something can be done about stigma and that it can be reduced through a variety of intervention strategies including information, counselling, coping skills acquisition, and contact. The preference given to community-based approaches in developing countries may reflect an understanding that stigma must be dealt with at both a collective and individual level (Brown et al. 2001).

One author raises the question of involving couples in prevention of mother to child transmission (PMTCT) "all the way from VCT through decisions on treatment and care, noting that "all arguments have been about mother-child … we have ignored the role of the father". In fact, studies have shown that providing HIV counselling and testing to both partners together can lead to greater acceptance and less abuse and abandonment of HIV-infected women. Thus, involving the fathers and couple counselling, or shared confidentiality, could promote the reduction of MTCT.

Good governance in the form of effective policies and laws that address gender inequality so as to bring about more democratic and stable social relations and enhancing the possibilities of social change to address HIV and AIDS. Good governance also includes political will and commitment that manifest in strong public voices on the epidemic, an effective government based on the rule of law, freedom from corruption, commitment to respecting, protecting and fulfilling human rights and human security, and the participation of a strong and active civil society, particularly the Greater Involvement of People Living with HIV/AIDS (GIPA) at all levels of policy formulation, programme implementation, monitoring and evaluation.

Mainstreaming gender as a cross-cutting concern of human rights and security would mean incorporating the gender and HIV and AIDS approach with that of the rights and security approach to transform relations between women and men that will eliminate gender inequality, reduce the risk of infection and foster an enabling environment that ensures true partnership in opportunities for both women and men to combat stigma, fears, denial, and discrimination in the workplace and communities.

However, no policy or law alone can combat discrimination against people living with HIV/AIDS. Be as it may, it has to be emphasised that the legislation must seek to ensure their right to employment, education, privacy and confidentiality, as well as the right to access information, treatment and support. The fear and prejudice that lies at the core of the HIV and AIDS discrimination needs to be tackled at the community and national levels. A more enabling environment needs to be created to increase the visibility of people living with HIV as a 'normal' part of any society, including the workplace. In future, the task is to confront the fear-based messages and biased social attitudes, in order to reduce the discrimination and stigma of people who are living with HIV.

Shared confidentiality is the pathway to the reduction of stigma, fear, denial, and discrimination in the workplace and community. Religious leaders can play a significant role in this regard.

Leaders can strongly encourage supportive attitudes and responses to all those living with and affected by the epidemic, by modelling honest and open discussion about HIV/AIDS. The active involvement of persons living with or affected by HIV/AIDS is central to the fight against stigma, fears, denial, and discrimination. Existing human rights instruments (notably international conventions, Treaties, Covenants and national legislation), should be used alongside complementary strategies within homes and communities, health care settings, religious organisations, and various communications media. This would help both to prevent prejudicial thoughts being formed and to address or redress the situation when stigma leads to discriminatory action, negative consequences or denial of entitlements or services.

Although public health mandates, and many AIDS organisations support the need for social, psychological, financial and legal ramifications of doing so, however, it should also be stressed that shared confidentiality leads to better strategies for prevention, increased support from health and social service providers, and enhanced care and support from family and community members. It should also be noted that people's fears of disclosure might not fully represent their experiences of sharing their HIV status with designated others. People exhibiting conduct problems and using substances seem to be at highest risk for contracting HIV as a result of risky sexual behaviour. Prevention interventions should target teens in high-risk environments during late elementary school or early middle school to encourage teens to delay intercourse, practise safer sex, and avoid drug and alcohol use. An interdisciplinary model of care in primary care settings is clearly indicated to provide these services to at-risk youths.

Preliminary data from research in rural Haiti suggest that the introduction of quality HIV care can lead to a rapid reduction in stigma, with resulting increased uptake of testing. Rather than stigma, logistic and economic barriers determine who will access such services. Implications for scale-up of integrated AIDS prevention and care must be explored.

Promoting hope and acceptance is a key response to stigma at all levels of society. In contrast, doing nothing about stigma can contribute to the growing death toll, as well as to distress and reduce quality of life for millions of people.

All those with influence and authority within society have a responsibility individually and collectively, to act in order to reduce stigma about HIV and AIDS within their sphere of influence. Accountability – based on transparency, honesty and openness – is a key component in improving HIV and AIDS prevention, care and support efforts, and to bring them to more people on an ongoing, sustainable basis. Clearly, it is essential that stigma and discrimination be monitored, and redress be provided when discrimination occurs in all of the areas discussed in this paper.

5.7.2 Sexuality, Gender Inequality, HIV and AIDS

Research shows that gender and sexuality are significant factors in the sexual transmission of HIV, and it is now known that these factors also influence treatment, care, and support. Both terms, nevertheless, continue to remain misunderstood and inappropriately used. The organisation of focus in this chapter is one of the major freight and logistics companies in Southern Africa. It is hard to overstate the scale of suffering that HIV has caused in Southern Africa. In order to reduce and manage the impact of HIV/AIDS in the workplace there is a need for gender-sensitive policy-making processes that require the partnership of women and men at all levels, and more importantly, to integrate these processes with the company's corporate strategic plan. It would be a major strategic move to align and integrate the development of a gender-sensitive HIV/AIDS policy with the re-branding process of the Company. A gender-sensitive HIV/AIDS Policy seeks to complement and strengthen the focus on gender equality in the Company's strategic plan. The policy will assist the organisation in integrating gender equity goals and objectives into all its operational strategies so that they become internally and institutionally accepted. Given the magnitude of the project, it is expected that the policy will be implemented within a period of six months with anticipation that modifications thereafter will be based on the Company's progress in implementation and will address emerging issues.

Goals and Strategies:

The gender-sensitive HIV/AIDS Policy and the Company' re-branding process establish an overall goal for the organisation in the conduct of its business and in all organisational matters. Critical to achieving this goal are strategies for implementation and measurable objectives set forth for the re-branding and the gender-sensitive HIV/AIDS policy therein. In addition, time-bound targets will be developed on an annual basis by the gender-sensitive HIV/AIDS Committee to guide the implementation process of the HIV/AIDS policy.

The goal seeks to be responsive to and promote gender equity and equality in the organisation and ensure that its operations and HIV/AIDS awareness interventions serve the needs and interests of both women and men, thus contributing to the elimination of discrimination against women.

Strategies for Implementation:

The following strategies will be adopted to ensure implementation of the gender-sensitive HIV/AIDS Policy in line with the organisational goals:

Endorsement of the gender-sensitive HIV/AIDS Policy by the Executive Board/ Senior Management of the Company, followed by advocacy for Organisation-wide commitment to the policy (Rau 2002).

Sufficient technical and financial resources should be committed for implementation of the policy. This will require identification of financial support both externally and internally, the sourcing of technical expertise in gender analysis and integration of gender into HIV/AIDS interventions (Rau 2002).

Development of special initiatives to raise awareness of gender issues and the gender-sensitive HIV/AIDS Policy at all levels of the organisation. This will require developing indicators for organisational awareness and monitoring progress (Rau 2002).

All internal policies, procedures and rules should be reviewed and revised in light of the gender-sensitive HIV/AIDS Policy (Rau 2002).

Women's representation should be increased in key decision-making bodies guiding organisational and programmatic issues (Rau 2002).

A gender analytical framework will be implemented to guide operations and HIV/ AIDS awareness and interventions (Rau 2002).

The main objectives are:

a) To introduce a gender-sensitive approach to formulating a workplace HIV and AIDS policy.
b) To ensure organisational commitment and the internal allocation of resources to ensure that the gender-sensitive HIV/AIDS Policy will be mainstreamed within the organisation.
c) Raise awareness and understanding of gender issues at all levels of the organisation to achieve gender equality, and thereby demystify the concepts of gender and sexuality with regard to HIV and AIDS in the workplace.

d) Create and maintain an enabling environment within which women's and men's needs can be openly and freely articulated and addressed.

Implementation and monitoring mechanisms and plans:

Responsibilities: The responsibility for the successful implementation of the gender-sensitive HIV/AIDS policy rests with each of the operational departments as well as the organisation's employees. Ultimately, the responsibility for implementation of the gender-sensitive HIV/AIDS Policy lies with the Group Chief Executive.

The same applies for the rollout of the new identity of the Company. Although brand champions will be appointed at each of the operational divisions of the Company, the ultimate responsibility for implementation rests with the Group Chief Executive.

Special Structures: While the responsibility for promoting equality is shared throughout the organisation, there is also a need for special resources and organisational structures to be put in place. The following steps may be used for the development of the policy:

The first step is to recognise that HIV/AIDS is a workplace issue, and it should be treated like any other serious illness/condition in the workplace. This is necessary not only because it affects the workforce, but also because the workplace, being part of the local community, has a role to play in the wider struggle, to limit the spread and effects of the epidemic (ILO Code of Practice on HIV/AIDS and the World of Work 2001; National Code of Practice for HIV/AIDS in the Workplace 2007; USAID Health Policy Initiative 2008).

An HIV/AIDS committee could be set up with representatives of top management, supervisors, workers, unions, human resources department, training department, industrial relations unit, occupational health unit, health and safety committee, and persons living with HIV/AIDS (if they agree) (ILO Code of Practice on HIV/AIDS and the World of Work 2001; National Code of Practice for HIV/AIDS in the Workplace 2007; USAID Health Policy Initiative 2008). The Gender-sensitive HIV/AIDS Committee should be chaired by the Chief Executive or her/his nominee. A Gender Specialist in the Human Resources Department should be Member-Secretary of the Gender-sensitive HIV/AIDS Committee.

Committee decides its terms of reference and decision-making powers and responsibilities; review of national laws and their implications for the enterprise (ILO Code of Practice on HIV/AIDS and the World of Work 2001; National Code of Practice for HIV/AIDS in the Workplace 2007; USAID Health Policy Initiative 2008).

Committee assesses the impact of the HIV epidemic on the workplace and the needs of workers infected and affected by HIV/AIDS. Any surveys or studies carried out in the workplace to determine this impact and the needs of its workers shall be with the workers informed consent, and maintain the autonomy of workers and the confidentiality of their medical records at all times (ILO Code of Practice on HIV/AIDS and the World of Work 2001; National Code of Practice for HIV/AIDS in the Workplace 2007; USAID Health Policy Initiative 2008). This step could also be aligned with the rollout of the Company's new identity in the following way: Internally, with immediate effect, there will be a kick off of a process to identify – across the Company – all the behaviours that are needed to support the values that must be lived by. This is part of promoting the emerging culture.

Committee establishes what health and information services are already available – both at the workplace and in the local community; committee formulates a draft policy; draft circulated for comment then revised and adopted (ILO Code of Practice on HIV/AIDS and the World of Work 2001; National Code of Practice for HIV/AIDS in the Workplace 2007; USAID Health Policy Initiative 2008).

Committee draws up a budget, seeking funds from outside the enterprise if necessary and identifies existing resources in the local community (ILO Code of Practice on HIV/AIDS and the World of Work 2001; National Code of Practice for HIV/AIDS in the Workplace 2007; USAID Health Policy Initiative 2008).

Committee establishes plan of action, with timetable and lines of responsibility, to implement policy. Policy and plan of action are widely disseminated through, for example notice boards, mailings, pay slip inserts, special meetings, induction courses, training sessions (ILO Code of Practice on HIV/AIDS and the World of Work 2001; National Code of Practice for HIV/AIDS in the Workplace 2007; USAID Health Policy Initiative 2008). This step could be aligned with the dissemination of the Company's new brand, which will be done through advertising campaigns in newspapers to promote our new brand to external stakeholders.

Committee monitors the impact of the policy; and committee regularly reviews the policy in the light of internal monitoring and external information about the virus and its workplace implications (ILO Code of Practice on HIV/AIDS and the World of Work 2001; National Code of Practice for HIV/AIDS in the Workplace 2007; USAID Health Policy Initiative 2008).

All steps described above should be integrated into a comprehensive enterprise policy that is planned, implemented and monitored in a sustained and ongoing manner.

Dissemination: After the gender-sensitive HIV/AIDS Policy is approved by the EXCOs, it will be translated into Zulu and Afrikaans. English, Afrikaans and Zulu versions will be disseminated at all levels. Various media will be used including industrial theatre, payslips, notice boards, peer educators, and briefings during shift changeovers.

Annual Plans: The Gender-sensitive HIV/AIDS Committee will develop annual work-plans to define steps for implementation of the Gender-sensitive HIV/AIDS Policy.

In due course, with regard to the re-branding process of the Company, the names of all the brand champions across the length and breadth of the Company will be announced. These champions will work very closely with the culture ambassadors. As one can imagine, changing the identity of a company as large as ours is an intensive process. It is anticipated that this process will take about two years.

Gender Analysis Framework: A gender analysis framework will be adopted with technical assistance from the World Health Organisation Gender Advisory Panel. It will be used for assessing whether gender concerns have been addressed in research and intervention proposals and for the review of training and services of the Organisation.

In the interim, with regard to the rollout of the Company's new brand, a professional project team has been appointed to assist with the rollout of the new identity. As with all projects, involving external parties, this remains the Company's own project, which it has to own.

Monitoring: The Human Resources Gender Specialist will be responsible for monitoring and documenting information related to the recruitment, training and promotion of female staff. In line with the Company's goal of becoming the employer of choice (attracting, developing and retaining talent), efforts to encourage women to take up leadership positions (Hunger Project 2002) should be intensified, including intensifying support for programmes for current and future women leaders and awareness-raising campaigns on the importance of women's participation in decision-making, including the formulation of workplace policies such as the gender-sensitive HIV/AIDS policy.

The Human Resources Department is responsible for carrying out performance reviews of implementation of the policy at the organisational level. On the other hand, the Communications Department is responsible for coordinating the rollout of the re-branding process.

The gender-sensitive HIV/AIDS Committee will review the performance reviews and submit progress reports to the Executive Committee (EXCO) on an annual basis. These ongoing reviews may lead to revisions of the gender-sensitive HIV/AIDS Policy. Similarly, the appointed project team responsible for the implementation of the Company's new brand will also review and submit progress reports to the EXCO on an annual basis, until the rollout process has been concluded. Thereafter, the brand champions through the Communications Department will be responsible for ongoing review and monitoring of the Company's brand and indicate areas that need improvement or modification where necessary, in order to promote and sustain the Company's image and success.

The gender-sensitive HIV/AIDS Policy should be a standing item in the EXCO and Level 2 (Senior Management and Labour unions) meetings.

Resource allocation for implementation of the gender-sensitive HIV/AIDS Policy:

Similar to the project for the implementation of the Company's new brand, a budget to cover costs associated with the implementation of the gender-sensitive HIV/AIDS Policy will be prepared and submitted to the Executive Committee of the Organisation.

The following conclusions can be drawn from the foregoing discussion:

Buy-in from senior management (people of greater power and influence) would ensure their commitment to and action on promoting gender equality goals in reducing and managing HIV/AIDS in the workplace.

The gender-sensitive HIV/AIDS policy should be sustained through a workplace environment that enables the mainstreaming (Rau 2002) of this policy with the overall organisational strategic plan.

Employers, workers and their trade unions shall cooperate in a positive, caring manner to develop a gender-sensitive workplace policy on HIV/AIDS that responds to and balances the needs of employers and workers.

Gender-sensitive training for all employees, in particular management personnel is highly recommended in order to create and maintain an enabling environment within which women's and men's needs can be openly and freely articulated (Hazelle 2002). Reducing gender inequality requires changing social norms, attitudes and behaviours through a comprehensive set of policies and procedures.

Sexuality should be recognised as a fundamental dimension of human relations in which gender inequality is often expressed and enforced at the workplace. The principle of zero tolerance for any form of discrimination at the workplace, should be enforced; particularly with regard to gender and sexuality. Therefore, more equal gender relations and the empowerment of women are vital to successfully prevent the spread of HIV infection and enable women to cope with HIV/AIDS at the workplace (ILO Code of Practice on HIV/AIDS and the World of Work 2001; National Code of Practice for HIV/AIDS in the Workplace 2007).

5.7.3 HIV and AIDS, Migration and Poverty

Southern Africa remains the epicentre of the global HIV epidemic: 32% of people with HIV globally live in this sub-region and 34% of AIDS deaths globally occur there (UNAIDS 2007). The multi-faceted relationship between migration and HIV is of particular significance in this region as the wide-ranging movement of people has been taking place for decades, beginning well before the arrival of the HIV epidemic in the 1980s (Health and Development Networks 2006). Mobility significantly increases HIV-related risk. Often, migrant workers move from low-prevalence rural regions to urban centres, where HIV prevalence is much higher and risk behaviours are more frequent (United Nations 2005). South Africa has experienced high levels of economic migration in recent decades, both between its provinces, and between itself and its neighbouring countries. Migration increases the extent of sexual networking, and thus facilitates the swift spread of the HIV/AIDS epidemic (Health and Development Networks 2006). The overall aim of this chapter is to identify the relationship between poverty, migration and HIV and AIDS with particular focus on mineworkers. The specific objectives are: To identify the economic, social, cultural and demographic profile of migrant mine workers in Southern

Africa; To identify the typical activities and movements, and vulnerabilities of migrant mine workers to HIV and AIDS; To formulate policy guidelines and strategies of how to deal with the risks and vulnerabilities to HIV and AIDS, and the needs the migrant mine workers have.

The interrelationship between poverty, migration and HIV and AIDS is complex. The following discussion reflects on this interrelationship with focus on the socio-economic, cultural and demographic aspects, as well as the risks and vulnerabilities to HIV/AIDS with regard to mine workers. Implications for policy guidelines and strategies are also highlighted. As is commonly accepted, in terms of numbers, males dominate the workplace at most mines. Therefore, the needs and preferences that are discussed in this paper are those of males and not necessarily those of their partners or spouses.

Socio-economic Profile

Mineworkers in South African mines predominantly come from poor rural areas from the neighbouring states and the former homelands of South Africa. The incidence of poverty is closely related to unemployment. In some rural areas, rates of migrant unemployment are as high as 60% males (Johnson and Budlender 2002). Although some studies report high prevalence of HIV in poor countries, the countries with the highest prevalence rates are not necessarily the poorest. Poverty is especially prevalent in rural areas, and particularly among Africans and Coloureds. The national data on poverty and unemployment indicate that, as a group, rural blacks have a high chance of being poor. Lack of access to employment is arguably the single greatest cause of rural poverty. It is hardly surprising that many economically active young men from these poor areas pack their bags and head for the mines in an attempt to escape the shackles of poverty and unemployment.

The main problem in the mineworker environment is the large dependency of households on a single income (Marais and Venter 2006).

Cultural Profile

The move to a different cultural context in search of work can also mean isolation from protective social rules, which can increase vulnerability to HIV. Behaviour is often different when people are away from home and away from the social norms that guide and control behaviour in stable communities. People who move from a conservative society to one perceived to be more liberal may be ill-equipped to deal with sexual freedom: they may not understand the norms or the limits in the new society, and how to protect themselves (Health and Development Networks 2006).

Migration stands for change: change of physical environment, of cultural traditions, of social norms, of power structures etc. Migrant mineworkers move between their home area, where they are located within familiar local structures and practices, and the mines, where they live in a new environment, often devoid of traditional social norms (Health and Development Networks 2006).

Demographic Profile

Although, the available literature indicates that approximately half of migrants in the world today are women (Health and Development Networks 2006), mineworkers are predominantly men.

The South African Migration Survey (SAMP) has been conducting numerous surveys focusing on immigration issues, and one such survey revealed that most of the migrants were in their economic prime, between 25 and 44 years. Only 15% were younger than 24 years, and 4% were older than 55 years (Maharaj 2004).

According to Marais and Venter (2006), the formal academic qualifications of mine workers are extremely low. Over 50% of the migrants are single (never married), and almost equal proportions who are married left their spouses in their home area (Maharaj 2004).

The International Organization for Migration (2005) indicates that over 90% of the mining industry's black employees are migrants.

Risks and Vulnerabilities to HIV and AIDS

The International Organisation for Migration (2005) reveals that much of the published research on migrant labour in Southern Africa has focused on the South African gold mines which have drawn large numbers of workers from all over the sub-continent. Because most of these migrant men live almost exclusively in single-sex hostels, without their wives or families, they are seen as being at high risk of contracting Sexually Transmitted Infections (STIs), including HIV.

Foreign workers on the mines (from Lesotho and Mozambique) generally return home less frequently than their South African counterparts, and their partners are less likely to be able to visit them on the mines. The prevalence of commercial sex and alcohol-related business supported by miners create conditions that render other groups in the surrounding communities more susceptible to infection as well (International Organization for Migration 2005).

Studies on temporary and permanent residents in the mining town of Carletonville, South Africa, the largest gold mine complex in the world, reveal the conditions that render miners and the communities around them susceptible to HIV infection. The high prevalence of HIV among men and women in the surrounding community demonstrates the high risk faced by all members of a mining community, not just the miners themselves (International Organization for Migration 2005). It is not uncommon for the mineworkers to have two wives, one in their home village, whom they see on rare occasions, and one near the mine.

In many cases the mineworkers may unknowingly infect their wives and partners when they return to their home communities. This has played a crucial role in the rapid spread of HIV in southern Africa (International Organization for Migration 2003). Evidence suggests that transmission in the opposite direction may also occur (Johnson and Budlender 2002).

Separation from home, sharing crowded rooms in large hostels, loneliness, and the harsh working conditions seem to add up to the feeling of helplessness in which the dangers of contracting HIV are outweighed by other pressing concerns and needs. Some mineworkers clearly express a fatalistic attitude towards their lives in general (Health and Development Networks 2006).

The lack of rights has been repeatedly recorded as one of the key factors increasing HIV vulnerability for migrant and mobile populations such as mine workers. Migrants' rights, including the right to work, to move within the country, to education or to access health care, are often directly related to the legal status of individuals. Foreign workers are generally not represented by unions, and often have weak negotiating and bargaining powers vis-à-vis their employers (Health and Development Networks 2006).

Policy Guidelines and Strategies

There is a need to formulate an HIV/AIDS policy, the plight of migrant mineworkers, including their housing and living conditions and the respective responsibilities of government and employers in addressing these issues. There is also a need to protect human and labour rights in relation to education, counselling, testing and treatment. The policy guidelines and strategies should include:

The response to HIV/AIDS in the mining sector should take into account the social, cultural and psychological pressures facing this group and the community contexts that facilitate the spread of HIV infection. A collaborative relationship needs to be established between governments, mining organisations and unions to ensure that the mechanisms for dealing with the epidemic are holistic and involve all stakeholders (International Organization for Migration 2003).

The mining sector should be integrated into national AIDS plans and include key representatives of the mining sector in multi-sectoral national AIDS councils (International Organization for Migration 2003).

It is essential that HIV and STI prevention programmes in mining communities include all sexual partners, including Commercial Sex Workers who are often excluded from such programmes due to the stigma and discrimination that surrounds them (International Organization for Migration 2003).

The cultivation of community cohesion via the membership of local voluntary associations such as sports clubs and youth groups should be promoted (International Organization for Migration 2003).

A range of tenure types should be offered to workers, including rental accommodation, home ownership and social housing. Housing options should include single and family accommodation, accommodation in nearby settlements where feasible, and accommodation in mineworkers' home areas. The principle of choice for mineworkers from a wide range of flexible housing options should apply (International Organization for Migration 2003).

Existing hostels on mines should be converted steadily into family units and into single units for mine workers without families or who choose not to live with their families. The provision of family housing should include community and education services and facilities (International Organization for Migration 2003).

Each mine should, in conjunction with representative trade unions, be required to draw up a five-year plan for the improvement of living conditions for workers, incorporating specific targets (International Organization for Migration 2003).

The management of hostels must be democratised so that residents participate jointly with mine management in all areas of decision-making around the running of hostels (International Organization for Migration 2003).

To reduce the HIV/AIDS vulnerability of mobile populations (such as mineworkers) in the long term, the socio-economic and political factors that drive mobility should be addressed, including the uneven distribution of resources, unemployment, socio-economic insecurity, economic instability and political unrest (International Organization for Migration 2003).

Similarly, the characteristics and underlying conditions of migration should be addressed. Programmes that train peer educators in the workplace and that distribute Information, Education and Communication materials and condoms are extremely important. But they do not address the root causes of vulnerability. Therefore, such programmes need to be implemented in tandem with efforts that protect basic human rights and improve the living and working conditions of mobile workers. If these workers feel valued and have their basic human rights protected, they would be likely to value their own lives enough to practice safe sex (International Organization for Migration 2003).

This section has examined the features (economic, social, cultural and demographic profile) of migrant mine workers, their typical activities and movements, and in particular the risks they are exposed to regarding HIV and AIDS.

From this description it is imperative to develop holistic policy guidelines and strategies that conceptualise HIV as a social and development issue that has to be addressed not only at the level of specific mines, but also at the level of the communities in which the mines are located.

To a large degree the paper confirms that the relationship between poverty, migration and HIV/AIDS is highly complex, and is likely to be obscured by a variety of other demographic factors. The crucial point is that the individual's risk of HIV infection is determined by both his socio-economic status, and the socio-economic profile of the community in which he is situated (Johnson and Budlender 2002).

Many of the factors that increase migrant mineworkers' vulnerability to HIV are cross-sectoral: dislocated social support structures, limited legal rights, poor access to health care services, sexual coercion, exploitation, violence, and, complex sexual networks that connect disparate communities (International Organization for Migration 2005).

Mineworker needs suggest that there are diverse needs, and that the hostel systems which keep the status quo in place are inappropriate for at least 50% of the mineworkers, while the living conditions are extremely poor and not to the satisfaction of the majority of mineworkers (Marais and Venter 2006).

5.7.4 A Labour Relations Perspective on HIV and AIDS

Joint Problem Solving
Evaluating whether an organisation meets the following conditions that facilitate a joint problem-solving approach for HIV/AIDS: A common objective or goal; appropriate attitudes; trust; constituency accountability; and information exchange.

A Common Objective or Goal

In the context of the particular organisation, joint problem solving through a common objective or goal is imperative to make sure that the internal stakeholders (including management, labour unions, people living with HIV/AIDS, and the rest of the employees) believe that there is likelihood that greater benefits will ensue from collaboration than from competition. Three types of goal offering this type of approach are described in Anstey (1999). These include: Common goals, shared goals, and joint goals.

Common Goals: the stakeholders share equal benefits that can be created only by collaborative effort. For example, in the face of a high prevalence of HIV among our workforce, a fully-fledged and practical HIV/AIDS strategy including the HIV/AIDS Committee could contribute towards making the business a success by reducing absenteeism and increasing productivity. Therefore, both management and labour could agree to an equal distribution of profits created by the joint efforts required to make the business a success. Although the particular organisation has had a documented strategy including working toward common goals regarding the management of HIV/AIDS, the approach has been very sporadic and inconsistent as each division was doing its own thing. Hence, there has not been clear-cut joint efforts by management and labour to effectively manage HIV/AIDS to make the business a success. This is one of the major challenges that the organisation faces.

Shared Goals: Anstey (1999) explains that the stakeholders involved work toward a common objective but benefit differently. For example, if the particular organisation could effectively manage HIV/AIDS through shared goals between management and labour, management would get higher incentive bonuses than labour unions and the people that they represent based on the profitability of the business. From the particular organisation's perspective, the intention of the joint management and labour involvement in the HIV/AIDS Committee was to work toward a common objective. However, the reality was that management and labour unions did not have shared goals. Most HIV/AIDS Committee meetings were not productive as there was often finger-pointing rather than having or addressing shared goals. Attendance at HIV/AIDS Committee forums was always poor, and meetings were often postponed because they could not form a quorum. This indicates that working toward a common objective through shared goals was not taken seriously, but rather as window-dressing.

Joint Goals: Anstey (1999) defines shared goals as a situation whereby parties have quite different goals but combine in a collective effort to attain a common objective. For example, employees living with HIV/AIDS, peer educators, labour unions, and safety representatives may unite their efforts in pressurising management to introduce a comprehensive disease management programme for employees infected with HIV, but who themselves have different goals in terms of the final shape of the structure of the organisation. In the particular organisation, there has not really been joint goals in this regard, as most decisions are unilaterally taken by management, based on budget and profitability of the business. The reality is that even though there may be various formal groups within the organisation, such groups do not carry enough vigour to challenge management and management decisions.

At this juncture, it is worth mentioning that before the major transformation ensued within the organisation, each sub-division was doing its own thing with regard to the management of HIV/AIDS. Such a practice was very sporadic and created a great deal of inconsistency and confusion for both internal and external stakeholders. In other words, the idea was there, but there was no clear common objective or goal in terms of joint problem solving.

Therefore, in line with the overall organisational turnaround strategy and new mission and vision, the process of developing a unified HIV/AIDS strategy with a common objective or goal as part and parcel of the emerging organisational culture, was underway.

Appropriate Attitudes

The following key beliefs must be shared by the stakeholders (including management, labour unions, peer educators, and employees living with HIV/AIDS) in order to enable the creation of integrative decision making, as suggested by Anstey (1999): a belief that mutually acceptable solutions are available; a belief that such solutions are desirable; a belief in cooperative endeavour versus competition; a belief that everyone is of equal value; a belief that the others' views are legitimate statements of their positions; a belief that differences of opinion are helpful; a belief that the other party could compete but has chosen to cooperate; and a belief in one's own problem-solving ability.

Trust and Firmness

According to Anstey (1999), trust is a prerequisite for open sharing of needs positions, underlying interests, fears and information. Joint problem-solving emerges from high-trust, high-limit situations. Similarly, rigid goals coupled with flexible means promote joint problem-solving. Where parties indicate commitment to their own needs but a willingness to engage in a search for a joint solution, this promotes trust in a relationship. The following factors emerging from research, contribute to the development of trust: perceptions of similarity; perceptions that a positive attitude is held toward one; perceptions of the other's dependency; perceptions of the other's desire to cooperate and make concessions; opening moves in a negotiation which are open and cooperative; and histories or patterns of cooperative engagement.

Constituency Accountability

In collective or representational situations negotiations are not participant on their own behalf but are mandated by and report back to constituencies. For example, in the context of the particular organisation, labour union representatives are mandated by and should report back to the employees that they represent. Anstey (1999) points out that low accountability may allow collaboration but not necessarily problem solving. On the other hand, high accountability tends to promote competition as negotiators try to meet their constituencies' demands and show strength in the bargaining process.

In the particular organisation there has been a long history of competition, whereby, employees have created very high demands, and because the labour representatives have not been seen to meet all these demands, the employees have already lost confidence in labour representatives even if reporting happens. The organisation's employees must, therefore, allow their labour representatives room for manouvre if problem solving is to occur, particularly on the issue of an HIV/AIDS strategy.

Information Exchange

Effective information exchange is a means of creating and promoting trust in a working relationship. In the particular organisation, information exchange has been one of the main deficiencies. In the HIV/AIDS Committee forums and other joint management and labour meetings such as Level 2 meetings, discussions or negotiations often reach a deadlock mainly due to the fact that one or all the parties concerned do not have all the information relevant to the matter at hand. However, one has to bear in mind that conflict may still be exacerbated even if there is genuine information disclosure, especially if there is a deep-seated belief that employees are being exploited by management.

Therefore, there is need to realise that building trust between management and labour is key to most avenues of success for the organisation, including information exchange. In this regard, it could be value-adding to organise monthly team building escapades for management and labour, with the understanding that building trust is a process that requires commitment and willingness from all parties concerned. And more importantly, also involve the rest of the employees in such team building exercises, particularly because the employees have not only lost trust in management but in the labour representatives as well. In other words, there is somewhat a need to start from scratch, and rebuild.

In conclusion, the re-branding (monolithic brand) for the said organisation is a major strategic move as it will provide an appropriate architecture to govern the relationship between the main brand and the sub-brands, and in the context of HIV/AIDS strategy provide a platform for joint problem solving with a common objective or goal, appropriate attitudes, trust and firmness, constituency accountability, and information exchange. Central to all this is to rebuild trust between management, labour representatives and the rest of the employees. Therefore, the organisation's new brand and the new emerging culture is an opportunity to achieve this objective.

Communication
Developing a practical internal communication strategy for HIV/AIDS in an organisation:

According to Swanepoel (1999), internal organisational communication can be defined as the presentation of messages by communicators to receivers in the same organisation, with the purpose of achieving the organisation's or the individual's purpose.

It is of paramount importance that the organisation establishes and maintains procedures for ensuring that pertinent HIV/AIDS management system information is communicated to and from employees. Employee involvement and consultation arrangements must be documented and interested parties informed (Swart and Kotze 2003:11).

First and foremost, Swanepoel (1999:330) emphasises that a clear distinction has to be made between an ongoing internal communication strategy to ensure good employment relations, and a strategy that has to be employed during a crisis. Based on the many factors influencing communication in the particular organisation, it may be impractical to suggest a strategic blueprint for an ongoing process, however, the key requirements for an effective internal communication strategy for HIV/AIDS with employees and labour representatives, will be discussed.

Proactive Approach:

The emphasis of effective communication on HIV/AIDS should be on creating positive employee attitudes. Management can invite labour union participation in broad business problem-solving, and in so doing can begin to develop a labour/management partnership. For example, labour unions should be invited to our monthly business review meetings.

Holistic Approach:

In order to ensure that HIV/AIDS related messages and signals are consistent and that a cohesive image is projected, the organisation needs to take a holistic view of communication. As the organisational transformation and turnaround strategy is completed, the company will no longer be a diversified Group. The re-branding is aimed at communicating that the company is now a focused and integrated freight transport company. Therefore, the organisation's internal communication on HIV/AIDS should have its roots in the overall new mission and vision of the company. The next step is to develop separate communication strategies for the various stakeholder groups of the organisation, including employees and labour representatives. The aim is to enable people at all levels of the organisation to appreciate the value of an integrated, holistic view of communication.

Communication Must Be Planned:

This means that the internal communication strategy on HIV/AIDS must be orientated to specific objectives. The results must be measured, and the plan modified if it is not meeting its goals. For example, it should be determined how, when, and what messages should be conveyed to employees, as well as the impact of the whole process.

Organisational Climate:

Management needs to devote particular attention to creating and maintaining an organisational climate characterised by openness and trust. The climate should be receptive to the upward transmission of employee ideas, suggestions and opinions. This is particularly critical when it comes to HIV/AIDS. For example, a conducive environment will enhance employee participation in Voluntary Counselling and Testing, disclosure and ready involvement with support groups such as employees living with HIV.

Communication Channels:

It is imperative for management to ensure that established formal channels of employee communication (upward, downward and horizontal) adequately meet the needs of employees including employees that have been diagnosed with HIV. This will enhance trust and openness between all the internal stakeholders in the organisation.

Support from the Top:

The Chief Executive must set the example if he or she desires substantial credibility and internal communication effectiveness on HIV/AIDS in the organisation. For example, during Voluntary Counselling and Testing campaigns, the Chief Executive must be the first to get tested for HIV.

*The Following Is an Internal Communication Strategy for HIV/AIDS in the Organisation in Times of Crisis or Great Change, as Adapted from Swanepoel (*1999):

Regular open two-way communication that is driven by employees is necessary to deal with cognitive and emotional needs during difficult times. The extent of the change must be communicated to all employees, as well as a clear vision of the direction in which the organisation is moving, and the implications of the changes in practical workplace terms regarding human resources, capacity and money.

Management should identify the most influential communicators or opinion leaders, including union representatives, peer educators and employee spokespersons in HIV/AIDS crisis communication.

Involving both management and peer educators in managing an HIV/AIDS crisis such as stigma could help the emotionally depleted employees to feel that they had recovered what they had lost – a sense of control over their futures and a belief that top management still value their input. Emotionally drained HIV infected or affected employees may need therapeutic messages via interpersonal communication channels, such as small group meetings with management and peer group counselling sessions.

Management must make sure that HIV/AIDS related messages are clear, consistent and realistic. For example, it must be made clear that Voluntary Counselling and Testing campaigns are not a means of identifying and getting rid of employees diagnosed with HIV. Using interpersonal communication channels such as memoranda, articles, payslips and DVDs or video tapes in conveying key HIV/AIDS related information to employees could be an effective way of conveying critical HIV/AIDS messages.

The foregoing practical internal communication strategy that has been developed for HIV/AIDS in the organisation was based on the guidelines for communication strategies on a continual basis, as well as for crisis situations and times of great change.

5.7.5 Developing an HIV and AIDS Workplace Policy: Content, Process, Challenges and Implementation

Impact of HIV and AIDS on the Workplace

The objective of this section is to describe the impact of HIV and AIDS on the QRST factory which is a medium to large sized motor manufacturing company in KwaZulu-Natal, South Africa, and to explain to the Executive Committee why it is essential to develop a workplace policy.

The impact of HIV and AIDS on the QRST factory is in two aspects: financial consequences, and the basic rights of the infected and affected employee. Together, these two factors determine what happens in the workplace with regard to ensuring effective labour supply and satisfying strategic labour demands (Government of South Africa 2000).

The end result is inevitably the evolvement of a smaller and active labour force and a greater dependency ratio. A climate of discrimination and lack of respect for human rights leaves employees more vulnerable to infection and less able to cope with HIV/AIDS because it makes it difficult for them to seek voluntary testing, treatment or support (ILO 2000).

HIV/AIDS is most likely to have profound effects on the quality of the labour force on the Rainbow factory as this enterprise is located in a high HIV prevalence country and province. Skilled and experienced employees may be lost to the epidemic. If more skilled and experienced people are lost, labour quantity could be preserved but the labour quality would not (ILO 2001).

As the rate of infection increases, so are the costs associated with the epidemic (Business Report 2003). These increasing costs may ultimately affect the level of benefits that the business is able to provide to its workforce. Demand for recruitment and training rises as a result of increased staff turnover and loss of skills. A situation like this would mean falling rates of return on human capital formation (UNAIDS 2000). Additional costs are incurred from frequent absenteeism (Business Report 2003) due to illness or attendance at funerals, as well as time spent on training. Losses in labour time and skills will reduce the quantity and quality (UNAIDS 2000) of cars produced and services by the QRST factory, leading to reputation losses and ultimately a reduction in customers.

It would be of great value to the QRST factory if the Executive Committee could realise the importance of developing a workplace HIV and AIDS policy. An HIV/AIDS policy sets the foundation for HIV/AIDS prevention and care programs; It offers a framework for consistency of practices within the business; It expresses the standards of behaviour expected of employees; It informs all employees what is available and where to get it; It guides supervisors and managers on how to manage HIV/AIDS in their work groups; It assures consistency with relevant local and national laws and statutes. There is growing recognition by businesses that economic benefits derive from care and treatment programs. There is growing body of evidence that prevention efforts reduce risk and contribute to lower HIV incidence (Rau 2004).

HIV and AIDS is a reality that affects productivity and profitability. Therefore, it is essential for the QRST factory's Executive Committee to realise the importance of implementing a workplace HIV and AIDS policy, as a policy embodies a commitment on the part of the company to proactively address the epidemic before the situation gets out of control.

Strategic Plan for Coordinating the Management of HIV and AIDS in the Workplace

The objective of this section is to outline a strategic plan for coordinating the management of HIV and AIDS at the QRST factory, a medium to large motor manufacturing factory located in the province of KwaZulu-Natal in South Africa.

Governance:

Workplace HIV and AIDS policy and strategy and ensure input from all stakeholders. Set clear roles and responsibilities of the HIV and AIDS Committee, peer educators and agree on sustainable strategy for the future. Have a specific budget for HIV and AIDS.

Management and Coordination:

Review the current representation of the HIV Committee members, ensuring realistic and sustainable approach with sufficient internal role players.

Prevention:

Develop a behaviour change communication strategy and identify the most effective media for ongoing employee communiqué. *Train the target groups such as* Management, Supervisors, Shop stewards and peer educators. Provide v*oluntary* counselling and testing (VCT)/HIV testing services (HTS) on an ongoing basis. Provide ongoing awareness and access to treatment for employees diagnosed with

Sexually Transmitted Infections (STIs). A workplace condom distribution programme will also be in place. Directly Observed Treatment Short Course (DOTs) programme for Tuberculosis (TB) will be provided as part of the worksite clinic services. A Post Exposure Prophylaxis/ Workplace safety procedure will be in place as per QRST factory's HIV and AIDS policy. Events based awareness campaigns: e.g. World AIDS Day (WAD) but move beyond awareness.

Treatment:

Ensure continuation of care for employees on disease management programme. Facilitate enrolment of employees testing HIV-positive onto the disease management programme. Clinical staging, monitoring and adherence of employees on the disease management programme.

Care:

Employees who are living with HIV and AIDS and who need help will be referred to the on-site Employee Assistance Programme for psychological support and counselling.

Monitoring and Evaluation:

Identify key process and outcome indicators to ensure ongoing monitoring and evaluation (Rau 2004) of programme uptake and effectiveness.

External Stakeholders, Partnerships and Communication Strategy:

Develop and strengthen supply chain networks and community partnerships. Develop an internal communication strategy (Rau 2004) with regard to QRST factory's HIV and AIDS strategy.

The workplace HIV and AIDS programme is the core of an organisation's response to HIV and AIDS. This programme will in turn be informed and sustained by a well-designed HIV and AIDS policy. It is critical to have a budget, Steering Committee, Policy and an HIV and AIDS Champion to ensure full implementation of the programme.

Steps and Timeframes When Developing a Workplace Policy:

The objective of this section is to describe the steps and timeframes that one would follow to develop the workplace policy at the QRST factory. The assumption is that process begins in July 2020.

By the 15th July 2020, the first step would be to involve all members of the QRST factory's workplace in an awareness-raising process where the outcome is the acknowledgement of HIV and AIDS as an issue affecting our workplace.

By the 20th July 2020, a presentation will be made at the QRST factory's Executive Committee meeting with the aim of getting full support and buy-in from top management of the factory. The support of management and of the company's leadership is vital to the process.

By the 31st July 2020, there shall be setting up of an HIV/AIDS committee with representatives of QRST factory's top management and management at all levels to ensure commitment to and leadership for the policies and programmes, supervisors, lower levels of employees as they are often extremely vulnerable to being affected by HIV and AIDS, trade unions, human resources department, training department, industrial relations unit, occupational health unit, health and safety committee, people with relevant skills for the policy-development process (such as communications skills and training in HIV and AIDS), employees active in HIV and AIDS activities in the community, and persons living with HIV/AIDS, if they agree (USAID Health Policy Initiative 2008). It will also be ensured that there is a representative balance between men and women.

By the 15th August 2020, the HIV/AIDS committee shall decide its terms of reference and decision-making powers and responsibilities (ILOAIDS): these must be approved by the Rainbow factory's Executive Committee.

By the 31st August 2020, a review of national laws and their implications for the enterprise would be done. This should go beyond any specific laws on HIV/AIDS and could include anti-discrimination laws, for example, and relevant International Labour Office (ILO) Conventions (ILOAIDS).

By the 8th September 2020, the HIV and AIDS Committee will gather relevant information which will enable the members to design an appropriate, manageable and cost-effective response. Information gathering includes finding out what are the needs and concerns of the employer, managers, supervisors, shop stewards, employees, and how these can be addressed (USAID Health Policy Initiative 2008). The HIV and AIDS Committee will also start to think about the nature of the Rainbow factory and how this may impact on the content of the HIV and AIDS policy. The HIV and AIDS Committee will also assess technical expertise and information that is available to assist them in their information gathering. There shall be benchmarking of the company's policy with other companies' existing policies and adapt these to the motor manufacturing business at the QRST factory, fitting it to the company's situation so that the policy is relevant and works for the company.

By the 30th September 2020, the HIV/AIDS Committee will have to discuss important issues and reach an agreement before they can begin the process of drafting an HIV and AIDS policy (USAID Health Policy Initiative 2008).

By the 8th October 2020, the HIV and AIDS Committee will formulate a draft policy. By the 11th October 2020, the Committee will establish a process of consultation at the workplace. On the 13th October 2020, the draft policy will be widely circulated for comment in the QRST factory. On the 20th October 2020 the draft will be revised and adopted – the wider the consultation, the fuller the sense of 'ownership' and support. The policy will be written in clear and accessible language (ILOAIDS). The policy will not only be written in English, but it will also be translated into isiZulu, given the geographical location of the QRST factory.

By the 25th October 2020, the HIV/AIDS Committee will draw up a budget. By the 30th October 2020, the HIV/AIDS Committee will establish a plan of action, with timetable and lines of responsibility, to implement policy. Alliances can be made with other businesses as well as links with NGOs in the surrounding community (ILOAIDS).

By the 15th November 2020, the HIV and AIDS policy and plan of action will be widely disseminated (Rau 2004) in such a way that it appeals and easily understandable to all sectors of staff (for example via notice boards, mailings, pay slip inserts, special meetings, induction courses, training sessions) and programmes of information, education and care put in place. The HIV and AIDS Committee will review this policy at regular intervals and conduct a formal review in the 1st Quarter of each year (Daimler Chrysler Workplace Policy 2002).

Developing a workplace HIV and AIDS policy requires full buy-in from all key stakeholders at the QRST factory, and rather more-so from top management. A wider consultation ensures a full sense of 'ownership' and support.

Roles and Challenges of Management in the Development and Implementation of an HIV/AIDS Workplace Policy

The purpose of this paper is to describe the roles and the challenges of management in the development and implementation of the workplace HIV and AIDS policy at the QRST factory.

Management must own, promote and communicate the policy to all staff (Rau 2004). Management must provide all the necessary resources to ensure that the policy is successfully developed and implemented (USAID Health Policy Initiative 2008). Senior management must make sure that the policy provides appropriate coverage of issues, encompasses all staff and addresses the issue of stigma and discrimination (Rau 2004). Consequently, senior management ensure that managers and supervisors both understand and exercise their responsibility to effective leadership if confronted by the risk of stigma and discrimination (Wellbeing 2008). Management must ensure that all new staff members, irrespective of location or duration of their appointments, have the company's HIV and AIDS policy and related support mechanisms explained to them early in the induction process (Wellbeing 2008).

Often the main challenge is reconciling the core business of the QRST factory and all that come with it (targets, profit, efficiency, and cost-effectiveness, among others, in a highly competitive world) with the demands of an effective, humane and socially responsible HIV and AIDS programme (USAID Health Policy Initiative 2008). Management is further being challenged to weigh up complicated cost-benefit factors (USAID Health Policy Initiative 2008).

The roles of management in the development and implementation of an HIV and AIDS policy indicate that management must be the key drivers if the whole process is to be successful. The challenges highlight the dynamics of HIV and AIDS and how this influences management's decisions regarding the core business of the company.

Importance of Involving People Living with HIV

The purpose of this section is to comment on the importance of involving People Living with HIV in the process of developing, monitoring and evaluating an HIV and AIDS workplace policy at the QRST factory, a motor manufacturing factory located in the province of KwaZulu-Natal in South Africa.

People living with HIV have directly experienced the factors that make individuals and communities vulnerable to HIV infection. Their involvement in policy development, monitoring and evaluation at the QRST factory will improve the relevance, acceptability and effectiveness of the policy. The participation of people living with HIV can change perceptions, as well as provide valuable experiences and knowledge. Disclosing one's status can be an empowering process if it starts by combating internal stigma and shame. It is essential that the role of HIV-positive employees in the HIV and AIDS policy task team should be part of decision-making. Their needs should be incorporated into the policy. HIV-positive employees can provide a wealth of information in terms of providing senior management with an understanding of the implications of an HIV-positive diagnosis for employees.

Employees living with HIV have an integral role to play in the development, evaluation and monitoring of a workplace HIV and AIDS policy. Therefore, the QRST factory can also derive great benefit from this group, in this regard.

5.7.6 Strategies for HIV Prevention

Nowadays, there are a number of options for HIV prevention, even though there might be variations in terms of priorities for a particular context and setting. Generally, the strategic interventions for HIV prevention is combination prevention, including: Social and behaviour change communication and demand creation; Condom distribution, access and use; Voluntary medical male circumcision; Elimination of mother to child transmission (EMTC); Pre-Exposure prophylaxis (PrEP); Post-Exposure prophylaxis (PEP); Economic empowerment; Prevention of sexually transmitted infections; Viral suppression; Harm reduction. It is a pity and missed opportunity that most current HIV prevention strategies have generally adopted a vertical "one-size-fits-all" approach that does not include a nuanced understanding of the context, needs, and motivations underlying the behaviour of different user types. The polarities between biomedical and non-biomedical interventions should be removed, as prevention, treatment and care are a continuum, and not silos. The importance of integration within prevention, within treatment, and between prevention and treatment and other services should be prioritised and practised, for effectiveness, efficiency, sustainability, and better health outcomes.

Social and Behaviour Change Communication (SBCC)

Social and behaviour change communication pays deliberate attention to creating social change as a necessary component to individual change. It responds and encourages underlying social factors that shape individual behaviour. As such, social and behaviour change communication interventions ensure that there is adoption of risk reduction behaviours and can improve the effectiveness of prevention, treatment and care interventions. Therefore, dissemination of information is not enough to change behaviour, as effective social and behaviour change communication must also involve change in the larger society in which individuals operate.

How to bring about such social change is still a matter for debate, but it can and must be done, and must be complemented by more participatory approaches.

An example of SBCC is USAID's flagship social and behaviour change communication (SBCC) project in Tanzania. This included health areas such as HIV (prevention, VCT, PMTCT, Treatment), family planning, malaria, maternal and child health. This project was led by the Johns Hopkins Center for Communication Programs in partnership with Media for Development International (MFDI), CARE Tanzania, and Tanzania Communication and Development Center (TCDC).

HIV/AIDS Prevention Model of Behaviour Change

An example of the application of the HIV/AIDS prevention model of behaviour change may be in the context of addressing risk and vulnerability, by explaining how the following factors influence an employee to decide to use a condom to prevent infection with HIV:

1) Information about HIV/AIDS
2) Past experiences
3) Social pressures
4) Risk perception
5) Personal concerns and motivations

Information about HIV/AIDS:

Providing information about HIV/AIDS is not enough. Merely informing an employee about the presence of a deadly disease, how it is transmitted, and how to protect him/herself from it is not sufficient to change behaviour (Brown et al. 2001). An employee would make decisions about using a condom to prevent HIV infection not only in response to information provided, but also in response to a variety of other factors.

Past Experiences:

Prior studies by Randolph et al. (Randolph et al. 2007), indicate that many people believe that condoms reduce sexual pleasure and that men, in particular, who believe that condoms decrease pleasure are less likely to use them. However, people who had used condoms in the past three months report higher pleasure ratings for condom-protected vaginal intercourse. This implies that an employee who has had past experiences of unprotected vaginal intercourse in the past three months is likely to decide not to use a condom, whereas if he or she had used condoms in the past three months is most likely to decide to continue using them. Moreover, if the employee had past experiences with venereal diseases, he or she is more likely to use a condom, especially after he or she has been educated about condoms.

Social Pressures:

Societal peer pressure may play a role especially where use of a condom is considered a sign of character weakness by macho peers (Health24.com 2008). As a result, the employee may be influenced to decide not to use a condom. Furthermore, the low status accorded to a woman without a male partner may put pressure on the female employee to end up engaging in risky sexual behaviour such as sexual intercourse without the use of a condom.

Risk Perception:

A study of South African couples found that women who considered themselves at risk of HIV because of their husbands were four times as likely to use condoms as women who did not (Prata et al. 2006). Therefore, an employee who perceives him/herself at high risk of HIV is most likely to decide to use a condom, whereas if he or she does not perceive him/herself to be at high risk of HIV he or she is unlikely to decide to use a condom.

Personal Concerns and Motivation:

If the employee has seen some of his or her close friends or relatives suffering or dying as a result of HIV/AIDS, this particular employee may be personally concerned about her own life, and may decide not to engage in risky sexual behaviour, and may always use a condom whenever she engages in sexual intercourse, to prevent infection with HIV.

The foregoing discussion highlights that there are a number of factors that influence an employee to decide to use a condom to prevent infection with HIV. These include information about HIV/AIDS, past experiences, social pressures, risk perceptions, and personal concerns and motivations.

How Barriers in the Workplace Can Increase an employee's Vulnerability to HIV/ AIDS

Even once individuals have made a decision to take protective measures, such as use a condom, a number of other factors or barriers may stand in the way. Many of these factors are part of the local environment in which risk behaviours occur or on the context in which the risk behaviours are undertaken. Collectively, they influence an individual's vulnerability to HIV infection.

The specific objective of this section is to describe how barriers in the workplace that are related to the following issues can increase an employee's vulnerability to HIV/AIDS:

1) Access to a condom
2) Skills to use a condom
3) Partner willing to use a condom

Access to a Condom:

A number of barriers may stand in the way of gaining access to a condom.

Legal Barrier: There is growing evidence that sex for money happens at our workplace, especially during night shifts. Therefore, a female employee may not be able to carry a condom if the workplace's security officers view condoms as presumptive evidence of sex work.

Social Barrier: The employee may be too ashamed to walk into the worksite wellness centre and ask for condoms. This may be escalated by fear of being perceived to be involved with multiple partners.

Economic Barrier: If free condoms are not provided at the workplace, an employee may not be able to afford condoms (Brown et al. 2001). As a result, he or she may be vulnerable to HIV/AIDS if she engages in unprotected sexual intercourse.

Time of Day: Sometimes, condoms just are not available when sex takes place (Brown et al. 2001), particularly bearing in mind the growing evidence that sex does take place at the workplace operational area, especially during night shifts.

Skills to Use a Condom:

Once the condom is obtained, the next question to be addressed is whether the employee possesses the skills to use the condom with his or her partner. Again, a number of barriers may arise.

Education and Training: The employee may never have been educated about condoms at the workplace. The employee may receive no skills training in use of condoms because management refuse to allow discussion of condoms, distribution of skills building materials, or demonstration of a condom use during work hours. Using a condom also requires negotiation and decision-making skills with partners, something often omitted from sexual health curricula not designed by those with HIV prevention experience (Brown et al. 2001).

Religion: Some senior managers who are influenced by their religious affiliation may oppose the teaching of condom skills or their distribution to any group of employees at the workplace.

Partner Willing to Use a Condom:

There is also the question of whether the partner is willing to use a condom (Brown et al. 2001).

Gender Roles: Societal gender imbalances may serve as a major barrier (Brown et al. 2001). Men are socialised to believe that women are inferior and should be under their control, and women are socialised to over-respect men and act submissively to them. The resulting unequal power relation between the sexes, particularly when negotiating sexual encounters, increases women's vulnerability to HIV infection and accelerates the epidemic.

Social Pressure: Societal peer pressure may play a role especially where use of a condom is considered a sign of character weakness by macho peers. Furthermore, the low status accorded to a woman without a male partner may put pressure on the female employee to end up engaging in risky sexual behaviour without the use of a condom (Health24.com 2008).

Norms: Societal norms or cultural beliefs often stand in the way of condom use, especially where there are negative attitudes towards condoms, as the use of condoms is felt to interfere with proper sexual functioning. Often there are difficulties negotiating and following through with their use (Health24.com 2008).

Education: Lack of knowledge and misconceptions about HIV/AIDS has been reported (Brown et al. 2001). The employee or employee's partner may refuse to use a condom because he or she has a misconception that condoms contain HIV.

Based on the foregoing discussion, it can be discerned that barriers such as lack of access to a condom, lack of skills to use a condom, and partner unwillingness to use a condom can sometimes be beyond the control of the employee. Therefore, effective workplace prevention programmes must address the multitude of factors which interfere with an individual's ability to protect himself/herself.

Condom Promotion
Strategies for condom promotion and distribution include: strengthening condom forecasting, procurement and supply management system; intensifying access, demand creation and distribution of condom using multiple approaches including integration in other health care services; intensifying and expanding condom distribution coverage for specific targeted groups at high risk; strengthening SBCC interventions in condom programming; strengthening monitoring and evaluation for condoms. It is worth highlighting that condom promotion is not without any challenges as some of the gaps are related to the predominant "push strategies" which are largely provider-driven, yet there should also be prioritisation of "pull strategies" which are consumer-demand-driven and are sustainable. Poor access and poor acceptability of condoms have been among some of the challenges in many parts of the world, and this points to the need to review the effectiveness of condom promotion approaches. The essence is to ensure that there is increased consistent and correct condom use among people engaged in risky sexual behaviour. Consistent and correct condom use has the added benefit of not only preventing HIV transmission, but also the advantage of preventing unintended pregnancies and further protect against other sexually transmitted infections. More importantly, condom promotion should be part and parcel of the combination prevention package and integrated with other health services.

Voluntary Medical Male Circumcision (VMMC)
Strategies for VMMC: Strengthen and decentralise VMMC services especially for neo-natals and males in health and non-health facilities; intensify education, awareness and community mobilisation to generate demand and increased benefits of VMMC for both men and women; address socio-cultural myths and misconceptions of VMMC that create barriers to service uptake; integrate VMMC services with other health services. The strategic objective should be increase targeted coverage of male circumcision, particularly, in HIV high burden settings. Some of the challenges in the implementation of VMMC were poor approach in the way VMMC was introduced; some implementing partners tend to chase targets at the expense of quality and sustainability; poor acceptability in settings where male circumcision is not part of culture. VMMC should not be an end in itself, but it should be delivered in the context of a combination prevention package and integrated with other health services.

Prevention of Mother to Child Transmission
PMTCT strategies are guided by four prongs: primary prevention of HIV infection among women of child-bearing age; prevention of unwanted pregnancies among women living with HIV; prevention of HIV transmission from women infected with

HIV; and treatment, care and support for women infected with HIV, their infants and partners, Strategic objective is to eliminate pre- and post-natal mother-to-child transmission of HIV, syphilis and hepatitis B and to keep HIV positive mothers, their partners and children alive and on treatment.

Pre-Exposure Prophylaxis

This is the use of antiretroviral medication to prevent the acquisition of HIV infection by uninfected persons. Strategic objective is to increase proportion of at-risk populations using PrEP especially adolescent girls and young women, key populations, and sero-discordant couples, among others.

Post-Exposure Prophylaxis (PEP)

This is a short-term antiretroviral treatment to reduce the likelihood of HIV infection after potential exposure, either occupationally or through sexual intercourse. Strategic objective is to reduce the risk of HIV infection among people who have been exposed to body fluids in occupational and non-occupational settings.

Viral Suppression

Evidence shows that effective antiretroviral therapy has the potential to reduce HIV viral load and can contribute to prevention of new infections by approximately 96%. This strategy is most effective and sustainable if implemented as part of the broader combination prevention strategy that involves biomedical, behavioural and structural interventions.

Management and Treatment of Sexually Transmitted Infections

Sexually transmitted infections (STIs) and HIV share the same transmission routes and the risk factors for each increase the risk of the other, persons infected with sexually transmitted infections are more vulnerable to HIV acquisition and genital inflammation attributed or resulting from gonorrhoea, chlamydia, trichomonas, and HSV-2 is reported to increase the risk of HIV infection among women, therefore, proper prevention, screening and treatment of STIs has several benefits for HIV prevention. Strategic objective is to reduce sexually transmitted cases and thereby control HIV transmission by minimising the risk factor.

Economic Empowerment

Economic empowerment focuses on addressing the vulnerability to HIV infection and mitigating the impact of HIV and AIDS vulnerable populations. Structural factors such as economic dependence and unequal economic opportunities, gender inequality, and poverty, render vulnerable groups susceptible to high risk sex. Strategic objective is to build self-esteem and promote empowerment opportunities to mitigate structural risk factors to HIV infection among young people. One of the main challenges is poor coordination of economic empowerment opportunities.

Harm Reduction

Harm reduction tools and strategies are aimed at preventing the spread of HIV and reducing other harms associated with drug use. Needle-syringe programmes reduce the spread of HIV, hepatitis C and other blood-borne viruses. Opioid substitution therapy and other evidence-informed forms of drug dependence treatment, curb drug use, reduce vulnerability to infectious diseases, and improve uptake of health and social services. People who inject drugs are among the key populations most at risk to acquire or transmit HIV. Yet they are also among those with the least access to HIV prevention, care and treatment services because their drug use is often stigmatised and criminalised. Few countries have achieved sufficient coverage of harm reduction services.

HIV Testing Services (HTS)
HIV testing services is an entry point to HIV prevention, and HIV treatment and care services. Strategic objective is to increase the proportion of people living with HIV who know their status (Tables 5.6, 5.7, 5.8, 5.9, 5.10, 5.11 and 5.12).

5.7.7 Therapeutic Management of HIV/AIDS – Challenges of Drug Therapy – Pharmacovigilance

Pharmacovigilance
Although many countries have documented national HIV/AIDS Clinical Care Guidelines, those documents often do not include a comprehensive pharmacovigilance programme.

First and foremost, the Coordinating Unit of the HIV and AIDS treatment programme in the country must have the following specific aims on the pharmacovigilance programme:

To determine the burden of drug-related morbidity and mortality in patients with HIV and AIDS, particularly associated with ARV use, and develop measures to minimise their impact.

To provide training and information to health personnel and patients on the safe use of antiretrovirals and other medicines commonly used in HIV-infected and AIDS patients.

To develop systems to assess the risks and benefits of treatment commonly used in patients with HIV, sexually transmitted infections (STIs), and tuberculosis (TB); including over the counter (OTC) medication or phytotherapeutic agents.

To identify, assess and communicate any new safety concerns associated with the use of ARVs and other HIV medicines.

To support regulatory and public health decision-making through an efficient, national post-marketing surveillance system, monitoring and quality, benefits and risk or harm associated with ARVs and other medicines currently used in the health sector.

To minimise the impact of misleading or unproven associations between adverse events and ARV therapy.

To detect, assess, and respond to safety concerns related to complementary and traditional medicines used in HIV-infected patients.

To establish an early warning system for resistance to antimicrobials commonly used in HIV, including, but not limited to, ARVs.

Table 5.6 Eastern and southern Africa, HIV Prevention Gap analysis, 2015

Gaps in HIV prevention	Low knowledge regarding HIV prevention.
	High levels of reported occurrences of transactional sex in some countries.
	High rates of sexually transmitted infections and teenage pregnancy.
	Insufficient financial allocation and programme implementation to address needs
	Inadequate programmes dedicated for key populations
	Inadequate protection from HIV and other sexually transmitted infections.
	Extremely limited data and information on transgender people.
	Challenging legal and social environment for key populations
	High HIV prevalence among key populations injecting drugs.
	Low condom uses and unsafe injecting practices exacerbate transmission.
	Increases in risky sexual behaviour and multiple concurrent partnerships.
	Low condom availability contributed to levels of condom use that were not high enough to significantly curtail rates of HIV, sexually transmitted infections or unintended pregnancies
	In countries such as Mozambique, South Africa, Uganda and Zambia, less than 35% of eligible men were circumcised.
	Uptake and impact of PrEP specifically with populations in high-incidence areas was a challenge.
	Extremely limited viral suppression data in the region
	Low rates of HIV testing weaken the links between prevention, treatment and care services in the region.
	Gaps still remain in the provision of treatment to populations who are affected by humanitarian emergencies, who face disruptions in HIV treatment, heightened exposure to HIV vulnerability and risks and limited access to quality health care and nutritious food.
	Unavailable viral load testing to the majority of people on antiretroviral therapy.
Challenges	High levels of HIV infections among adolescent girls and young women aged 15–24 years
	Extremely high levels of sexual abuse and violence against female children
	Marginalisation, stigma and discrimination towards key populations
	Lack of strategic information for a number of countries in the region.
	Lack of or ineffective coordination of the HIV response in some countries
	Heavy reliance on international resources to fund responses to HIV
Opportunities	**Investments and sustainable financing:**
	Important to conduct financing analyses to explore the fiscal space for health and HIV and innovative options for financing HIV and AIDS responses.
	Using evidence to inform programming:
	It is increasingly important to gather and use strategic information to guide the efficient delivery of services to the locations and populations in greatest need.
	Engaging communities: Civil society and communities are vital to the region's achievement of the targets in the 2016 political declaration on HIV and AIDS.
	Integrating sexual and reproductive health and HIV services

Source: UNAIDS 2016 Prevention Gap Report

Table 5.7 Western and central Africa, HIV Prevention Gap analysis, 2015

Gaps in HIV prevention	**Young women and girls and their male partners:**
	Alarmingly low knowledge about HIV among young people in the region.
	Very low school completion rates and low literacy especially among girls
	Significant gap in service availability on sexual and reproductive health.
	Lack of targeted, youth-friendly HIV prevention services for young people
	Population growth among young people and adolescents in western and central Africa was also the highest in the world, creating an additional burden on health and education services.
	Key populations:
	Needle and syringe programmes and opioid substitution therapy were only nationally available in Senegal.
	Condom programmes:
	Few countries had comprehensive condom programming plans, however, and often where they did cist they were not implemented.
	Condom use among men who have sex with men remained low in countries such as Sierra Leone (32%)
	Viral suppression:
	Very low viral suppression (12%) in the region, and only 2% of the total population of people living with HIV on antiretroviral therapy had a viral load testing result.
	Uptake of HIV testing services in the general population is low.
Challenges	**Human rights:**
	Stigma and discrimination against people living with HIV remained high.
	Limited funding
	Women and girls:
	Women and girls in the region were more vulnerable to HIV – In part due to laws and policies that maintain traditional gender roles – And that women in key populations had limited access to services.
	Rates of gender-based violence were high
	The responsiveness of HIV programmes and strategies to women's needs was uneven.
Opportunities	***Fast-track cities initiative:***
	The overall goal of the initiative is to contribute to more sustainable, secure, smart and healthy cities in which every individual and every company will do better.
	Improving the efficiency and sustainability of HIV programmes:
	Commitment for efforts to improve HIV programmes efficiency, effectiveness and sustainability.

Source: UNAIDS 2016 Prevention Gap Report

Table 5.8 Asia and the Pacific, HIV Prevention Gap analysis, 2015

Gaps in HIV prevention	**Key populations**:
	There are multiple challenges to reaching sex workers with HIV prevention services.
	In several countries where HIV prevalence is higher among people who inject drugs, the coverage of needle-syringe programmes was still low, with fewer than 100 clean needles and syringes provided per person in need per year.
	Low coverage of opioid substitution therapy in 2015.
	For the region as a whole, only 55% of people who inject drugs reported using a condom the last time they had sex.
	Viral suppression:
	Considerable gaps in the treatment cascade remained in many countries.
	The gaps in diagnosing and treatment led to just 34% of all people living with HIV in Asia and the Pacific achieving viral suppression necessary to prevent HIV transmission.
	Out of the 39 countries in the region, just 15 reported data on viral load testing in 2015. The percentage of people among those tested who were virally suppressed ranged from 57% in Pakistan and 63% in Viet Nam, to more than 90% in Cambodia, China, Mongolia, Nepal, the Philippines and Thailand
Challenges	Challenges that need to be overcome include the criminalisation of key populations, stigma and discrimination (particularly in healthcare settings), a lack of innovation in service delivery models, and the slow pace of introducing and adapting new technologies at a scale that will make a difference.
	Strong dependence on international financing for prevention – And the limited fiscal space and political will of countries to invest in effective combination prevention programmes for key populations – Remains a major impediment to the response.
Opportunities	A fast-track response in Asia and the Pacific will require countries to seize key opportunities. This includes introducing and scaling up new approaches and technologies like task-shifting, active case finding and management, reanimating combination prevention including community-based treatment alternatives and services for people who use drugs, and the smart use of social media for HIV prevention.
	Achieving targets will require innovation and a mix of strategies to expand HIV testing for key populations and their intimate partners. Efforts to support countries to protect and sue trade-related aspects of intellectual property rights (TRIPS) flexibilities to ensure sustained access to affordable medicines, diagnostics and commodities – Including second- and third-line antiretroviral therapy regimens, and tuberculosis and hepatitis C medications – Must be intensified.
	It is important to promote an investment approach that supports countries in the implementation of evidence-based programming, including the development of transitional financing plans and the use of universal health coverage schemes to ensure the sustainability of the AIDS response.
	The Asia-Pacific regional framework for action to end AIDS by 2013 – The regional framework adopted by 53 member states of the United Nations economic and social Commission for Asia and the Pacific – Continues to guide national efforts towards accelerating action and investment in the HIV response to end the AIDS epidemic as a public health threat by 2030.

Source: UNAIDS 2016 Prevention Gap Report

Table 5.9 Latin America and the Caribbean, HIV Prevention Gap analysis, 2015

Gaps in HIV prevention	Prevention was inadequately funded and did not reach sufficient percentages of key populations.
	Condom use among key populations was as low as 40% in some countries.
	Percentage of people living with HIV had been diagnosed was lower among people who inject drugs and men who have sex with men
	Low uptake of PrEP among potentially eligible people
	Young people, especially among key populations were disproportionately at risk of HIV infection, and they faced greater barriers to accessing prevention services.
	Multiple sexual partners and inconsistent condom use compounded the risk of age mixing
	Estimates of viral load suppression were much lower in the Caribbean
	In the Caribbean, 11 out of 16 countries were highly dependent on external funding
Challenges	There were still high rates of violence against LGBTI across the region
	Eleven Caribbean countries had discriminatory laws against same-sex sexual acts
	Key populations and women living with HIV were subject to practices such as forced sterilisation and denial of health services
	Nicaragua and Paraguay had restrictions on the permanent stay of people living with HIV and who had been in the country longer than three months in both countries.
	In the Caribbean, small island states faced challenges in ensuring the confidentiality of people living with HIV.
	Across the region, there were a number of barriers preventing adolescents and young people, especially key populations, from accessing sexual and reproductive health and HIV services and commodities
Opportunities	Self-testing
	Regional approach for a fast-track approach, including prevention targets for 2020 and 2030, with an emphasis on combination prevention packages for key populations
	Ensuring respect for the rights of people living with HIV, women at risk and key populations

Source: UNAIDS 2016 Prevention Gap Report

To respond to unfounded and unsubstantiated claims of efficacy of untested products and treatment modalities (Department of Health 2003).

Plan of Action:

The national pharmacovigilance programme should pursue a phased plan of action over the coming three years, reflecting short, medium, and long-term goals:

Priorities

Training and information support for health care teams and strengthening of the existing spontaneous reporting system. Advocacy on pharmacovigilance and ADR

Table 5.10 Middle East and North Africa, HIV Prevention Gap analysis, 2015

Gaps in HIV prevention	HIV testing coverage figures were as low as 17% in countries such as Sudan
	In Tripoli, Libya, where the HIV prevalence among people who inject drugs was reported to be above 80%, the current conflict situation has made it difficult to establish any programme for this population
	For most of the countries in the region, transgender people had not been acknowledged as a separate key population
	An estimated 37% of people living with HIV in the Middle East and North Africa in 2015 knew their HIV status, about 17% were on antiretroviral therapy and only 11% had achieved viral suppression
Challenges	In all of the countries in the Middle East and North Africa, members of at least one of the key populations could face criminal charges because of their sexual orientation, gender, identity, occupation or behaviours
	Prevention programmes for gay men and other men who have sex with men and sex workers rarely received support from domestic resources or through public services
	Several of the countries in the region were challenged by conflict or humanitarian emergencies, with rapidly changing environments, violence, displacement of people - within and across borders, resource constraints, and disruption of already stretched health and social services. These situations also disrupted responses to HIV
Opportunities	Leadership commitment and partnerships
	Domestic financing, shared responsibility and regional solidarity

Source: UNAIDS 2016 Prevention Gap Report

reporting can be initiated as part of enhancing spontaneous adverse event reporting.

Strengthening regulatory infrastructure and further provision of online support, including the development of a database that will be functional in 2009.

Initiation of focused surveillance and novel pharmacovigilance methods for addressing key research questions, including maternal and peri-natal surveillance and phytovigilance (Department of Health 2003).

Activities

Enhance national spontaneous reporting system with active feedback to decision-makers, prescribers, reporters, patients and the public.

Develop and improve regulatory procedures to support the defined objectives.

Further development of sustainable, functional, user-friendly database to support the national spontaneous reporting system.

Provision of unbiased, evidence-based information on the safety profile of ARVs, the safe and effective use of ARVs and the management of potential complications.

Introduce targeted sentinel surveillance systems to evaluate signals of safety issues of potential public health importance (e.g. high-risk groups such as pregnant women, infants, HIV/TB co-morbidity). This will include resistance monitoring and documentation of trends to facilitate an early warning system.

Table 5.11 Eastern Europe and Central Asia, HIV Prevention Gap analysis, 2015

Gaps in HIV prevention	The scale of prevention programmes for key populations was insufficient to curb the region's surging epidemics
	Capacity to provide opioid substitution therapy remained low as part of harm reduction for people who inject drugs
	Needle-syringe programmes in prisons were not widely available in most countries
	Condom use was inconsistent, and it was as low as 36% in some countries
	A very large number of people living with HIV remained undiagnosed
	Only 19% of all people living with HIV in eastern Europe and central Asia had achieved the viral suppression necessary to prevent HIV transmission
	Coverage of antiretroviral therapy in the region remained significantly low at 21%.
	A major barrier to expanded antiretroviral therapy coverage was the lack of continuity between treatment in the community and prison system
	The price of antiretroviral medications and the full unit costs for treatment-related services remained high in several countries with large numbers of people living with HIV, impeding scale-up
Challenges	Lack of national commitments to combination prevention
	Legislative barriers to access for key populations
	High prevalence of HIV, and large numbers of key populations in urban centres
	Access to prevention of mother-to-child transmission and other HIV services was still insufficient for the most vulnerable and socially marginalised groups of women, including regular migrants and pregnant women who used drugs
	Children in the region who were living with HIV continued to need support as they became adolescents to attend school and ensure a smooth transition from paediatric to adult care
Opportunities	Significant gains could be made through more efficient use of existing resources
	The increasing number of people living with HIV will require innovative strategies that focus on key populations who may feel uncomfortable or even afraid to access services at public health clinics

Source: UNAIDS 2016 Prevention Gap Report

Develop novel pharmacovigilance methods to complement and support spontaneous reporting and sentinel surveillance systems.

Develop key indicator(s) for estimating the prevalence of drug-related morbidity and mortality.

Develop a phytovigilance programme for safety monitoring of complementary and African traditional medicines (Department of Health 2003).

Adherence to ARV Therapy

Adherence is probably the single most important factor in determining success of ARV therapy, starting therapy should be delayed in situations where there are serious concerns about adherence (Ministry of Health and Social Welfare 2003). Every effort should be made to deal with these concerns to maximise adherence. The

Table 5.12 Western and Central Europe and North America, HIV Prevention Gap analysis, 2015

Gaps and challenges in HIV prevention	In the United States of America, heroin use increased among men and women in most age groups and across all income levels. This trend coincided with an increase in hepatitis C virus infections and new outbreaks of HIV associated with injecting drug use
	Increases in the annual number of cases of sexually transmitted infections such as gonorrhoea, syphilis and HIV diagnoses in the European Union and the United States of America suggest that levels of condom use among gay men and other men who have sex with men had not improved
	In the United States of America, of the 1.2 million people who were eligible for PrEP, only an estimated 30,000 were prescribed in in 2015
	National health systems viewed the relatively high cost of PrEP as the biggest barrier to full adoption of this HIV prevention option
	Nearly half of all people living with HIV in western and central Europe and north America had achieved the viral suppression necessary to prevent HIV transmission
Opportunities	Early studies of the care Act's effect on the health care of people living with HIV in the United States of America suggest that many people have used the systems established under the act to find more affordable and comprehensive health insurance coverage
	Decriminalisation and de-penalisation of drugs for personal consumption, similar to Portugal and Czech Republic, would reduce the pressures on people who inject drugs to avoid engaging with HIV prevention and treatment services.
	Decriminalisation of sex work could empower women and men engaged in commercial sex work to seek and utilise HIV prevention and treatment services
	The widespread use of mobile dating apps among gay men and other men who have sex with men, offers opportunities for collaboration to engage with men, to inform users of the locations of HIV testing or prevention services
	Increasing levels of official recognition of same sex marriages and other steps toward improved integration of the LGBTI people community needs can reduce stigma and discrimination of community members, aiding access to needed HIV services

Source: UNAIDS 2016 Prevention Gap Report

national HIV/AIDS Coordinating Unit in Eswatini would be advised to implement the following strategies to promote adherence:

Spend time and have multiple encounters to explain goals of therapy and need for adherence.

Consider monitoring of medications such as Cotrimoxazole or other surrogate prior to ARV initiation.

Negotiate a treatment plan that the patient can understand and to which he/she commits.

Encourage disclosure to family or friends who can support the treatment plan.

Inform patient of potential side effects – severity, duration, and coping mechanisms.
Establish 'readiness' to take medications before ARV initiation.
Provide adherence tools where available: written calendar of medications, pill boxes.
Encourage use of alarms, pagers or other available mechanical aids for adherence.
Avoid adverse drug interactions; full disclosure for over-the-counter drugs and traditional medicines.
Anticipate, monitor and treat side-effects.
Include adherence discussions in support groups.
Develop links with community-based organisations to support adherence.
Encourage links with support groups.
Create links with patient advocates (Department of Health 2003).

The foregoing discussion highlights the fact that side effects are real and must be closely monitored and regimens must be changed if necessary. In order for the treatment to be effective it is of utmost importance that the patient adheres strictly to the treatment instructions, namely what, when and how to take the drugs on a daily basis.

It is therefore imperative for the Coordinating Unit of the national HIV/AIDS treatment programme in my home country to develop and implement a comprehensive pharmacovigilance and adherence programme to ensure the safe and effective use of ARVs and other medicines commonly used in patients living with HIV/AIDS. Ultimately, the pharmacovigilance and adherence programme should improve patient well-being and public health in my home country.

5.7.8 Using Life Skills Training and Education in an HIV/AIDS Context

The purpose of this section is to develop a life-skills training programme for risk and harm reduction in HIV/AIDS among adolescents in the community which is the main feeder area for an organisation that one worked for. Since adolescents are on the threshold of adulthood, they are often faced with the dilemma of coming to grips with their sexuality and responsibility with little or no support from the outside world. The dilemma is all the more pronounced in cultures where traditional values, consumerism and mass media tend to project machismo as sexual precocity and adventurism, but frown upon any attempts at preparing the young adults for responsible adulthood by making information and services for adolescent education accessible and equipping these adolescents with life skills.

Life skills training and education focuses on the development of abilities for adaptive and positive behaviour that enables individuals to deal effectively with the demands and challenges of everyday life. The acquisition of life skills can greatly affect a person's overall physical, emotional, social, and spiritual health that, in turn, is linked to his or her ability to maximise upon life opportunities.

The specific objectives of the life-skills training programme that is planned to be implemented in the community of focus are:

a) To increase self-esteem
b) Increasing young people's ability to resist pressure
c) Encouraging sexually inexperienced young people to delay the onset of sexual intercourse
d) Encouraging sexually experienced young people to decrease the incidence of unprotected sexual intercourse and to reduce the number of sexual partners.

Content:

There must be focus on the main goal – promoting sexual health by increasing youth's ability to avoid and/or reduce sexual risk behaviours. Program objectives should focus on key behaviours and the conditions that are linked to achieving the main goal.

The content of the Life Skills training program should emphasise information, attitudes and skills based on their relevance for promoting healthy behaviours and for preventing risk behaviours. Health promoting behaviours include acquiring accurate information, clarify personal values, developing peer support for safer behaviours, and using condoms correctly and consistently. Risk factors for teen pregnancy and STIs, including HIV, may include being aware of risks, feeling or facing gender bias, having multiple sexual partners, and having sexual intercourse with casual and/or commercial partners.

Ensure that youth understand sexual and reproductive health, the behaviours that place individuals at risk, and the social context and interrelationship of these factors. The program should address values, attitudes, and behaviours in individuals and the community of focus and provide basic facts about preventing pregnancy and Sexually Transmitted Infections (STIs), including HIV.

Training Logic

To be effective in supporting quality-learning outcomes, life skills education must be used in conjunction with a specific subject or content area. Therefore, it is important for skills-based approaches to be accompanied by activities that focus on the target group's knowledge and attitude.

In addition, skills-based education emphasises the use of learning activities that are culturally relevant and gender-sensitive. To achieve this, the learning activities offer numerous opportunities for participants to provide their own input into the nature and content of the situations addressed during the learning activities (e.g., creating their own case studies, brainstorming possible scenarios, etc.). This approach ensures that the situations are realistic and relevant to the everyday lives of participants. It is critical that the skills youth build and practice in the classroom are easily transferable to their lives outside the classroom.

A growing body of research has documented that skills-based interventions can promote numerous positive attitudes and behaviours, including greater sociability, improved communication, healthy decision-making and effective conflict resolution. Studies demonstrate that these interventions are also effective in preventing negative or high-risk behaviours, such as use of tobacco, alcohol and other drugs, unsafe sex, and violence. It is important to note that research has also found that programs, which incorporate skills development into their curricula, are more effective than programs which focus only on the transfer of information (e.g. through lecture format).

Skills-based training should aim to:

Increase providers' knowledge around the content of what is being taught or learned;
Increase providers' familiarity and level of comfort with using participatory and interactive teaching methodology in the classroom;
Increase providers' understanding of developmental issues in learning; and
Strengthen providers' skills in the management of classroom behaviour, given that skills-based education is used primarily in a large group setting and often deals with sensitive topics.

Effective training on skill-based education teaches providers how to:

Establish an effective, safe and supportive program environment;
Access resources for health information and referral;
Address sensitive issues;
Model the skills addressed in the program;
Apply interactive teaching methodologies in the classroom;
Provide constructive criticism, positive reinforcement and feedback;
Manage group process.

Whichever agency plays the primary role in the implementation of life skills training and education, it is equally important for program providers to collaborate with other local stakeholders and community members in all stages of planning and delivery. For example, providers may want to invite parents to attend training programs to enhance their own skills for communicating with their children or for coping with difficult personal circumstances. Likewise, other community members (e.g., health care workers or police officers) might be invited to participate in specific learning activities both in and outside the classroom.

Effective life skills program providers should be perceived as credible, trustworthy, high status, positive role model, successful, and competent. Life skills program providers should have the following qualities: Competent in group processes, able to guide and facilitate, respectful of children and adolescents, warm, supportive, enthusiastic, knowledgeable about specific content areas relevant to adolescence, knowledgeable about community resources.

Program providers may need help, building assertiveness, stress-management, and/or problem-solving skills for themselves before being able to teach these skills in the classroom. Therefore, an important component of any training program is the inclusion of activities in which potential providers can also address their own personal needs.

Skill-based health education encourages participation by all students, and as a result, can create classroom dynamics with which some teachers are not familiar. Research, however, has found that teachers who were initially uncomfortable with the idea of using participatory methodologies in their classrooms overcame their reluctance after practising these methods during training sessions. Provider confidence is essential to the success of skills-based education.

Some providers may feel unprepared to communicate with their students about sensitive topics such as sexual and reproductive health, violence, and relationships. They also may not know where to go to access additional information on these topics. Again, training teachers prior to implementation on how to best address and respond to questions or comments about sensitive topics is key to overcoming this challenge. Providers should also be encouraged to interact and meet with one another throughout the school year to share ideas and suggestions.

Therefore, providers need to understand how skills-based education can have immediate and long-lasting benefits not only on their students' lives but also on their own personal and professional lives. Training programs should include activities which help teachers build skills that they can use in their daily lives, e.g., to improve relationships, avoid sexual violence or harassment, or overcome alcohol or drug use. Studies have shown that skill-based education programs can indeed improve attendance and morale among providers.

A lack of coordination between school administrators, curriculum coordinators and health and education sectors can result in a number of competing curricula. This can prove to be frustrating to overworked teachers who may start to view new programs as just another addition to their existing workload. Key to overcoming this challenge is a close collaboration between all involved including teachers so that there is a clear understanding of how new curricula can realistically be used to complement what is already being implemented.

Strategy for Implementation

Since the objectives, content and training logic, have already been stipulated, the next step would be to craft and implement the *strategy*. At the heart of implementation is a planning process that begins with the end in mind. Ensuring a fit between the program, the interests and needs of providers and young people, local conditions and resources is essential. Nothing can be implemented without the enthusiasm, buy-in and involvement of the providers.

Providers, i.e., trainers, health workers, counsellors, and volunteers, are perhaps the most critical component to the implementation process, due to the talent and commitment of local level people. Examining, taking into account, and responding to the concerns, interests and needs of providers' personal working conditions is a major factor in program success.

From the earliest stages of program development, there shall be use of advocacy to influence leaders, mobilise the community, and secure the commitment of policy makers. Frequently, policy makers and other leaders lack knowledge of adolescent sexual health issues and of current rates of adolescent pregnancy, STIs, and HIV infection. Accurate, timely data can help to convince leaders of the importance of early and comprehensive sexual health and of scaling up successful programs.

It would be essential to do a community profile or the evaluation of the community's internal and external environment. This will enable us to succeed in crafting a strategy that is an excellent fit with the community of focus' situation.

In terms of the community's internal environment, there is need to understand the demographics or *structure* of the community. In terms of the external environment, there is need to consider influences from outside the community, which may include external Non-Governmental Organisations (NGOs) that are currently doing work in the community, the political landscape of the community, and other external factors. This kind of evaluation is critical because it will inform the approach that will be followed in order to add value to the community of focus. Moreover, this evaluation will ensure that there is no duplication of work that might already have been done by other service providers in the community.

There is also a need to take into account the *systems* within the community of focus. From the first, there is need to use advocacy to influence the community leaders or authorities, mobilise the community, and get their buy-in. All stakeholders involved with the community shall be sensitised about the importance and benefits of life-skills training. This means that there must be proper communication channels about the whole project.

The next thing is to ascertain the *resources* available within the community. For example, do the teachers have any skill in life-skills training and HIV/AIDS? If so, how many teachers are skilled? And also, how many teachers need to be trained on life skills-training and HIV/AIDS?

It is also important to understand the lifestyle or way of life in the community of focus. For example, youth's abilities, feelings, and beliefs shall be respected. Respect and understanding will ensure that a program is acceptable to and appropriate for participants. Focus on risks that youth actually confront and respect youth's feelings and beliefs regarding risks. Recognise what individuals can and cannot do with respect to tasks. This will help in addressing young people's motivations for behaviour change.

Ensure that the programme's objectives, teaching methods, and materials are appropriate to the age, gender, sexual experience, and culture of young people and the community of focus in which they live. Encourage participants to learn from each other, as well as from educators, family, and community, thus integrating the knowledge and experience of everyone involved.

More importantly, it is essential to uphold and inculcate the principle of *shared values*, in order to ensure that the young people as well as the community of focus take ownership of the programme, so that it can be successful and sustainable.

Coordinate educational programmes with other effective components, such as positive public health policies, youth-friendly health services, social marketing, condom and contraceptive availability, community development, and media campaigns. The determinants of sexual behaviour are varied and complex; and a coordinated, multi-pronged, long-term approach, is critical to promoting sexual health among youth.

Involve students, parents, out-of-school youth, and community members in all stages of programmes design, development, implementation, and operation. Involving youth and adults will ensure that programmes meet the specific needs and concerns of a community's youth in a culturally and socially appropriate way. Participation fosters a sense of ownership that, in turn, enhances sustainability.

Ensure that the programme continues in an orderly sequence and progress over time, building on earlier efforts. For example, young people need to hear messages about sexual and reproductive health from an early age. The messages should continue – regularly, in a timely fashion, and from credible sources. Education and other health promotion efforts must persist over time to ensure that successive cohorts of children and youth achieve sexually healthy adulthood – including themselves from HIV, other STIs, and unintended pregnancy.

Provide a safe and supportive environment for all youth, including teenage parents and children and youth living with, or affected by, HIV/AIDS. These young people need the care and protection of adults they can trust. This is a role for which teachers and other adults in the community may need training and support.

Work to meet the special needs of children and youth in unstable and crisis situations. Instability and adversity are normal conditions for many young people, and their vulnerability to sexual health risks can increase significantly during crises.

Consider the full range of available strategies that may contribute to the main goal. Conduct research to identify credible sources and pertinent data, choose the most effective and relevant strategies, and adapt effective programs whenever possible.

Evaluate program objectives, processes, and outcomes using realistic, relevant indicators. Allow enough time for results to be accurately observed. Choose appropriate monitoring and evaluation processes that will assess knowledge, attitudes, skills, and behaviours.

Anticipated Benefits

Evaluation shows that life skills programs can contribute to the reproductive and sexual health of young people around the world.

Despite the challenges that may accompany the implementation of skills-based education, the rewards and positive outcomes which may result from such programs are immeasurable. By creating a coordinated effort between stakeholders, both local and national, program planners and advocates can help to ensure an educational program that is both effective and sustainable.

Competence building through Life Skills education may be the single most effective way of addressing concerns in most communities. Developing your interpersonal skills training programme is very important to the employer. It can also greatly reduce stress, increase productivity and morale within the firm. Life Skills acquisition should thus become an integral component endorsed by the employer as part of the process of lifelong learning towards self-actualisation (Taute 2007).

The foregoing steps have enabled an accomplishment of the main goal of developing a life-skills training programme for the community of focus, in order to increase self-esteem, increase youth's ability to resist pressure, to encourage sexually inexperienced youth to delay the onset of sexual intercourse, and to encourage sexually experienced youth to decrease the incidence of unprotected sexual intercourse and to reduce the number of sexual partners.

Creating a collective responsibility is of paramount importance when it comes to life skills for risk and harm reduction in HIV/AIDS among adolescents. Since parents and teachers are the main stakeholders, effort is to be made to involve them in the process.

The potential strengths of a school setting are that children have a curriculum, teachers and a peer group and the school teaches them not only information but also skills and attitudes. Partnering with schools provides an efficient and organised way to communicate with large sections of population.

Young people have great energy and commitment. They also exert a great influence on one another. They can be worthy agents of change if life skills are inculcated and developed. As a result, their self-esteem can improve, and they can be able to resist pressure.

Given the vulnerability of young people to HIV/AIDS, society needs to do more to help children protect themselves, primarily by educating them and providing a supportive and understanding environment.

Care should be taken when designing a school education program between school knowledge and outside knowledge, as these can become a source of mistrust and conflict.

Community involvement contributes to a sense of collective responsibility and provides support.

Programmes on sexuality and adolescent education are more effective if given before onset of sexual activity. The behaviours concerned are highly individual and intimate and it is therefore crucial to seek opinions and suggestions of students themselves about program content.

Parents should be first educators because they can grade information according to the age and development of their children and link it to the values they want to instil.

Every effort should be made to provide facts of life and education for life while youth are at school, as this might be their only chance to learn vital information for their protection even after they have left school.

Schools are ideal places for promoting and supporting initiatives such as life skill camps in non-threatening environments, which could be facilitative to effect behaviour change in students, such as delaying the onset of sexual intercourse or decreasing the incidence of unprotected sexual intercourse and to reduce the number of sexual partners.

5.7.9 Scaling up of HIV Prevention, Treatment and Care in South Africa

The mere fact that South Africa carries the heaviest burden of HIV/AIDS in the world is an indication that urgent interventions are required to scale-up the HIV prevention, treatment and care, as the burden of HIV/AIDS is already compromising the already overburdened health care system. What complicates the whole picture of scaling up HIV interventions is that there are so many constraints including lack of political will and commitment, lack of capacity, poor harmonisation of stakeholders, medical laboratory challenges, poor infrastructure, poor integration of TB and HIV services, challenges of paediatric care and treatment, and poor monitoring.

Political Will and Commitment:

One of the biggest challenges is lack of political commitment, as some commentators regard the period prior to 2001 as a period of political inaction, largely because the government did not commit to mass roll-out of antiretroviral therapy with regard to the fight against the huge burden of HIV. Since the more focus on prevention was a strategic direction that the South African government had taken with the notion that prevention is cost-effective than cure, civil society groups such as the Treatment Action Campaign backed by Western countries were beginning to put more pressure on the government to put more focus on antiretroviral therapy, instead of the prevention posture.

In that sense, it seems to me as if policymakers in South Africa have for over an extended period been grappling with the challenge of the dichotomy between prevention and treatment. According to Nattrass, contrasting the cost-effectiveness of prevention over treatment is wrongly headed especially if political decision-making power is ceded to technical arguments, whilst the implicit social injustice of not addressing the real issue such as mass roll-out of antiretroviral therapy is overlooked. This vindicates claims that making antiretroviral therapy widely available is not only cost-effective but is also sustainable especially in the context of developing countries such as South Africa.

Maybe the government's HIV prevention posture was informed by the principles that guide the implementation of essential health packages (EHPs), whereby cost-effectiveness is a factor when prioritising the delivery of health services, but of course one needs to bear in mind that EHPs are interpreted differently. However, sometimes, the challenge is not really about analysing the technical merits and demerits of cost-effectiveness of prevention versus treatment of HIV or whether to implement EHPs or not, but it is about policymakers' lack of understanding and awareness about the whole issue.

It seems as if the South African government ultimately succumbed to the pressure from Western countries and to civil society groupings such as the Treatment Action Campaign, and hastily did a mass-roll-out of antiretroviral therapy, which is like a "quick-fix" because it was poorly planned. The acute shortage of antiretroviral therapy in parts of South Africa has compounded the challenge of poor adherence to HIV treatment. Another issue is that even if the antiretroviral drugs are available, poor leadership and poor management of the HIV programmes has unfortunately been a huge negative factor in this regard.

South Africa's general approach of providing antiretroviral therapy in hospitals has been a challenge because it somewhat puts access out of the reach of the majority of people who live in the rural areas. In fact, the abject poverty that grips the majority of South Africans makes it difficult to travel to and from the hospitals, largely because they cannot afford transport costs. Moreover, even if the patients receive antiretroviral therapy, the challenge is that they often take them on an empty stomach due to poverty, to such an extent that some of the people who receive antiretroviral therapy end up having to sell these therapeutic drugs just to buy food. Actually, there are often reports of antiretroviral drugs being stolen from those who are sick or from hospitals and used as a concoction with other illicit drugs, such as the creation of the new illicit drug known as Whoonga. As such, poverty, desperation and criminal elements are really becoming a huge threat to South Africa's scale up of HIV treatment.

Much as it is important to use policies and standards that have worked in other settings such as developed countries, it is of paramount importance to ensure that the policies and strategies are specific and applicable to the South African context. So much money has been spent on scaling up the HIV prevention, treatment and care, but the reality is that money alone is insufficient to address the burden of HIV. This raises the issue of lack of good governance as there is no efficiency, no effectiveness, and decision-makers are not accountable to the public.

As such it is imperative that policymakers are empowered before they assume positions of power, and one option of doing this is to include leadership as part of the curricula at institutions of higher learning as part of health workers' training so that there could be an expanded pool of competent and qualified potential decision-makers in healthcare.

Stakeholder Involvement:

Sometimes policies and strategies are developed at high level without the involvement of key stakeholders such as the public. Even if the stakeholders such as non-governmental organisations, private sector, and the community are involved in the fight against HIV, sometimes it becomes a challenge if their involvement is not well coordinated, as this ends up in duplication, fragmentation and confusion of efforts, perhaps due to lack of trust both within the government itself and between the government and other stakeholders. This challenge is quite common in South Africa as there are so many different organisations operating in the communities, and each doing their own thing in terms of efforts to address the burden of HIV.

For example, in the remote rural area of South Africa known as Lusikisiki, the charity organisation known as The Doctors Without Borders has done a sterling job by delivering an almost complete package of HIV services, which have rapidly scaled up HIV prevention, treatment and care services. Various non-governmental organisations have also made such a huge positive impact in one of the HIV hardest hit informal settlements of South Africa known as Khayelitsha.

However, it is still a challenge that the activities of such organisations are not part and parcel of the national strategy to scale up HIV prevention, treatment and care, and such uncoordinated efforts are not sustainable. A systematic incorporation of non-governmental organisations and other providers into the national HIV strategy could add value in terms of being a source of technical expertise and finance.

Human Resources for Health:

The scale up of HIV prevention, treatment and care has put a huge burden on health services and increased pressure on health professionals to deliver these services under challenging conditions, thereby resulting in health worker burnout, demotivation and turnover. Health worker shortages pose a serious challenge here in South Africa, and the issue is even more acute in the rural areas where the majority of the population live and where the burden of HIV is even more pronounced. Infact, the shortage of human resources for health is regarded as the main constraint with regard to the scaling up of HIV prevention, treatment and care.

Sometimes the issue of staff shortages is attributed to the brain drain or migration of health personnel from the public health sector to the private health care sector, and also the emigration of health personnel to other countries. However, merely attributing health worker shortages to brain drain is not enough as there are deeper issues that need to be identified and addressed such as low morale and demotivation due to a number of reasons including burnout as a result of heavy workload.

Studies show that the migration of health personnel is also influenced by financial and non-financial incentives. As such, policymakers and decision-makers need to take these issues into account as they have a huge bearing on the success or failure of any efforts to scale-up HIV treatment and care services in this country. In fact, the brain drain can be so severe as it is in South Africa such that so many years of investment are lost, leaving the country with another challenge of spending more resources to try and fill the gap which could end up being a vicious cycle and leaving the country with loss of hope.

It is worth highlighting though that the South African government and other neighbouring governments in the Southern African Development Community (SADC) have tried to address the issue of brain drain by implementing policies that prevent other African countries from recruiting health professional from fellow developing countries in the sub-Saharan Africa region. However, this seems to have had little impact as most of the South African health professionals migrate to developed countries in Europe, North America and Australian and New Zealand, and this compromises whatever gains have been made in scaling up the HIV prevention, treatment and care services in this country.

The power of financial and non-financial incentives is one aspect that policymakers should not take lightly, as studies show that a mix of financial and non-financial incentives could stem the tide against the brain drain as financial incentives will attract health workers and non-financial incentives will make the health workers stay. Financial incentives may include among others salary hikes, medical aid, bonuses, rural allowances, night shift allowances and overtime pays, whereas non-financial incentives may include praise and recognition for sterling performance, workload reliefs, flexible working time, and career development.

Another way of addressing the issue of health worker shortage is by increasing enrolments of students who want to be trained as health workers in institutions of higher learning and to ensure that the training curricula is modified to suite the real health challenges facing South Africa.

Other creative ways of addressing health worker shortages include decentralisation of services and task shifting which is a way of enabling the nurse to initiate treatment as opposed to the physician, thereby decreasing the heavy load on the physician.

Medical Laboratory Services:

Medical laboratory services are often overlooked when it comes to the implementation of essential health packages and this poses serious challenges in the scaling up of HIV programmes. The following laboratory challenges are an issue because they compromise the quality of laboratory tests and negatively impact patient management:

- Weak laboratory infrastructure
- Lack of human capacity
- Lack of or poor laboratory policies and strategic plans
- Limited synergies between clinical and research laboratories.

According to Walley and Wright (2010), medical laboratory services are a key element in the control of infectious diseases such as HIV, and they even serve as a source of information or evidence on the presence and distribution of particular infectious diseases such as HIV. The execution of effective laboratory services at all levels of the health system including at primary, secondary and tertiary levels underpins the success of any prevention and care programme and is crucial for addressing the status quo but future infections as well.

If laboratory services or systems are weak or non-existent, scaling up HIV prevention, treatment and care would be compromised and unsustainable. As such it is of paramount importance to ensure that national laboratory systems are strengthened because such strengthening could have had a positive impact on the achievement of the Millennium Development Goals (MDGs), such as MDG 6 which focused on combating HIV/AIDS and other diseases.

Infrastructure:

Poor infrastructure stifles many aspects of the fight against HIV in South Africa, specifically in the public health sector where many health facilities are in a sorry state despite the fact that the public sector delivers services to at least 80% of the population.

Although it may be attractive to politicians to form public-private partnerships to assist with the upgrades of infrastructure including the building of hospitals, this could also backfire, as the private investor may be more interested in reaping the profits while compromising the public health budget, which could negatively affect the sustainability of scaling up the HIV programme.

Integration of TB and HIV services:

In the context of the coexistence of TB and HIV there are operational barriers to integrate care and treatment of these two diseases, and such barriers include the following:

- The fact that South Africa's national TB and HIV programmes are separate creates challenges such as the following:
  - Separate personnel
  - Separate funding streams
  - Separate facilities
  - Separate responsibilities
- The growing burden of the coexistence of TB and HIV raises concerns because it disrupts and overburdens the already strained public healthcare services.
- Often, the personnel or providers that were trained on TB are not familiar with HIV infection diagnosis and treatment strategies.
- There are limitations with regard to diagnosing both TB and HIV, largely exacerbated by the issue of stigma, limited capacity for conducting pre-test and post-test counselling for HIV, and also due to challenges related to strategies for accurate diagnosis of smear-positive or smear-negative TB.
- In South Africa, there is also the challenge of treating both TB and HIV concomitantly as this raises the issue of immune reconstitution syndrome, increased drug toxicity and the fact that there is an increased pill-burden on the patients.
- We cannot ignore the fact that there are separate cultural issues between TB and HIV, and this also poses a challenge on its own.

Given the above-mentioned operational barriers and the many interactions of TB and HIV infections at the community level and at the clinical level, this influences the design, and implementation of policies and programmes aimed at addressing the needs of people living with both TB and HIV.

Paediatric HIV Care and Treatment:

It is worth highlighting that paediatric care and treatment poses another challenge in the sense that the compartmentalised roll-out of the antiretroviral therapy programme hinders the prevention of mother to child transmission and also makes it difficult to identify children who are infected with HIV. Further, even if the children are identified, the lack of adequately trained staff on paediatric care and treatment, as well as poor facilities makes it difficult to effectively address the issue of HIV in children.

Monitoring:

In theory the monitoring tools may be available as they may have worked in other countries, but practically there is a glaring inability to monitor the scale up of HIV interventions in South Africa.

In conclusion, the magnitude of the policy and programme challenges of scaling up HIV prevention, treatment and care in South Africa should not be viewed in isolation, but should be viewed in the context of a sector-wide approach based on a foundation of strong leadership. In that context, scaling up of HIV interventions could act as a catalyst to stimulate wider achievement of an effective and responsive health system. However, policymakers need to guard against unsystematic rapid expansion of HIV prevention, care and treatment services to the detriment of other health care services, as this underpins the gap between policy intentions and implementation actions.

5.7.10 A Business Perspective on HIV/AIDS

Determining the Extent to which an Organisation Is Affected by HIV/AIDS

The natural tendency for most senior managers in the private sector is to adopt an actuarial approach when it comes to addressing the impact of HIV/AIDS in their organisations. To illustrate this point, an impact assessment was performed at a southern African transport and logistics firm, and the approach solely followed a financial scope of the impact of HIV/AIDS on the company. However, in this discussion, the focus is on the broader scheme of things, that is, it employs an institutional audit.

According to the UNAIDS (2002), two concepts inform the institutional audit: susceptibility and vulnerability. In the context, the idea of susceptibility describes those features of an organisation that make it more or less likely that its workers will contract HIV infection. In contrast, vulnerability describes those aspects of an organisation that make it more or less likely that usual levels of illness and/or death will have negative effects on organisational performance. The institutional audit consists of the following components that form a series of linked steps in the process:

- Personnel profiling
- Critical post analysis
- Assessment of organisational characteristics
- Estimate of organisational liabilities
- Productivity
- Organisational context

In the following discussion, each of these steps is examined in turn, as per the UNAIDS (2002) study at Debswana. Debswana is a diamond-mining company in Botswana. It is worth mentioning that the management of HIV/AIDS at Debswana has now come to be recognised as a global benchmark.

Step 1: Personnel profiling:

What kind of people are employed?

This question is addressed in relation to two sub-questions: which groups (if any) among employees are most likely to be susceptible to infection? What different skill levels exist in the organisation; what are their characteristics and what is their strategic importance to the organisation?

Susceptible groups:

Are there particular groups among employees who may be particularly exposed to infection?

Why are they exposed?

Can/should the organisation do anything to reduce this exposure?

Will understanding such programmes benefit the organisation?

Should all employees be included or only those who are most difficult to replace?

Skill levels:

What skill levels are there in the organisation?

How many people are there at each level?

What are the costs of training/replacing these people?

Given the known and predicted rates of sero-prevalence, how many people might be expected to become ill or die each year over the next five years in each category of employment?

Ease of training and replacement:

How easy will it be to train or recruit personnel at each skill level, considering costs and time for training and also the state of the national and regional labour market?

Step 2: Critical post analysis:

Are there key personnel whom it will be particularly difficult to replace, and on whom a production or administrative process depends (for example, the 'institutional memory' or the person who knows how to use the computer?

Step 3: Organisational characteristics

Size of organisation and flexibility of employees

- How easy will it be to replace or retain within the organisation
- Are there sufficient people to allow for internal training?
- Should the organisation introduce 'shadowing' of key employees (i.e. employ an additional staff member for every critical post)?
- Does it have sufficient internal resources to be able to undertake replacement and/or training or replacement of personnel?
- Is it big enough to move people around to take over other people's jobs?
- What is the lead time for training or recruiting a replacement for different skill levels?

Step 4: Liabilities

The potential or actual liability of an organisation will be determined by some or all the following factors:

- Level and type of employee benefits. This relates to contracts of employment and considers the benefit packages.
- Level of labour value added. In our production organisation, this measures the part of gross profit attributable to the work done by labourers. Variable considered here are quantity of labour/quality of labour (seen in levels of pay); and labour as a proportion of all inputs to product.

Step 5: Productivity

There may be a reduction in the quality and quantity of labour supplied by employees who are sick or are caring for sick dependants. Absenteeism may result in a slow and barely detectable decline in output in the particular organisation. How is this going to be detected and managed?

Labour/capital substitution:

- Can capital be used to replace people who are sick or have died?
- Could larger numbers of unskilled workers replace the lost skilled workers?

Out-sourcing and 'multi-skilling':

- Can non-core functions (for example, security and cleaning) be outsourced?
- Can staff be trained to have multiple skills enabling them to do their own and others' jobs, should the situation demand it?

Step 6: Organisation context:

- What is the legislative and industrial relations framework?
- What must the particular organisation do for its workers in the way of invalidity benefit, keeping them at work while they are HIV-positive but are not ill, or when they have AIDS but are not too sick to work?

The lesson learned from the foregoing discussion is that the impact of HIV/AIDS could not be considered only, or even most importantly, in financial terms. The impact of HIV/AIDS on an organisation is too complex to be considered only in these terms. In addition to the bottom line, HIV/AIDS, affects, among other elements, staff morale, public perceptions of the organisation, institutional memory, labour relations, and the community in which the organisation is situated. Therefore, determining the impact of HIV/AIDS on an organisation should encompass the abovementioned aspects, and not only from an actuarial point of view.

Strategy to Ensure there Is Enough Staff to Run an Organisation over the Next Five Years

Strategy is all about combining choices of what to do and what not to do into a system that creates the requisite fit between what the environment needs and what the company does (Thompson et al. 2007). Studies have emphasized the analysis and options that go into matching a company's choice of strategy to industry and competitive conditions and its resource strengths and weaknesses, competitive capabilities, opportunities and threats, and market position. But there is more to be revealed about the how of matching the choices of strategy to an organisation's circumstances. For the purpose of this discussion, a synthesis of two of the good HIV/AIDS strategies for companies, shall be employed. This includes the HIV/AIDS strategy for Gold fields and also that of Debswana.

Before developing an HIV/AIDS strategy for the organisation, it would be imperative to do a situational analysis. For instance, an impact assessment or institutional audit will enable forecasting. In other words, the institutional audit will identify the need to develop a separate strategy on HIV/AIDS in order to give the issue the attention it deserves. A task team must be put together to develop the strategy. The following mission and vision should be adopted:

Mission: To reduce the impact of HIV/AIDS on our employees, their families and the company through the prevention of new infections, the care and support of those infected and the containment of costs.

Strategic vision: To become the global benchmark company in the fight against HIV/AIDS in the workplace.

Furthermore, six strategies should be identified:

Epidemic containment – a strategy for prevention of new infections among employees and their families.

This may be achieved through the following activities:

- Awareness campaigns
- Education, training, counselling, and voluntary testing
- Condom promotion and distribution
- Treatment of sexually transmitted infections (STIs); syndromic treatment of STIs; periodic presumptive therapy for employees at high risk

Economic impact containment – a strategy for minimising the financial impact of HIV on the company to ensure its survival. This will be done through proactive planning for the various HIV-associated impact indicators such as deaths, sickness, ill-health retirements, and targeted succession planning, particularly for those jobs that have been identified as critical to the business.

Living with HIV - a strategy for minimising the negative impact of HIV on employees living with the virus, through enabling policies, and by improving the quality of their lives and their productivity. The emphasis will be on the promotion of a healthy lifestyle through a balanced diet, physical, mental and spiritual well-being and the provision of antiretroviral therapy to employees and their spouses who are infected with the virus.

Where an employee gets to a point where early ill-health retirement must be considered, it will have to be done in accordance with current practice/policies.

Where it becomes necessary to remove the employee permanently from his/her job due to HIV or any disability related thereto, Human Resources would effect the re-deployment. All reasonable endeavours will be made to re-deploy such an employee for as long as possible.

Palliative or home-based care should be made available to affected employees and their families.

Shareholder engagement – a strategy for engaging those stakeholders who are important to the success of the company's HIV/AIDS programme by setting standards and guidelines for such stakeholders to follow, and through collaboration and partnerships.

Public/private partnerships should be strengthened to ensure continuity of care, as well as access to dependents for care in the community.

Evaluation measurement and monitoring - a strategy for the regular evaluation of effectiveness of the company's HIV/AIDS programmes and the constant measurement and monitoring of HIV impact indicators such as death, absenteeism, ill-health retirements, costs and benefits.

Communication – a strategy to support the HIV/AIDS programmes and to improve awareness of these and other initiatives internally and externally with relevant stakeholders. This strategy is also aimed at promoting the vision of the particular organisation becoming a global benchmark company in the fight against HIV/AIDS in the workplace.

Managing HIV/AIDS in the workplace requires proactive management of the epidemic by seeking to understand it, managing it and mitigating its impact as part of every organisation's response to the HIV/AIDS epidemic. There is broad acceptance that HIV/AIDS is having and increasingly will have a significant impact on the workplace. Ideally HIV/AIDS should be managed in the same manner as other long-term threats to an organisation. This implies that organisations should have a management plan to support their workplace HIV/AIDS response.

If an organisation wants to successfully manage the impact of HIV/AIDS, the impact of the pandemic must be considered during strategy formulation and must be implemented as part of the organisation's business plan.

Even the most successful company HIV/AIDS prevention programme can become outdated in time or stand as a single effort in a surrounding wilderness, unless there is a concerted effort to build a united HIV/AIDS response. Businesses should seek opportunities to collaborate with each other, with their suppliers and with other organisations – locally, nationally, or globally – to offer HIV/AIDS programmes and services.

Strategy to Counter the Erosion of Organisational Skill

The business impact of HIV/AIDS is already visible in workplaces in many parts of the world – something that worries managers, from the shop floor to the top management.

HIV/AIDS takes its toll in the workplace in a number of ways:

- The loss of experienced personnel
- Absenteeism through HIV-related illnesses, to care for others, and to attend funerals.

- Increased recruitment and training costs – in many developing regions, finding qualified top management and skilled line workers to replace those who die, or can no longer work can be extremely difficult
- Increased labour turnover – productivity suffers during the time it takes to replace workers, particularly among more skilled or senior workers
- Lower productivity of new recruits – often it takes weeks for new employees to become as productive as those whom they replaced (ILO 2000).

It is important to mention that there is not a current best practice on how to utilise training and development to curb the impact of HIV/AIDS on the organisation's skilled workforce.

The challenge is to put heads together and to design training and development policies and strategies in such a way that the adverse effects of HIV/AIDS on the organisation's skilled workforce could hopefully be neutralised.

In that regard, the following strategy shall be developed to counter the erosion of skill in the organisation.

Strategic Vision:

The company seeks to achieve sustainable growth in order to become the leading transport and logistic company in Africa.

Strategic Mission:

The company seeks to achieve this by improving productivity and profitability, and by providing appropriate capacity to our customers ahead of demand.

Strategic Objective

The objective is to counter the erosion of skill in the organisation by implementing a training and development strategy that focuses on multi-skilling.

Environmental Scan

According to the Quick MBA (2008), the environmental scan includes the following components:

- Internal analysis of the firm. Need to consider the training in the context of the rest of the organisation. What are the training implications of the organisation's strategy? What will be the result if training is not undertaken? How does this training programme fit in with the organisation's future plans and goals? Where in the organisation is training needed? How are various departments performing in relation to expectations or goals? In which departments is training most likely to succeed? Which departments should be trained first? Can the organisation afford this training? Which training programmes should have priority? Will this training adversely affect untrained people or departments? Is this training consistent with the organisation's culture? Will this training be accepted and reinforced by others in the organisation, such as trainees' superiors, subordinates and clients?

- Analysis of the task environment. According to Nel et al. (2005), it must also be borne in mind whether or not the training is commensurate with the organisation's mission, strategy, goals, and culture.
- External environment (PEST analysis). The PEST analysis involves the political, economic, social, and technological aspects of the external environment in which the organisation operates.

Crafting the Strategy

The job: Conduct a thorough task analysis of an incumbent. The purpose is to find out if an individual's task is of importance to the organisation, and whether training is to be executed.
The individual: training can only be executed if it has been determined which employees should receive training and what their current levels, knowledge and skills are.
Devise instructional objectives. An instructional objective is a description of a performance learners must be able to exhibit before they can be considered competent.
Prepare test items based on the objectives and desired outcomes. This enables the trainer to establish whether the learner has mastered behaviours that a training programme has been designed to teach.
Select or design instructional content: the decision what to teach, is based on the test items and instruction objectives.
Choosing delivery methods: The method of teaching is dependent on what to teach.
Offering instruction: training can be offered either on the job by the supervisor, off the job by in-house trainers, or outside the organisation.
Transferring learning back to the job: The main purpose of off the job training is to give employees the knowledge and skills they need to perform effectively on the shop floor.

Evaluation

Training and development can never be effective if not properly assessed. The evaluation of training is a continuous process (Nel et al. 2005).

Loss of human capital as a result of HIV/AIDS burdens the capacities of organisations in unpredictable ways. It is essential that skills and competencies be sustained if organisations are to move towards fulfilment of their business goals. From an organisational perspective, emphasis should be placed on training and development to minimise the loss of skills. Training and development should move away from a primary focus on teaching employees, specific skills, to a broader focus of creating and sharing knowledge. That is, to use training to gain competitive advantage, training should be viewed broadly as a way to create intellectual capital. Intellectual capital includes basic skills, advanced skills, an understanding of the customer and self-motivated creativity.

Report on how to Determine Level of Awareness about HIV/AIDS in the Workplace

The purpose of this section is to report briefly, on how to determine the level of awareness about HIV/AIDS within an organisation. The KAPB survey can be used to determine the level of awareness about HIV/AIDS within the organisation. KAPB is an acronym for Knowledge, Attitudes, Practices and Behaviours.

Workplace HIV/AIDS programmes need to be monitored and evaluated according to their stated objectives. Such evaluations are important in improving the programme and measuring the effectiveness of the interventions. Examples of indicators that might point to the success or effectiveness of a programme include: a decrease in Sexually Transmitted Infections (STIs) among the workforce; a decrease in alcohol and drug use; increased involvement of employees in workplace activities; and an increase in activities – such as community service – resulting from educational programmes.

How to Ensure that Managers and Supervisors Are up to Date with the Management of HIV/AIDS in the Workplace

The purpose of this section is to indicate how one would ensure that managers and supervisors are up to date with the management of HIV/AIDS in an organisation.

In addition to participating in information and education programmes that are directed at all employees, supervisory and managerial personnel should receive training to:

- Enable them to explain and respond to questions about the workplace's HIV/AIDS policy
- Be well informed about HIV/AIDS so as to help other workers overcome misconceptions about the spread of HIV/AIDS at the workplace
- Explain reasonable options to workers with HIV/AIDS so as to enable them to continue to work as long as possible
- Identify and manage workplace behaviour, conduct or practices, which discriminate against or alienate workers with HIV/AIDS
- Enable them to give advice about the health services and social benefits, which are available.

The management of HIV/AIDS should be seen as an intrinsic part of the management of human and financial resources. All managers are required to have a level of competence in managing costs and human resources. Therefore, a level of competence in HIV-related issues for all managers is a natural part of this. The following areas of competence have been identified (UNAIDS 2002), and it is imperative that these standards are also applied in the context of the organisation:

- Medical facts and basic epidemiology and data sources
- HIV/AIDS epidemic determinants
- Impact of HIV/AIDS on the individual, the company and society
- HIV/AIDS workplace issues
- The organisation's policies and practices on HIV/AIDS and the rationale behind them.

From an organisation's perspective, implementation of these standards should be carried out as part of the five-year organisational strategic objectives and standards should be used during the selection process to determine the competence of new managers joining the organisation at particular levels.

Workplace education and training programmes are essential to combat the spread of the HIV and to foster greater tolerance for workers living with HIV. Effective education for managers and supervisors can contribute to the capacity of workers to protect themselves against HIV infection. It can significantly reduce HIV-related anxiety and stigmatisation, minimise disruption in the workplace, and bring about attitudinal and behavioural change. It can also enhance productivity, because it can improve the morale of HIV-infected and affected employees to know that the company cares about them especially with regard to the available option of reasonable accommodation to enable them to continue to work as long as possible.

5.7.11 The Individual: Differences and Behaviour; Psychological Variables and HIV/AIDS; and Career Management

Management of an employee's Career at the Workplace in the Context of HIV Status

The purpose of this section is to draw up brief notes for the management of an employee's future career at the workplace, in order to allow him to perform at a psychologically optimum level, given the fact that the employee lives with HIV.

One of the primary concerns of present-day employees is the concern for the management of their careers.

Workplace accommodation for people living with HIV

People living with HIV can be productive for many years. Even in the best of circumstances, the challenges associated with HIV can be significant.

There is no simple formula for the accommodation of employees living with HIV

The dual goals of accommodation are to ensure that work assignments are accomplished, and that the individual living with HIV continues working for as long as possible. Effective accommodation does not require the lowering of the expectations of the employee. Rather, it requires ongoing negotiation and creative problem solving to determine alternative means of accomplishing work assignments. This negotiation process may result in different outcomes in similar circumstances.

Providing accommodation to employees living with HIV is a team effort with impact on a company's workforce, managers and policies

Because of the fear and stigma still associated with HIV/AIDS, accommodating people living with HIV affects virtually everyone in the workplace. A fearful work environment is not a productive one. In the process of providing accommodation of employees with HIV infection or AIDS, Dynamic Stores might consider addressing co-worker attitudes. In order to dispel unwarranted fears and to ensure cooperation in the accommodation process, managers need accurate information about HIV infection and AIDS.

If co-workers become suspicious of preferential treatment, it may be helpful for a manager to discuss with the employee, what, if anything, they want to do about the situation, and offer support for whatever decision is made.

Psychological optimisation

It is the responsibility of a manager to create a climate in which the needs of the total person, their uniqueness, are met. Only then will such an employee be able to experience psychological optimisation – optimising their physical, psychological and mental potential in the workplace.

To conclude, leadership is an important part of effective accommodation in order to allow an employee living with HIV to perform at a psychologically optimum level.

Manager's Personal Responsibility to Manage the Psychological Contract

The objective of this section is to take a personal responsibility to manage the psychological contract that exists between an employee living with HIV, and the organisation.

Psychological contract

The psychological contract represents a set of unwritten mutual expectations – what the employee expects to give and receive from the organisation and what the organisation expects to give and receive from the employee.

It is at this interface where the employee and the organisation start to experience difficulty in sustaining the psychological contract. During the initial stages of infection, the employee may still be able to maintain a high level of involvement, motivation and commitment. As "communication" is considered the root of the psychological contract between the employee and the organisation – communicating mutual expectations, the contract needs to be renegotiated after the revelation of the illness. However, a large number of unknown and unpredictable issues hamper this re-negotiation.

Although the psychological contract is established between the employee and the organisation, employees regard their immediate manager, as the "organisation". Therefore, the employee's manager needs to appreciate this phenomenon. Re-negotiation of the psychological contract therefore becomes the direct responsibility of the manager. Through proper performance management systems, it is the manager's task to continuously manage individual workers, especially by staying aware of the needs and expectations of each person, including their emotional and psychological needs.

In the context of the brief notes above, a psychological contract represents the mutual beliefs, perceptions, and informal obligations between an employer and an employee (in this case the employee lives with HIV). So long as the values and loyalty persist, trust and commitment will be maintained.

A Plan to Assist an Employee Deal with Challenges Associated with Living with HIV

The objective of this section is to draw up brief notes to assist a worker living with HIV (with the stress that he experiences as a result of his HIV status). In this respect the plan would be to assist him to utilise his generalised resistance resources (GRRs) in order to develop a strong sense of Coherence.

In the event of an employee becoming HIV positive, any existing distress they may have had to cope with now becomes even more acute and amplified. Antonovsky introduced the concept of GRR (generalised resistance resources) within the Salutogenic model that can facilitate effective tension management in any situation of demand.

Antonovsky described a range of such GRRs. All GRRs have in common that they facilitate "making sense" out of the countless stressors with which one is constantly bombarded. However, through repeated experiences of "sense making" a person may develop over time a strong "sense of coherence" (Tan et al. 2014).

This is a global orientation that expresses the extent to which one has an all-encompassing, enduring, though dynamic feeling of confidence that: The stimuli deriving from one's internal and external environments in the course of living are structured, predictable and explicable – it is clear, ordered, structured and consistent. It is therefore comprehensible. In the event of HIV infection, the stressor (as stimuli causing severe stress) is perceived as structured (it has certain structural properties regarding its origin, development, treatment, prognosis) – it makes cognitive sense. The resources are available to one to meet the demands posed by the stimuli. It is therefore manageable – it can be coped with; challenges can be met. These demands are challenges worthy of investment and engagement – it makes sense emotionally, rather than cognitively. In some way it is felt that the challenges are welcome, motivating one to invest energy. It is therefore meaningful (Eriksson and Lindstrom 2008).

In the context of the brief notes above, it remains of the organisation's manager to facilitate the coping abilities of the said worker. A strong sense of coherence without the appropriate ability, skills, training and development (accommodating) would be of no avail. The organisational environment needs to be conducive to assisting and facilitating employees in their attempts to cope with the stressors they experience (The Healthy Employee 2008).

5.7.12 *Ethics in the Management of HIV/AIDS*

Ethics is the discipline that deals systematically with the nature of obligation, including with the issues, judgements, theories and possible answers pertaining to the question: when are our actions right or wrong, and what things are good or bad?

The HIV pandemic has revealed a remarkable array of ethical problems that occur in the effort to identify HIV-positive people and to treat patients suffering from AIDS appropriately, and, eventually, to vaccinate the population against the disease, should a vaccine eventually be successfully developed. The purpose of this discussion is three-pronged. Firstly, to identify an ethical problem related to HIV and AIDS in the workplace. Secondly, to explain why the problem is ethical, and to develop possible approaches to think about it. Thirdly, to suggest solutions on the basis of thorough moral reflection. In this discussion, the issue of lack of will by workplace leadership to effectively manage HIV and AIDS has been identified as an ethical problem. The spotlight will be cast on Company F2F, where this ethical problem has been specifically identified. The author prefers to refer to the company of focus as Company F2F in order to protect its identity. Company F2F is one of the major retail companies in its home country, located in the Southern African region.

HIV and AIDS is a serious problem in the workplace, but it can be managed in an affordable way. The most serious impediment to its humane and effective management is not a lack of knowledge, the unavailability of antiretroviral drugs, the infrastructure to make them available or their unaffordability. It is the lack of will and the denial of the seriousness of the problem on the part of the workplace leadership, particularly at Company F2F. Once this leadership assumes its rightful responsibility, all the indications are that aid from government or pharmaceutical companies, will be forthcoming, and a very significant reduction in HIV transmission can be expected. It is for the leadership in companies such as Company F2F to seize the day: cooperate with both government and pharmaceutical companies who are willing to come to their aid, accept their offers, make the infrastructure available for the distribution of these drugs and do what is now possible to prevent an almost unspeakable tragedy.

It is incumbent upon leaders to accept the moral responsibility for choices and the consequences of not effectively managing HIV and AIDS at the workplace.

5.7.13 Cost Impact of HIV/AIDS on a Company

Background

Perhaps, one wonders what the cost impact of HIV/AIDS is on the company that one works for. Due to the sensitivity of the topic, and for the purpose of this paper, the company will only be referred to as "Company X". Judging by the high absenteeism rate, the worsening skills shortages and the high staff turnover rate within the organisation, there is no doubt that there are huge cost implications to the company as a result of HIV/AIDS. Although there is a disease management programme in place, there has not been a specific study to determine the cost of HIV/AIDS to the business in "Company X". And very little industry-specific research has been done.

"Company X" is one of the major transport and logistics companies in Southern Africa. The company is made up of five operational divisions, and the total staff complement is currently 60 thousand employees. It is noteworthy to mention that the company comprises five operational divisions and most of the main worksites or business units are spread across three provinces, which are KwaZulu-Natal, Eastern Cape, and Western Cape. The bulk (65%) of our workforce is located in the province of KwaZulu-Natal, and approximately 70% of the work force, are male. The average age of the work force is 45. The total staff complement is approximately 60 thousand employees.

The purpose of this discussion is to assess “Company X’s” vulnerability to the cost implications of HIV/AIDS. The research will be based on data regarding skills, absenteeism, cost of healthcare and labour turnover at “Company X”.

With HIV prevalence and AIDS deaths on the rise in South Africa (including “Company X”), the disease presents challenges to the public and private sectors alike. In the business environment such as in “Company X”, HIV/AIDS is manifested in higher production costs, which are expected to continue over the next decade. The magnitude of HIV/AIDS cost to business is determined by workforce and industry characteristics. Workforce characteristics include size, skills profile, prevalence/incidence rates, and demographic factors such as age, race and gender. The industry characteristics include location, terms and conditions of employment, salary scale, level of skill required and replacement costs (Njobe and Smith 2004).

The impact of this epidemic on business operations in South Africa has taken precedence in HIV/AIDS research over the last 4–5 years. Large businesses have begun to address the epidemic through prevalence testing, estimating costs and implementing workplace HIV/AIDS programmes, which vary from knowledge, awareness and prevention to treatment. The emergence of models to estimate the cost of HIV/AIDS has enabled corporations to examine their vulnerability to increased costs (Njobe and Smith 2004). These analyses are typically restricted to in-house use and have not been made available to the public. As such, few studies provide a cross sectional view of business vulnerability to HIV/AIDS. This paper aims to accomplish this. The overall objective is to assess the relative risk of exposure to inflated HIV/AIDS costs at “Company X”.

HIV/AIDS: A Strategic Business Imperative

The HIV/AIDS pandemic is real. The situation requires a strategic response from top management, intensive planning, immediate action and non-traditional strategies and collaborations to minimise the impact on companies (Metcalfe 2004).

It has been estimated that 40% to 50% of the current South African workforce will die of AIDS within the next ten years. Every sector of the economy is vulnerable to the HIV/AIDS threat (Metcalfe 2004).

According to the UNAIDS (2006) report, more than five million South Africans are estimated to be HIV infected, representing almost 25% of South Africans of working age.

This makes South Africa the worst affected country in the world and it is estimated that the South African GDP could be reduced by more than 17% by 2010 as a result of the disease (Metcalfe 2004).

These estimates are corroborated by the International Labour Organisation (ILO) recently released international research results, which estimates that HIV/AIDS has already cost the South African economy more than $70 billion in the 10 years between 1992 and 2002 (ILO 2005).

This translates into 2% of GDP or more than $7 billion per year, for the years up to 2002, and income per capita has dropped by 1.3% (Metcalfe 2004).

The ILO places South Africa's HIV prevalence rate at 21.5% and states that the costs to the economy were mainly due to workforce deaths and labour absenteeism. These are only two ways in which companies will be affected in the HIV/AIDS epidemic and many companies are realising that not taking action will affect their bottom line (ILO 2005).

Anglo American PLC, for example, estimates that 24% of its 125 00 employees in South Africa are infected with HIV and started its own AIDS treatment and prevention program in 1994, which includes administering anti-retroviral drugs. The company reports that decline in employee mortality and absenteeism offset the treatment costs (Brink 2003).

The problem, however, is not confined to human resource costs in individual companies. Former UN Secretary-General Kofi Annan called on businesses to think globally about.

AIDS and said that the micro-economic effects in the developing world (*absenteeism, decline in a skilled workforce, higher payments for sickness and death benefits*) will lead to macro-economic effects worldwide (Metcalfe 2004).

In addition, HIV poses a huge threat to companies' markets, both in terms of future customers and the societies in which companies operate, source labour and seek investors and shareholders (Metcalfe 2004).

The sheer scale of the pandemic will affect entire nations and economic systems, as the effects filter through to economic growth, income levels and poverty levels worldwide. These effects include pressures on governments' social healthcare systems, decreased industrial productivity and an overall decrease in consumer demand. All these factors will reverberate in all sectors, including foreign investment and tourism (Metcalfe 2004).

In June 2004, the Global Economic Initiative of the World Economic Forum released the results of a survey, which found that almost two thirds of African businesses believe that AIDS will affect their bottom line. Of the 1620 African businesses surveyed, most reported that they were already seeing the negative effects of HIV/AIDS, including higher costs relating to increasing absenteeism, rising healthcare costs, higher operating costs and in some instances, even a reduction in revenue (Metcalfe 2004).

Recent research conducted by the Bureau for Economic Research on behalf of the South African Business Coalition on HIV/AIDS showed that almost 33% of the 1006 companies surveyed said that their profitability had been negatively affected. The surveyed companies were operating in the manufacturing, construction, motor, wholesale and retail sectors. A further 43% of the companies expected a "significant adverse impact" on their operations and profits within five years (Ellis and Terwin 2004).

The research further showed that HIV/AIDS has had the most impact on the manufacturing sector, while the retail sector has seen less of an impact, as did the construction sector, which relied more on part-time semi-skilled or unskilled workers (Metcalfe 2004).

Small businesses are also at risk and perhaps even more so, as they lack the resources to respond comprehensively to the issue. Yet, strategic planning for the future and collaborations with other companies may result in less costly but still effective steps taken to minimise the impact of HIV/AIDS in smaller companies (Metcalfe 2004).

The South African Business Coalition on HIV/AIDS research further revealed that over 45% of medium and large companies reported an adverse effect on profits, while 30% of small companies said they had lower profits due to HIV/AIDS (Metcalfe 2004).

In excess of 40% of companies in Gauteng and KwaZulu-Natal, the worst affected provinces, reported lower labour productivity and increased absenteeism due to HIV/AIDS (Metcalfe 2004).

The Impact on Human Resources

The authors of the ILO report say that HIV/AIDS destroys human capital built up over years and weakens the capacity of workers to produce goods and services for the economy. They add that the situation might worsen if more treatment is not provided and might lead to a 20% loss of labour force by 2010 (ILO 2005).

The research report from the South African Business Coalition on HIV/AIDS revealed that over 33% of companies experienced reduced productivity or more absenteeism. Nearly 40% reported that their demand for labour had increased, as they required replacements for employees that were sick. Less than 15% of the companies said they were reducing their dependence on labour through investments in machinery or equipment (Metcalfe 2004).

According to Journ AIDS, a study of six large enterprises in the retail, agriculture, media, mining and heavy industry sectors in South Africa and Botswana, found that the direct costs associated with HIV/AIDS varied considerably. The cost per HIV infection of an unskilled worker ranged from \$2094 to \$15,000 (2001 prices), while the cost of a manager ranged from \$8736 to \$65,000. Companies' human resources will be affected in several direct and indirect ways (Metcalfe 2004).

As HIV/AIDS sufferers begin to see the effects of the disease in their lives, companies are likely to be faced with an increase in sick leave and absenteeism. According to a USAID publication, a sugar mill in South Africa reported that 26% of all tested workers were infected with HIV. Infected workers incurred, on average, 55 additional days of sick leave during the last two years of their life (Metcalfe 2004).

Additional leave days will be required even for employees who are not infected, as they attend funerals, take compassionate leave and care for family members who may be infected. This places additional pressure on the rest of the employees to fill in for and carry the workload of those not at work. The resulting overtime, exhaustion and stress could lead to reduced job satisfaction and a reduction in productivity. But productivity could suffer in many other ways. Employees living with HIV/AIDS may be less productive when at work due to ill health. Even in good health, these employees are likely to experience stress of living with HIV/AIDS, discrimination and uncertainty (Metcalfe 2004).

The productivity of those employees not infected may be affected as they watch their colleagues and family members die, and their fears and concerns for their own safety and health increases. This stressful environment can damage staff morale and lead to further decrease in productivity. Indeed, the atmosphere may become fatalistic. Discrimination against employees living with HIV may further cripple company cohesion and destroy any teamwork in the company (Metcalfe 2004).

Companies cannot afford not to respond to the issue, as employees may construe a lack of response as an indication that management does not care – a serious threat to communication, labour relations and productivity. This implies a further cost as management resources are used to plan, respond to and manage HIV/AIDS policies and problems (Metcalfe 2004).

As employees die or become too sick to work, new employees must be recruited. This may become increasingly difficult as the supply of skilled labour is affected by HIV/AIDS, which is predominant in the working age group. This may not present an immediate problem in terms of semi- or unskilled labour, but some companies have already been forced to find expensive foreign management expertise as the disease compounds the lack of skills (Metcalfe 2004).

Once recruited, employees must be screened, interviewed, selected, oriented and trained. All these activities increase costs, while also placing additional strain on the employees who must assist the new employees during their training and learning and learning curve. A further problem arises as the new recruits find it increasingly difficult to "fit in" as they replace friends and colleagues who have passed away (Metcalfe 2004).

The constant stream of new employees disrupts the continuity of the workflow process and destabilises the balance between new, inexperienced employees and experienced employees. A great deal of unspoken know-how is lost, as is the knowledge or institutional memory gained through years of company-specific experience (Metcalfe 2004).

Companies must have a strategic plan, including detailed policies on how the issue of HIV/AIDS will be handled in the company, creating a succession plan for replacing employees, and looking at strategies to move ill employees to less-demanding jobs. Consideration must be given to the rights of the employees in terms of various legislation and ways to address the company's liability in terms of discrimination (Metcalfe 2004).

Costs and profitability

In addition to the labour costs discussed above, companies will face increased costs in other, related areas. The costs of, for example, medical aid and health insurance, group life and disability insurance, employee benefits and pension fund contributions, funeral expenses and severance pay, will increase as the effects of HIV/AIDS is felt in both the company and the economy. Further costs relate to management and staff resources and direct costs involved in planning, implementing and participating in HIV/AIDS prevention, training and treatment (Metcalfe 2004).

Bill Lacey, an economic consultant at the SA Chamber of Business (SACOB), was quoted in the media saying that a crude survey, comprising 18 of SACOB's members, showed an HIV prevalence rate of between 3% and 30%. Most of the companies surveyed provide treatment for their employees at a cost varying between R100 000 and R20-million. The cost was directly related to the size of the company and how many people were being treated. *"This cost is said to increase, in some instances threefold,"* Lacey said in a media report. But, according to the survey, the cost of doing nothing was even more. *"This varies between R1-million and R30-million,"* he said (Metcalfe 2004).

In 1995 already, research in Canada estimated that HIV/AIDS had resulted in $8 billion in lost productivity and it was predicted to increase to $15 billion by 2000, while the cost to the employee benefit plans was $100,000 per HIV/AIDS case (Metcalfe 2004).

The 2004 South African Business Coalition on HIV/AIDS research found that 8% of the companies surveyed projected passing some of the costs they incurred as a result of the epidemic to their customers, to avoid profit margins coming under pressure (Metcalfe 2004).

The combination of increased costs and reduced productivity could result in companies seeing a decrease in their profitability and their competitiveness in the global economy (Metcalfe 2004).

Hypothesis

The stated hypothesis to the above investigation is that HIV/AIDS is having a significantly negative effect on the cost to the business at "Company X".

Research Design

The Deutsche Securities Hybrid HIV/AIDS Cost Model will be employed. This model was developed in-house and integrates elements from previously developed models, with some new assumptions. The model was used to estimate the costs of HIV/AIDS to companies in four South African industries, given prevalence rates, employee costs, size of the workforce and the distribution of the workforce between the different levels – or grades. The analysis is conducted using company level data, which is representative of the industry benchmark (Njobe and Smith 2004).

This model is a useful tool for company specific evaluations of costs imposed by HIV/AIDS. Specific knowledge about HIV prevalence, workforce demographics, uptake, attrition and benefits offered would enable a thorough assessment of individual company risk to HIV/AIDS costs (Njobe and Smith 2004).

The sample group will include all the five operational divisions of "Company X".

The methodology to arrive at the cost estimates for the organisation is as follows:

Employee profiles by gender, grade and age would be input to an AIDS projection model – ASSA SELECT. Projections of HIV prevalence and AIDS cases would be produced for the organisation, by gender, age and grade level (Njobe and Smith 2004).

An average prevalence rate would be computed for 2008–2023. This rate would then be used as the standard prevalence rate for the organisation by grade. Prevalence by grade is not expected to vary much over the 15-year period; therefore, average prevalence would be an appropriate benchmark (Njobe and Smith 2004).

The total cost to the employer will be computed using the average prevalence rate. Note that hostel dwellers will not be considered as a separate grade but will be treated as such in this model because their risk of HIV infection is much higher than that of employees living with their families.

The number of employees infected in the organisation by grade level would be computed from the average prevalence (Njobe and Smith 2004).

The number of employees would be based on permanent workers. The quantitative analysis would not include costs attributed to infection rates among contract workers (Njobe and Smith 2004).

The cost of HIV infection would be computed by grade level for the organisation, as a multiple of the number infected the annual adjusted salary and per employee cost of HIV/AIDS, which is estimated to be 3.2 times the annual salary. This methodology assumes that all who are infected will eventually become sick and the costs will be borne by the employer. In reality there is attrition over time, transition to ART and staggered stages in which employees develop full-blown AIDS. Therefore, the employer will not face the costs from all their infected employees at the same time. In the absence of sufficient data to estimate attrition and transition to ART within workplaces, the method described above is used. It is representative of the worst-case scenario, given current knowledge about HIV prevalence (Njobe and Smith 2004).

The costs would be computed in present value terms assuming a corporate long bond rate of 10%, plus 5%, which is the long-term estimate of the equity risk premium (Njobe and Smith 2004).

The research will be carried out over a period of three months.

Subjects

The sample group will include all the five operational divisions of "Company X". This means that the sample size will be 60 thousand employees.

The methodology to arrive at the cost estimates for the organisation is as follows:

Employee profiles by gender, grade and age would be input to an AIDS projection model – ASSA SELECT. Projections of HIV prevalence and AIDS cases would be produced for the organisation, by gender, age and grade level (Njobe and Smith 2004).

An average prevalence rate would be computed for 2008–2023. This rate would then be used as the standard prevalence rate for the organisation by grade. Prevalence by grade is not expected to vary much over the 15-year period; therefore, average prevalence would be an appropriate benchmark (Njobe and Smith 2004).

The total cost to the employer will be computed using the average prevalence rate. Note that hostel dwellers will not be considered as a separate grade but will be treated as such in this model because their risk of HIV infection is much higher than that of employees living with their families.

The number of employees infected in the organisation by grade level would be computed from the average prevalence (Njobe and Smith 2004).

The number of employees would be based on permanent workers. The quantitative analysis would not include costs attributed to infection rates among contract workers (Njobe and Smith 2004).

Expected Results

Distribution of Costs: The bulk of the costs would be expected to be incurred at the lower grade levels (Njobe and Smith 2004). These costs would contribute to over half the total costs. It would also be expected that the proportion of total costs by grade would decline with increasing grade level.

Cost escalation: The nature of the AIDS epidemic is such that the direct costs to the employer increase per employee infected, by an amount that is directly proportional to the earnings of that employee (Njobe and Smith 2004). There is no declining rate of increase in total costs as infected rates rise.

Demographics: Workforce demographics, specifically age and gender, influence prevalence rates, which in turn drive costs (Njobe and Smith 2004). It would be expected that HIV infection rates at "Company X" would be typically highest in the 20–39 age group, in accordance with the national population of South Africa.

HIV infection is expected to be higher among male employees than women at "Company X". HIV/AIDS among the male workforce is expected to have higher cost implications to the business.

Implications

With higher prevalence among lower grades, the costs contribute to over half of the total costs. This indicates that notwithstanding significantly lower costs per employee at this level, the prevalence rates are high enough to inflate costs to a level that far exceeds costs at higher grades, where the per employee cost is significantly higher (Njobe and Smith 2004).

Infection rates of nearly 6% at the skilled level which includes professional staff raises concern about the loss of specialised skills at "Company X". Unlike the financial and industrial sectors, these skills are not easily replaceable making the cost of AIDS at these levels even higher than can be estimated. Similarly, the expectation that the skill level among management is even more highly specialised, highlights the vulnerability of the sector to losing intellectual capital that is scarce and, no doubt, difficult to replace.

Workforce demographics, specifically age and gender, influence prevalence rates, which in turn drive costs. Among the general population HIV infection rates are typically highest in the 20–39 age group. A similar trend is expected at "Company X", whereby this age group is the most severely affected by HIV/AIDS. The implications to the organisation are that productivity is compromised, and this adds to the cost to the company.

The gender composition of workforce is also a determinant of prevalence. HIV infection is believed to be higher among men in workforces than women. The higher proportion of men to women at "Company X" increases vulnerability to high prevalence rates and hence higher costs.

Since the majority of our employees are migrant labour forces, the conditions in which these labourers reside perpetuate behaviours, which exacerbate the spread of HIV/AIDS. The hostel situations attract commercial sex-workers and drive the spread of HIV/AIDS. These labourers then become the conduit through which HIV is transmitted back to their communities.

"Company X" has embarked on vigorous educational programmes to inform employees of the dangers of HIV. However, these education programmes must not only be limited to employees but must be extended to the community at large as these will be the communities where the particular organisation is most likely to recruit new staff members.

With HIV/AIDS prevalence rates among South African workforce estimated at nearly 15% in 2001, business vulnerability to increased costs from the disease is unquestionable. In recent years, company assessments of the impact of HIV/AIDS among workforces have revealed prevalence rates of 3 to 33%. This implies the cost impacts will vary by business and sector, largely driven by prevalence rates and the size of the workforce. At these levels of infection, there is no question that it is in the interest of South African businesses to assess their vulnerability to the cost implications of HIV/AIDS. This is particularly important since HIV/AIDS affects the production input that gives them their competitive advantage – human capital (Njobe and Smith 2004).

As the infection rate for the workforce are higher than for the population as a whole, the labour force will be disproportionately affected by the epidemic (Van den Heever 2002).

Conclusion

The hypothesis provides that HIV/AIDS will have a significantly negative impact on the cost to the company's business.

Workforce size matters with HIV/AIDS costs. Therefore, larger workforces like in "Company X" imply higher costs. The quantitative costs present one level of vulnerability to business. However, these future costs are based on existing and future levels of HIV prevalence. Little is known about the latter and, at best, companies such as ours can use forecasts of prevalence to estimate costs (Njobe and Smith 2004).

Given that costs of HIV/AIDS to business do not increase at a declining rate as more employees become infected, companies such as ours (that is, "Company X") are better off developing interventions to address the epidemic among their workforce. Stigma is a significant driver in exacerbating the spread of HIV/AIDS. Business can therefore play a role in reducing stigma through various initiatives including knowledge awareness and prevention programmes, voluntary counselling and testing, and treatment care and support programmes through private health insurers, or onsite HIV/AIDS clinics (Ellis and Terwin 2004). Workplace prevention programmes are significantly less costly than the costs incurred through absenteeism, lost productivity, benefit pay-outs and turnover (Njobe and Smith 2004).

Provision of ART to extend the lives of sick employees is an intervention option available to business and has been shown to be cost-effective (Njobe and Smith 2004).

While the provision of antiretroviral therapy (ART) to employees is viewed as the ultimate HIV/AIDS intervention for businesses, it raises the question of whether the benefit should be extended to dependents of employees. Evidently this has cost implications for business regardless of whether ART is provided through an in-house company clinic or private medical care. Studies have shown that in cases where ART was not provided to dependents, employees share their dosage with spouses and other family members. This is detrimental to the effectiveness of ART, as 95% adherence level is required to prevent against the build-up of resistance. This puts both the employee and the dependent at risk of building up resistance (Njobe and Smith 2004).

5.7.14 Community Mobilisation

Community Mobilisation on HIV/AIDS Intervention

HIV/AIDS is giving organisations and communities new challenges. It is of utmost importance that all people should be mobilised against HIV/AIDS. This means that one must look beyond only the world of work but look at the environment where workers come from. The battle should not only be fought in the workplace, but also the communities where the workers come from.

The purpose of this section is to develop a community mobilisation project on HIV/AIDS intervention in the Lubombo District, in Southern Africa.

Planning session with the community:

It is worth mentioning upfront that the Lubombo District Council elected NGO-X as the catalyst given its experience in the field of HIV/AIDS and in its networks in the community. Therefore, NGO-X will be coordinating the community mobilisation project in the Lubombo District.

Firstly, it is crucial to begin with basic planning steps that will help give the assessment specific goals and objectives to be met.

The community mobilisation project will be approached from multi-sectoral coordination at district level. A group will be gathered together, those who will do the assessment and those who have some knowledge or interest in prevention activities and/or the community. The gathering would involve Non-Governmental Organisations (NGOs) and Religious organisations, District Council (Sectoral services), The Community leaders and other community representatives including People living with HIV/AIDS. At this meeting, the project team will be selected, and the big question would be determined.

Each participant should write down on post-it notes or cards areas that she/he would be interested in exploring. Every idea should be written on one card and each card should have an idea. At this stage, participants should not be limited on what they want to know, they must just write it down.

The participants will share their ideas by taping or attaching them to a wall or a large sheet of paper. If an idea is already posted, similar ideas should be taped or pasted over the top of the previous one.

Participants should then discuss what they see on the board. After the discussion, each can vote on one to three areas to explore. The top three to four areas can then be used as points for discussion on how to do the exploration. The group can do this immediately after deciding on topic areas, if the participants have already looked through the manual and are familiar with some of the concepts in it, or they can take time to choose methods that would best answer the questions and come back together to decide.

Each topic should be listed together with a general idea as to how to address it, including an estimate of the amount of time the group thinks it will take; barriers/obstacles to doing the investigation and why it would be important to address this particular topic. After that, the group can prioritise by using one of the ranking exercises, or by simply taking a vote or coming to consensus.

Once the questions have been determined, the project form for community-based assessment will be filled out. This form is intended to assist in planning the community assessment.

Therefore, based on the project form, the following information would be generated:

Team members: X, Y, Z, A, B, C, D, E, F, G, H, I, J, and K.

Goal for completion: 01/12/2020.

1. The Big Questions:

   A. What are the factors behind relapse from safer sex?
   B. What do men trust for information and support?
   C. What do men know about HIV and other sexually transmitted infections?

2. Defining the population: Men, above 15 years of age, who are sexually active. All ethnicities.
3. Goals and Objectives:

   A. To engage in a meaningful dialogue with communities about gender, sexuality and HIV/AIDS vulnerability in order to promote change in community norms.
   B. To promote behaviour change for HIV/AIDS prevention.
   C. To strengthen community capacity to deal with HIV/AIDS-related psychosocial problems.

4. Data collection methods: Community mapping
5. Observation sites:

A. Geographic description of area (boundaries, etc.): The present study focuses on the community mobilisation project in the district of Lubombo, which is the main feeder area for the major industries along the north coast of KwaZulu-Natal. The project covers five chiefdoms, reaching out to a population of some 50,000 people living in the town of Mbazwana and in villages near the town.
B. Anticipated observation sites (e.g., bars, parks, etc.): Sexually transmitted disease clinics.

6. Individual interviews (estimated): 500

   A. Purposeful sampling plan: Extreme case sampling
   B. Characteristics of participants: Men who practise safer sex consistently; Men who used to practise safer sex but do not anymore.
   C. To be completed by 30 October 2020.

1. Focus group interviews:

   A. Number of groups (estimated): 10
   B. Purposeful sampling plan: Extreme case sampling
   C. Characteristics of participants: Men who practise safer sex consistently; Men who used to practise safer sex but do not anymore.
   D. To be completed by 15 November 2020.

Specific steps will be followed to implement community identification:

Step 1: Defining and Describing the Population. The goal for this step is to organise knowledge of the Lubombo district population. Write down everything that is known about the target population, with a goal of developing the population taxonomy – a listing, defining, and categorising of all segments of the population.
Step 2: Survey of internal knowledge. Step two involves finding out what other staff members know about the Lubombo district population. This is especially helpful because some of the temporary staff is not directly on the project team. To save time, this shall be done in a group session.

Here, there is expansion on the information learned in step one, furthering understanding of the target population. Areas of interest in this stage are: a description of the population, ways to access, ways to enhance access/eliminate barriers, locations for potential interventions, perceived risk, actual risk, factors for risk, referrals to gatekeepers and informal networks within the population, internal resources, and other outside groups operating within/serving the population.

These internal knowledge interviews will be carried out until no new references within our own systems are obtained (that is, redundancy is reached in the network), and all indicated staff have been interviewed. After each interview or short series of interviews the supervisor will debrief the interviewer. The focus of this interaction is on interview content, context of the interview, responsiveness of the interviewee, clarity of response, and interview completeness. The purpose of these debriefings is to obtain information not spontaneously reported and to sharpen observation, interviewing, reporting, and debriefing skill in preparation for future steps.

Step 3: Summary of Internal Knowledge. Now, one will organise what one has learned. Begin to identify patterns. Piece the elements together, paying particular attention to individuals identified as members of the target population. It should be possible at this stage to begin making an actual geographic map of where segments of the population can be found. It would be good to set aside space to plaster the walls with all the information collected, including any maps.

Step 4: Creating an External Knowledge Base. Now it is time to get out of the office and access other sources of information identified as relating to the Lubombo district population. There are three categories of information sources:

(a) Materials – any items that deal with the population or segments of the population including books, videos, articles, reports, etc.
(b) Systems people with knowledge of the population – These people would include members of service agencies and community-based organisations providing services to the Lubombo district population, law enforcement, judicial systems, healthcare providers, etc.
(c) Interactors who are not part of formal systems or part of the population itself – This would include such people as shopkeepers, taxi drivers, hotel clerks, bus drivers, etc.

All non-interview material available shall be collected and reviewed, realising that this collection may continue throughout the remainder of this process. If more than one person at any given agency is identified as being knowledgeable on the community, a group interview shall be conducted. List all the names mentioned in association with the Lubombo district population and keep track of how many times they are mentioned. The people named numerous times may be key information sources. The saturation point would have been reached when the other systems or interactor persons to whom the investigators are referred are people with whom the investigators have already spoken and information begins to be repeated – no new information is being gained. The forms used for interviews at this stage are the same as those used in the "Big Questions" as indicated earlier (that is, Project Form for Community Assessment). Debriefings are continued in this step.

Step 5: Integration and Refinement. There will be new pieces of the puzzle to add, and there will be discrepancies that will warrant further research. This is a good sign. It is better to identify problem areas now instead of tackling them after an outreach programme has started.

See where strengths and weaknesses are in the information collected so far. What areas of the puzzle are blank? Has there been identification of access points into the community for the next stage of the process? If not, what has kept this from happening? There is need to constantly challenge the reliability and validity of the information that is received. This is still an etic perspective so far.

Step 6: Gatekeeper Interviews. In step 2 and 4, respondents may have mentioned people that serve as intermediaries into the target population. In this step, these individuals shall be interviewed. Again, beginning to work in areas where the population exists, it is important to approach each person with a reference to the person who referred the investigators to them.

This is a critical phase. Often, gatekeepers can serve as access points into the community. Gaining their trust and respect can make or break our program. It is important to familiarise them with the project and its goals. Try to let them know that they are a significant part of the plan or programme. How this first interaction is handles is vital to the success of the rest of the programme. It will be like "feeling each other out" and establishing the trust relationships that are necessary. These gatekeepers may be the project's most valuable supporters. Remember to follow through on the leads provided at this stage. This will be testing in many ways and this ability to follow through will be one form of testing one's sincerity and consistency. There is no need to skimp at this stage. There must be the time to do it well.

If conducting gatekeeper interviews in areas where the actual intervention may take place, observations will begin to be made. As one enters and leaves the area, one will keep notes on what is seen and heard. It must be remembered to assume an attitude of complete ignorance and never to assume one has an idea of what is valuable. Each time one returns to the office, one will immediately conduct a debriefing on observations made. One must get into this practice! Create an actual written and narrative picture of what was seen on that trip and add this to the records. Pay attention to the details of the site and subtle nuances of behaviour. This helps with understanding networks and mobility or access patterns.

Step 7: Observation. This step can actually take place along the previous one. Now, one needs to devote time to nothing but observations of the sites where interventions may take place. No matter what one does, one must expect to draw attention to oneself now. This attention can be good if one handles it well. Let the people that one will be contacting see one and get used to one's presence. One must go out at all times of the day, and all days of the week, so that one will get a complete picture of the activity that takes place.

Step 8: It is time again to meet with the project staff and look at all the information collected. It should be possible to create a very accurate and full description of the target population.

It is important to look for gaps in the information collected so that these can be filled. Also, it is time to start seeing what the information tells about interventions concerns. Are the reasons for intervening still valid? Is an intervention possible? Can the community mobilise to help? What are all the components needed to make the intervention work?

Can several agencies form cooperative efforts? As these questions begin to be asked, the second phase of the process is entered. This is the initial creation of an intervention programme.

Step 9: Individual Interviews. Finally, the emic perspective is reached where the Lubombo district population is directly interviewed. For a programme that is true to the needs of its clients, this is the most important step of all. Who is the target population? What are the informal networks that they have established? What are their concerns and needs? What do they know or not know about these issues in question? These and other questions are what one asks as one holds these interviews. Conduct the interviews in a group format or individually. This is another one of those critical areas where the interviewer simply must not be stingy. This must be given time to conduct as many interviews as possible using both the individual and group approaches.

Step 10: As one proceeds through the Community Identification steps, summative statements about information obtained in each step should be created. It is requested to complete the summation for each step before undertaking the next step. After the internal analysis is completed, all subsequent summative steps are developed individually and then integrated with the preceding summative information. This results in an evolving etic picture of the entire risk population.

For each of the segments identified within the risk population, a narrative is developed, which includes at a minimum: Estimates of the number of individuals in the target population; Specific locations where members of the target population may be found; Barriers to accessing members of the Lubombo district population; How to access members of the Lubombo district for individual interviews; Values of the Lubombo district population as currently known (these could change or be based on conjecture depending on information then currently available); General trends that appeared in the information for this target population; Respondents' approaches to interventions;

Anomalous information obtained and how it has been accounted for in the data reduction.

For the key participant interviews (KPI), interviews with those with a great deal of knowledge about the population, a new analysis scheme is offered that includes specific information about working with the interview data. The KPI analysis can include such issues as (du Toit and Freeman 2002): demographics of the population, mobility of the population, daily activities and relationship patterns, drug and needle behaviour, sexual behaviour, condom information and use, use of and comfort with health care services, and intervention-related information.

Results

Communities have generally welcomed the opportunity to discuss gender and sexuality issues, which they have rarely had the chance to do before. But there have been gender differences in their reactions (International HIV/AIDS Alliance 2003).

Women have usually responded well to the discussions of gender inequalities, but men have been more resistant. By contrast, it is men who have been more open than women in talking about issues of sexuality. However, women have become more open as they have learned to trust NGO-X and the value of talking about these issues directly.

Community leaders have varied in their reactions to NGO-X's work on gender and sexuality. Some chiefs and religious leaders have supported the work while others have been more resistant. The strong relationships which already exist between community leaders and NGO-X have proved very helpful to the work.

As community members themselves, staff have also had their own reactions to using the tools. Some have been uncomfortable in using the tools which deal more directly with issues of sexuality. It is clear that building people's capacity to use such tools and do this work must also involve helping people to think about and discuss their own attitudes and values (International HIV/AIDS Alliance 2003).

There are a number of reported changes as a result of the gender and sexuality tools being used. These changes have not been formally evaluated and are, of course, influenced by many factors besides the work of NGO-X. But there are reasons to believe that NGO-X's use of the gender and sexuality tools is having an impact on changes that are already underway within communities in Lubombo district. These changes include:

A greater acceptance of the fact that young people are having sex and more and more willingness to talk about their sexuality. Young people seem more realistic about the risks of HIV infection, as indicated by an increased demand for condoms from youth-friendly corners and more young people coming for information about VCT/HTS and HIV/AIDS from the resource centre. Some of the young men among the peer educators are saying that they no longer feel entitled to sex from young women and were accepting of the women's right to say no (International HIV/AIDS Alliance 2003).

Some changes in gender role, as indicated by a greater reported sharing of household tasks and family responsibilities between husbands and wives. The silence that used to surround men's violence against women is being broken. People are more willing to talk about this violence, and there are signs of an increased willingness to report such violence (International HIV/AIDS Alliance 2003).

A greater openness in talking about sex, as indicated by some married couples reporting that they are communicating more openly about sex and now have a better understanding of their own and their partner's sexual pleasure. Women in the community are also saying that they are now more able to refuse sex if they do not want it. There are still problems, however, in women being unable to talk openly about their own sexual desires. This may be changing for married women, but unmarried women continue to be stigmatised if they propose sex to their boyfriends. Men's sense of entitlement to sex seems to be changing slowly, and both women and men say that men are showing more respect for women's wishes and rights (International HIV/AIDS Alliance 2003).

Discussion

Discussing gender and sexuality can bring up many sensitive issues. So, when the tools are used with groups of adults or young people, NGO-X staff and peer educators try to create a relaxed and safe atmosphere. Sometimes, this is done by working with men and women separately, or by dividing the group according to marital status or age. It is important to make these discussions relevant to the community concerns.

Starting discussions about gender and sexuality issues with communities can lead to controversy and conflict. It is essential to create and maintain strong relationships with formal and informal community leaders in order to get their support and reduce resistance to the work. This includes explaining carefully, and continually, why this work is important and what it involves (International HIV/AIDS Alliance 2003).

Men can be resistant to certain aspects of this work, especially in relation to issues of gender equality. But this resistance lessened when they could see facilitators practising what they were preaching. It also became clear that talking about sexual satisfaction was a good way to get men interested in the discussion, and that it was important to target the most resistant men (International HIV/AIDS Alliance 2003).

It is important to 'practise what we preach'. Organisational policies and culture must reflect the gender equality work that the organisation is doing. NGO-X staff felt that one of the reasons they had been effective in this work was the quality of relations between men and women on the staff (International HIV/AIDS Alliance 2003).

Building the capacity of staff and peer educators to use the tools requires attention to both skills and attitudes. Skills in group facilitation and talking about sensitive issues are needed. But facilitating discussions of gender and sexuality issues also challenges staff and peer educators in terms of their own attitudes and values. It is important to create opportunities and support for them to reflect on and discuss these attitudes and values (International HIV/AIDS Alliance 2003).

It is helpful to target this work at pre-existing groups in the community in order to improve the continuity and intensity of the work (International HIV/AIDS Alliance 2003). NGO-X faced difficulties in being able to work intensively with a single group of people over a period of time using a sequence of tools. It was often unable to control who came to its community group meetings, meaning that there was little continuity in group membership from week to week. Better targeting of this work at community groups with a consistent membership would help to improve continuity and enable more intensive work to be done using a sequence of tools (International HIV/AIDS Alliance 2003).

Regular supervision and follow-up are critical to maintain quality of work (International HIV/AIDS Alliance 2003). It was observed that regular supervision of peer educators and follow-up visits to them 'in the field' played a critical role in monitoring and maintaining the quality of their work. These follow-up visits were also important in maintaining key relationships with community leaders and their support for the work.

Conclusion

In this study, the main goals and objectives were achieved, and they included conducting a meaningful dialogue with communities about gender, sexuality and HIV/AIDS vulnerability in order to promote change in community norms; promoting behaviour change for HIV/AIDS prevention; and strengthening community capacity to deal with HIV/AIDS-related psychosocial problems in the Lubombo district, through the use of community mobilisation techniques and tools.

When communities decide on behaviour change actions, they will address needed actions for women, men, and youth. Besides, they will decide on actions that will create a more supportive environment for behaviour change in their own community (Schapink et al. 2000).

It is generally accepted that a true community-based initiative is one in which local people will say, "We did it ourselves." The assessment and planning of an initiative must take into account the need for community feelings of ownership to be created. This may require more resources or simply more time than is necessary to meet the technical requirements of the initiative; it may also require better communications with community opinion-makers or informal leaders.

Therefore, creating collective responsibility is of paramount importance when it comes to community mobilisation.

An organisation's Use of the Community Mobilisation Manual in Fight against HIV/AIDS

The purpose of this paper is to determine how an organisation can successfully use the community mobilisation manual in its fight against HIV/AIDS to identify new projects.

In the manual, there are various methods of learning about a community, whether it is using snowball sampling to disseminate a survey or employing visual techniques to understand community attitudes and barriers to change. There are also tools here for the educator to assess what participants know about issues related to HIV and STIs in general. Other methods use problem-solving activities so that a prevention team can develop the most effective ways to change risk-taking behaviour in partnership with the affected communities.

Using these techniques can give credibility to what you know, taking it beyond merely anecdote. Exploring issues this way allows HIV prevention workers to separate out what may be based on a chance encounter with someone engaging in a certain practice from the practices that are common in the community. In this manner, prevention workers can determine what intervention strategies are necessary to target the behaviours that are truly a problem in a given community. Systematic assessment may also help to convince funders that resources need to be dedicated to solving the problems identified, or to justify the amount of time being spent on addressing the issues that were heard while doing the work.

One important thing to keep in mind is that assessment is not just a process of finding out needs. It should also be a way to find out about the community's assets – what are the strengths, talents, and/or resources that the community holds? Another way of looking at this is to examine community resilience, "the capacity of an individual (or group or community) to withstand negative influences and/or to bounce back after experiencing adversity" (du Toit and Freeman 2002).

The foregoing process is intended as a step-by-step guide to what is called "community-based assessment." It defines community-based assessment as a way to examine the community's HIV prevention workers encounter in their work. It starts with setting up the basic questions the assessment team wants to address, then gives them several alternatives to choose from that best fit why they are trying to find out.

There are two broad ways to gather information. One is to understand how common something is – for example by using a questionnaire – and another is to understand why something is occurring. A questionnaire filled out by enough people can answer the questions, "How many people are doing this?" or "How many people believe this way?" But questionnaires are not the only methods of understanding all the factors behind why a community is doing something or why they think the way they do. Understanding some of the dimensions of behaviours can often be accomplished using other techniques. And these same techniques, when carried out as a first step, can help with developing a survey so that the most relevant questions are asked.

5.7.15 *AIM-B: AIDS Impact Model for Business*

Using the AIM-B Model to Explain the Impact of HIV/AIDS on a Company

According to van den Heever (2002), a Business Day article announced dramatically as follows: "Almost 9% of SA's highly skilled labour force and about 19% of skilled workers are expected to be HIV-positive by 2015, slowing the country's economic growth by worsening the skills shortage. This is according to the research reported by ING Barings on the effects of the AIDS epidemic on the SA economy. … For every 100 normal deaths in the same year, 88 highly skilled workers and 176 skilled workers will die of AIDS. A further 308 semi- and unskilled workers will die for every 100 normal deaths. … Although the number of the latter is far greater, the cost of supporting and replacing a highly skilled worker suffering from HIV/AIDS will be far greater than those who are semi- or unskilled."

An important question arising from the above is: what do we actually know and understand about the impact of HIV/AIDS on the workplace?

In recent years a number of studies have attempted the complex task of estimating the potential impact of HIV/AIDS on South Africa's economy. The result has been a wide variety of results derived from a sometimes quite different assumptions and methodologies (Van den Heever 2002).

The AIDS Impact Model for Business (AIM-B) is an economic and demographic model designed to help managers analyse how HIV/AIDS is affecting their businesses and project how it will affect them in the future (USAID 2010). The benefit of the AIM-B Model is the utilisation of strategic planning processes to improve health and wellbeing of communities (USAID 2010). The process effectively integrates both quantitative and qualitative data for decision-making.

This simplified on-line version of AIM-B estimates the main direct costs of HIV/AIDS in health, recruitment and benefit costs (USAID 2010). It does not estimate the epidemic's effect on productivity, labour relations, workforce morale or absenteeism. The objective of this section is to employ the AIM-B Model to explain what impact HIV/AIDS will have on Company-X. For the purpose of this discussion, the entire workforce of the company will be taken into consideration.

How to use AIM-B

This model is designed to help human resources managers and medical personnel assess the effects of HIV/AIDS on particular sections of the workforce.

The model works by calculating averages within particular groups of employees. You many choose to input data for the entire workforce within a particular country. However, wage levels, benefits and recruitment costs often vary greatly between different sections of the workforce so you may prefer to calculate averages within particular sub-sections, such as mangers, skilled workers or unskilled workers (du Toit 2008a, b).

You may find it necessary to repeat AIM-B several times for different groups of employees until you build up a complete picture of HIV/AIDS impact on your workforce.

You will have to go to the internet and do this exercise while you are online. It will be handy to gather the information before you connect because that way you will spend less time on the internet. Follow the following steps (du Toit 2008a, b):

Gather all the following information:

How many of your employees may be infected with HIV?

This section asks you to estimate how many people within a particular group of employees are likely to be infected with HIV. For the purposes of this paper, the group will be the entire workforce at Company-X.

You may have some indication of prevalence in your workforce from company records or local research. If not, the pull-down list gives the averages within particular countries. These averages are based on UNAIDS estimated from 1999 and apply to the general population aged 15–49. It is important to note that prevalence within particular workforce may differ from that found within the population as a whole.

You are then asked for the average annual salary of the workers in the chosen group.

Recruitment costs

As HIV-positive workers become sick and die, the costs of finding and recruiting new staff will begin to escalate. This section asks you to think about how much it costs to recruit a new employee. Your estimate should include:

Cost of advertising for new staff
Agency fees (if appropriate)
Administration
Staff time spent selecting and interviewing candidates
'Down-time', when the vacancy is not filled
Administration to fill the post
Training costs

Once recruited, how much does it cost to train new employees? Your estimate may include some or all the following:

Fees to external trainers
Associated costs (travel, lodging, hire venue, etc.)
Lost output during training (note: include lost output for trainers/supervisors as well as trainers)
Death benefits

What is the total cost to the employer when an employee dies? Your estimate may include some of the following:

Death benefits payable to the deceased's family
Funeral costs
Transport to the funeral for workers and their families
Compassionate leave for co-workers
Transport of the body to the family home
Health care

What do you estimate is the current additional cost to the company of health care per individual HIV-positive worker? You may know this from your existing records. If not, you could develop a broad estimate by calculating the costs of treating a package of two or three opportunistic infections, such as TB.

If employees are covered by health insurance, you may either leave this section blank or input any additional contributions or surcharges you would be expected to make. You should be aware that companies may have to pay an increased rate for insurance that includes treatment of HIV-related illnesses. The cost of health insurance generally will also increase as HIV/AIDS prevalence increases.

If you do not have this information, leave it blank, the model will still make other projections without this information.

Once you have all the information, connect to the site at: http://www.futuresgroup.com/aim/
Now follow the steps. Once you have entered the information go to *Continue*
The impact on the workforce at Company-X

The staff complement is 5600, and 1400 (25%) are female and 4200 (75%) are male.

Responses

5600 are in the group to be analysed
R201 600,000 is the average annual salary of this group
15 is the percentage of the workforce which is estimated to be infected with HIV
R358 056 is the total cost of recruiting a new worker
R50 128 is the total cost of training a new worker
R15 000 is the total cost of death benefits
R20 000 is the additional cost of health care per AIDS case

Calculation of HIV Infection and Annual Number of New AIDS cases.

Estimated number of HIV-positive employees	840
Estimated number of employees presenting symptoms of AIDS per year	82
Cost of health care	R3 280,000
Productivity losses	R4 756,000
Cost of death benefits	R225 000
Cost of training and recruitment	R6 122,760
Annual cost to company-X	R14 383,760

It is evident that the effect that HIV/AIDS will have on the core business of Company-X will be adverse. Firstly, the operational cost will increase dramatically, and the cost of health care will increase. It is estimated that one-sixth of the staff compliment is HIV-positive, and this relates to 840 HIV-positive employees. This will have adverse effects on the morale, absenteeism and productivity of the company and these factors will continue to have an impact of the delivery of services in Company-X. Citing UNAIDS the life expectancy of persons with HIV is currently 59 years. With the onset of the disease, a person's life expectancy would be reduced to between 39–49 years. Cost for health and death benefits would escalate by 300%. The cost for training would also escalate (Classen-Hoskins 2005).

Recruitment cost

Recruitment in Company-X over the past three years has been attracting the youth (20–35 years). The disease would have the greatest impact on the young adults who are in their productive years of their lives. As the HIV-positive workers become sick, temporary staff would be needed ore the recruitment of new staff. For entry-level posts, Company-X would normally first advertise internally. Therefore, cost for advertising in local media, such as newspapers would be reduced substantially. Agency and administration fees would be minimised. With the entry posts, normally, preference is given to school leavers who can be trained to do various administrative roles. But for the more skilled occupational categories such as accountants, economists, engineers, health practitioners and other professions, the criteria for entry is different as they need to have minimal qualifications in their specific occupations.

Based on the AIM calculation it is estimated that 840 employees will be HIV-positive. This represents 20% of the age group 20–29 and 15% of the total staff. It is further estimated that 82 employees will be presenting with the symptoms of AIDS per year. The cost of health care was previously R20 000 but will increase to R3 280,000. Here death benefits would include time off for other staff members to attend funerals, memorial services and just time spent arranging some of the mentioned events. Productivity losses would cost R4 756,000. This would be both direct and indirect productivity losses.

The age structure of the labour force will change – the proportion of young people will increase, which reduces the average experience and productivity of the labour force (Van den Heever 2002). In situations where important skills are in short supply, the loss of skilled workers will have a strongly negative impact on productivity (Van den Heever 2002).

In conclusion, the objective of this discussion was to employ the AIM-B Model to explain the impact of HIV and AIDS on Company-X. HIV/AIDS will have an increasing impact on businesses. One of its first impacts is that it increases operational costs. As employees become sick the cost of providing health care rises. Death benefits increase, and recruiting and training costs grow, as the company tries to replace lost personnel. At the same time, it reduces company income by lowering worker productivity and increasing absenteeism.

Uncontrolled, HIV/AIDS will also damage businesses in ways that are harder to quantify. One of the epidemic's most damaging features is its impact on morale. HIV/AIDS usually affects people who are young. Watching numbers of colleagues die before their time is depressing and difficult. Often, workers are afraid of colleagues who are infected, not least because they fear they too might be infected by it. The result is an atmosphere of tension, suspicion and recrimination within the workplace. This loss in morale is not, however inevitable (du Toit 2008a, b).

Overall, it appears as though HIV/AIDS has had the largest impact on labour productivity, worker absenteeism, followed by employee benefit costs at Company-X. Company-X is also experiencing higher labour turnover rates, lost experience and skills and higher recruitment and training costs due to the epidemic, but these seem to be slightly less concerning than the impact of the epidemic on productivity and employee benefit costs. HIV/AIDS related illnesses and deaths are clearly taking their toll on the labour force in Company-X.

From a provincial perspective, companies such as Company-X, which are located in KwaZulu-Natal appear to be the worst affected by the epidemic.

The global spread of the AIDS epidemic and increasing evidence of the economic impact of HIV/AIDS has highlighted the need for business to take action against the epidemic. Although Company-X has stepped up the challenge, the results from the AIM-B Model show that there is still more work to be done.

AIDS-related illnesses and deaths of managers, employees and their family members will have a significant impact on business. It is expected that companies such Company-X will need to increase their contributions to pension, life, disability and medical benefits on account of the AIDS epidemic.

Should Company-X succeed in restructuring their risk benefits so that employees carry a larger share of the responsibility, a proportion of the direct costs of HIV/AIDS will be absorbed by employees who will have to increase their own benefit contributions (and hence reduce their personal savings or expenditure on other consumer products and services), accept lower benefits or opt out of schemes altogether.

Finally, to try and estimate the exact impact and costs is no easy task. The difficulty arises in part because prediction of the disease itself is fraught with known and unexpected difficulties. Nonetheless, it is a task worth considering and pursuing urgently. The information shall not only support the management of business enterprises, it will also guide national and regional policies in mounting the necessary responses and fostering sustained economic growth and social development (Tawfik and Kinoti 2003).

In order to avoid huge costs spent on recruitment of new staff, death benefits and health care, serious interventions should be made with regard to prevention of further spread of the disease. Company-X should have the following four elements in their programme:

Prevention Strategy

A prevention strategy that includes awareness campaigns among staff and also their families. It would be futile if only the staff members benefit from the awareness campaigns but not their partners or their children (Classen-Hoskins 2005). Therefore, Company-X should venture into an integrated and multifaceted approach. This implies that all the stakeholders that have dealings with Company-X, including clients, labour supply agencies, and the greater community of the north-coast of KwaZulu-Natal, which is the main feeder area for Company-X, should also be involved.

The prevention strategy should include awareness campaigns on sexually transmitted infections (STIs) and tuberculosis (TB) infections. Behaviour change, health promotion, food security and HIV testing and services (HTS) should also be key areas of focus in the prevention strategy.

Wellness Management Strategy

A broad approach which integrates HIV/AIDS and health and wellness should be implemented. A health and wellness programme could also address issues such as disability, gender equity, disease management and also the implementation of an employee assistance programme (Classen-Hoskins 2005). An on-site wellness centre could be established which will focus on primary health care, occupational health care, and rehabilitation.

Management Strategies

Management strategies to deal with the direct and indirect cost of HIV and AIDS are critical as this will give managers a broader understanding of how resources should be allocated and how an integrated approach can be introduced through proper resource allocation. HIV and AIDS should form part of the core business strategy of Company-X.

The first step would be to include everyone in the strategy (unions, management, supervisors and team leaders, wellness champions and employees). Reviving the HIV and AIDS committee and modifying all managers and committee members job descriptions to include roles relating to HIV and AIDS responsibilities. A holistic approach should be noted by including the families of staff members into the awareness programmes.

Management, unions and the committee members should be held accountable and responsible for regular feedback and also serve as an advisory committee. They should also be able to understand the adverse effect of the especially in the workplace (Classen-Hoskins 2005). Supporting the communities where the workers come from, would be of great benefit to Company-X, in the sense that it would have a dualistic effect, because the employees, their families and larger population in the particular community will be empowered on the subject of HIV and AIDS.

A periodic impact assessment should be done to ensure short- and long-term planning for both budgetary and human resource related issues. Budgetary aspects would include calculating direct cost of absenteeism and sick leave, medical cost, disability and ill health retirement, pension and dependent benefits and funeral costs. Human resource costs such as replacement, recruitment, reduced productivity and training should not be ignored (Classen-Hoskins 2005).

Partnership Strategy

Partnership will always be an important link in the management of HIV and AIDS in the workplace. Partners have various links to other resources and expertise in the field and this expertise can aid in organisations where limited and scarce resources need to be utilised (Classen-Hoskins 2005).

5.7.16 Strategic Human Resource Management in the Context of HIV/AIDS

Formulating a Strategic Approach for HIV/AIDS Management

Introduction

When a pandemic like HIV/AIDS impacts on society, it is inevitable that the business community and all the institutions within that community will be adversely affected. In this regard, it is imperative that the leadership of these businesses and institutions make a commitment to confront the pandemic through the implementation of an integrated response strategy (Manser 2005).

Therefore, the purpose of this section of the paper is to formulate a strategic approach for Hospital Z regarding the management of HIV/AIDS.

Discussion

The following discussion spells out the vision, objectives, practices and approach for Hospital Z regarding the management of HIV/AIDS. It also refers to the use of the balanced scorecard, KAP studies and the Human Resource Management Rapid Assessment Tool for HIV/AIDS Environments, to evaluate the effectiveness of the programme.

Vision: To manage the impact of HIV/AIDS on Hospital Z, to enable the institution to remain globally competitive for the benefit of shareholders, employees and South Africa.

Objectives:

To prevent more employees from becoming infected with HIV

To extend the lives of those infected for as long as possible to the benefit of the company and society at large

To establish a workplace free from discrimination and stigmatisation

To ensure the impact of HIV/AIDS on the hospital is managed to enable Hospital Z to grow and contribute to South Africa's developing economy

Best Practices:

The workplace programme at Hospital Z should address the following: leadership and management, prevention and awareness programmes, as well as care and support programmes.

Leadership and Management Framework

The leadership and policy framework should consist of (Sampson 2004):

- Top management, including the board, executive committee and Chief Executive of Hospital Z should take complete ownership of the HIV and AIDS problem to get results.
- HIV and AIDS management structure – functional HIV and AIDS manager in the human resources management department, HIV and AIDS Committee, support groups and social dialogue sessions
- HIV and AIDS policy, in accordance with the International (ILO and ISO) and National Code of Practice/Conduct, including information management and the confidentiality thereof
- HIV and AIDS strategy – HIV and AIDS determinant identification and risk assessment, mitigation and management (goals, objectives, targets, plans, implementation strategies, monitoring and evaluation of conformance methods)
- HIV and AIDS audit system to determine compliance with the organisational strategy and the impact of HIV and AIDS on the organisation
- Appropriate HIV and AIDS information management system (including documentation control)
- Updated HIV and AIDS-related legal and other requirements
- Conditions of Service to benefit employees living with HIV and AIDS – reflecting reasonable accommodation of access to benefits, such as opportunities for rest breaks, time off for medical appointments, flexible sick leave, part-time work and return-to-work programmes
- Appropriate HIV and AIDS-related workplace procedures
- Appropriate risk management programmes for occupational and non-occupational exposures (proactive, continuous and reactive)
- Appropriate communication structures and strategies
- Research programmes and/or the support thereof
- Annual reporting, in accordance with the principles of corporate governance – nature and extent of strategy, plan and policies adopted to address and manage the potential impact of HIV and AIDS on the hospital's activities
- HIV and AIDS management system review

Prevention and Awareness Programmes

Prevention and awareness programmes for Hospital Z focus on the following (Sampson 2004):

- Education and awareness programmes in the workplace, utilising the models for Science Education for New Civic Engagements and Responsibilities (SENCER)
- Skill development programmes to ensure competence in prevention, mitigation and management of HIV and AIDS in the workplace
- Participatory education programmes, referred to as Peer Group Education
- Programmes to facilitate behavioural change
- Condom distribution
- HIV testing services (HTS) programmes, crucial to all employees who should be encouraged to use testing services to determine their status in a context of informed consent, confidentiality and non-discrimination

Care and Support Programmes

Care and support programmes in the workplace should focus on at least the following (Sampson 2004):

- Wellness management, such as Employee Assistance Programme for employees living with HIV and AIDS, including psychosocial support
- Access to treatment and drugs, both therapeutic and palliative, such as antiretroviral therapy and treatment for opportunistic infections and Sexually Transmitted Infections (STIs)
- Nutritional support for People Living with HIV (PLHIV)

Approach:

Hospital Z acknowledges the seriousness of the HIV and AIDS; seeks to minimise the economic and developmental consequences to the institution and its employees, and commits itself to providing resources, training, education, support and leadership to implement an HIV and AIDS and STI programme in the workplace.

Hospital Z affirms that:

- HIV and AIDS programme will be implemented and maintained in consultation with employees and employee representatives and will be reviewed from time to time.
- HIV and AIDS is a shared responsibility by the employer and employees
- Employees living with HIV and AIDS have the same rights and obligations as all employees and will be protected against all forms of discrimination
- The hospital will assume a non-judgemental position
- HIV status will not constitute a reason to preclude any person from employment or participation in any benefits unless there are known compliance issues

Current employees who contract the virus while in the employ of Hospital Z and are concomitantly unable to effect their work, must be dealt with in the appropriate manner consistent with the recommended procedures for any employee who becomes unfit for whatever reason. Where an employee gets to a point where early ill-health retirement must be considered, it will be done in accordance with current practice or procedures (Global Business Coalition on HIV/AIDS (GBC) 2005).

The process of temporarily removing an employee from his/her post to an alternative post due to disability caused by HIV/AIDS will always be done in consultation with the relevant employee and/or trade union representing the employee. Where it becomes necessary to remove the employee permanently from his/her job due to HIV/AIDS or any related disability, Human Resources will effect the redeployment of employees in consultation with the employee and his/her trade union representative. There will be no exceptions to the rule. All reasonable endeavours will be made to redeploy such an employee for as long as possible (Global Business Coalition on HIV/AIDS (GBC) 2005).

People living with HIV/AIDS will fall under the normal rules of the Benefit Schemes. These may or may not have exclusions or specific rules for medical conditions, including HIV/AIDS. With that in mind, the hospital should create a viable non-discriminatory approach to benefits, such as medical aid and health-related benefits, pension, housing and bursaries, training and study subsidies (Global Business Coalition on HIV/AIDS (GBC) 2005).

Employees living with HIV/AIDS will be allowed to work for as long as they are reasonably capable of performing a full day's work. The institution will conduct regular analyses in order to understand the evolving epidemic and how it will impact on the future of the hospital, its structure, operations and functions (Global Business Coalition on HIV/AIDS (GBC) 2005).

The hospital will at all times endeavour to create a work environment conducive for employees to disclose their HIV status. However, the rights of each employee will always precede any disclosure made by any employee.

The hospital is committed to ensure a holistic wellness programme to interlink with the HIV/AIDS programme. A wellness strategy will be put in place.

Evaluation of the HIV and AIDS Programme

Monitoring and evaluation of the effectiveness of the HIV and AIDS programme at Hospital Z will occur by means of criteria stipulated in the Balanced Score Card, such as (Government of Malaysia 2001):

- The number of employees that have attended HIV and AIDS Education and Training
- The targets achieved with regard to HIV testing services (HTS)
- The completion of surveillance reports such as KAP (Knowledge, Attitudes and Practices) Survey and Prevalence Assessments, and
- Enrolment onto the disease management programme

The Human Resource Management Rapid Assessment Tool for HIV/AIDS Environments is another tool that could possibly be used to evaluate the effectiveness of the Hospital's HIV and AIDS programme. The Human Resource Management Rapid Assessment Toll for HIV/AIDS Environments is an adaptation of Management Sciences for Health (MSH's) Human Resource Management Assessment Tool that health managers can use to assess both their organisation's Human Resource Management (HRM) system in general and their HRM policy and practice in response to the impact of HIV/AIDS on the workforce. In particular, they can strengthen their capacity to (Management Sciences for Health 2003):

- Develop adequate human resource plans
- Strengthen retention and recruitment of staff
- Minimise the rate of infection among the healthcare workers
- Improve overall organisational morale and performance
- Adapt human resource strategies to changing service delivery needs

Conclusion

The context of the forgoing discussion was elucidated focusing on the vision, objectives, practices, and approach for the strategic management of HIV and AIDS at Hospital Z. It also referred to the evaluation of the effectiveness of the HIV and AIDS Programme, using the balanced scorecard, KAP studies and the Human Resource Management Rapid Assessment Tool for HIV/AIDS Environments.

It can be concluded that an HIV and AIDS strategy should be integrated into the overall business strategy of the organisation, in order for it to be effective and sustainable. In this regard, top management of the organisation should take complete ownership of the HIV and AIDS programme.

Work Analysis and Work Design in Identifying the most Critical Jobs

Introduction

The purpose of this paper is to describe how one would utilise the notions of work (job) analysis and work design in identifying the most critical jobs in Hospital Z.

Job analysis is such an important activity to Human Resources managers that it has been called the building block of everything that personnel, does. This statement refers to the fact that almost every human resource management program requires some type of information that is gleaned from job analysis: selection, performance appraisal, training and development, job evaluation, career planning, work design, and human resource redesign, and human resource planning (Muller et al. 2006).

Job analysis and job design are interrelated. Job analysis refers to the process of getting detailed information about jobs. Job design is the process of defining how work will be performed and the tasks that will be required in a given job (Muller et al. 2006).

Discussion

The development of guidelines for the identification of critical jobs, which are core to the business, is one of the major outcomes of an institutional audit. The identification of these positions will assist in targeting them for specific risk-reduction strategies, including recruitment, training manpower and succession-planning strategies.

The starting point in the process of critical job identification is the definition of the business objectives for all operations. It is out of the business objectives that the critical paths are derived, together with their functions (UNAIDS 2002).

The actual identification of critical jobs starts with categorisation of all the organisational functions into the three broad groups, as follows (UNAIDS 2002):

Important functions – those that are operationally necessary for the efficient running of the organisation;
Essential functions – those that provide service support or are a legal requirement in an operation; and
Critical functions – those that are core to the critical path of the business process.

To qualify for criticality, functions are subject to a 'critical job selection instrument'. This is the first stage of the test. The instrument involves three questions, as follows (UNAIDS 2002):

Does the function have a high potential to:

- Stop production?
- Disrupt the production process?
- Have an impact on the quality of the product?

If the answer is 'yes' to at least one of the above questions, the job qualifies as critical (UNAIDS 2002).

The above could also be achieved by using the various methods for analysing jobs and there is no "one best way." These methods include the following: the position analysis questionnaire, the task analysis inventory, and the job analysis system (Noe et al. 2008).

For the purpose of a focussed discussion, only the position analysis questionnaire (PAQ) method will be described because it is one of the broadest and most well-researched instruments for analysing jobs. Moreover, its emphasis on inputs, processes, relationships, and outputs is consistent with the work-flow analysis approach.

The PAQ is a standardised job analysis questionnaire containing 194 items. These items represent work behaviours, work conditions, and job characteristics that can be generalised across a wide variety of jobs. They would be organised into six sections (Noe et al. 2008):

- *Information input* – Where and how a worker gets information needed to perform the job.
- *Mental processes* – The reasoning, decision making, planning, and information processing activities that are involved in performing the job.
- *Work output* – The physical activities, tools, and devices used by the worker to perform the job.
- *Relationships with other persons* – The relationships with other people required in performing the job.
- *Job context* – The physical and social contexts where the work is performed.

- *Other characteristics* – The activities, conditions, and characteristics other than those previously described that are relevant to the job.

The job analyst would be asked to determine whether each item applies to the job being analysed. The analyst would then rate the item on six scales: extent of use, amount of time, importance to the job, possibility of occurrence, applicability, and special code (special rating scales used with a particular item). These ratings would be submitted to the PAQ headquarters, where a computer program will generate a report regarding the job's scores on the job dimensions. This may assist in identifying the critical jobs in the organisation (Noe et al. 2008).

So far, the focus has been on understanding what gets done, how it gets done, and the skills that are required to get it done. Although this is necessary, it is a very static view of jobs, in that jobs must already exist and that they are already assumed to be structured in the one best way. However, a manager may often be faced with a situation in which the work unit does not yet exist, requiring jobs within the work unit to be designed from scratch. Sometimes, workloads within an existing work unit are increased, or work group size is decreased while the same workload is required, a trend increasingly observed with the movement toward downsizing. Finally, sometimes the work is not being performed in the most efficient manner. In these cases, a manager may decide to change the way that work is done in order for the work unit to perform more effectively and efficiently. This requires redesigning the existing jobs (Muller et al. 2006).

Research has identified four basic approaches that have been used among the various disciplines that have dealt with job design issues. Although these four approaches comprehensively capture the historical approaches to this topic, one still needs to go below the category level to get a full appreciation of the exact nature of jobs and how they can be changed. All jobs can be characterised in terms of how they fare according to each approach, thus a manger needs to understand the trade-offs of emphasising one approach over another. The work design questionnaire (WDQ), a specific instrument that reliably measures these and other job design characteristics is available for use by companies wishing to comprehensively assess their jobs on these dimensions (Noe et al. 2008).

The last step would be to test for the level of criticality with an understanding that all the jobs that passed the above test were critical but did not necessarily have the level of criticality. In addition to being used for the identification of critical jobs, the job analysis and job design instruments mentioned above could also be of relevance in determining the level of criticality of the identified jobs. A 'post evaluation form' with some predetermined critical factors could be used for this purpose. Each of the critical factors would be multiplied by a 'recovery time weighting', which is the degree to which it is difficult to resume normal duty when people performing that particular duty are away. The level of criticality of the jobs would be the summation of the product of critical factors and the recovery time weightings (UNAIDS 2002).

Conclusion

The foregoing discussion has highlighted how the notions of job analysis and job design would be utilised in identifying the most critical jobs at Hospital Z. It can be concluded that using the instruments of job analysis (such as the Position Analysis Questionnaire) and job design (such as the Work Design Questionnaire) could assist in identifying the most critical jobs in an organisation. A manager needs to understand the trade-offs of emphasising one approach over another, in order to weigh the level of criticality of the identified critical jobs.

It is important to note that all jobs in an organisation are required; most of them are important and some are a legal requirement. The critical jobs are core to the business objectives, and they can only be found in the determined critical paths. However, for an organisation to run efficiently the critical jobs alone are insufficient, and important and essential jobs are necessary to give a complete and functional organisational picture (UNAIDS 2002).

Importance and Necessity of an Institutional Audit

Introduction

The purpose of this paper is to discuss the importance of an institutional audit and the necessity of such an audit in the management of human resource planning, recruitment and selection and placement.

For most senior managers, the questions that they have to address in the face of HIV/AIDS epidemic seem very straightforward (UNAIDS 2002):

- What is the effect of this disease?
- How do we measure it?
- What can we do about it?

Their natural tendency is to adopt an accountancy approach, using either the wage bill or operating profit as the main indicator of impact. But the impact of HIV/AIDS on an organisation is too complex to be considered only in these terms. In addition to the bottom line, HIV/AIDS affects, among other elements, staff morale, public perceptions of the organisation, institutional memory, labour relations, and the community in which the organisation is situated (UNAIDS 2002).

Discussion

The importance and necessity of an institutional audit in the management of human resource planning, recruitment and selection and placement will be discussed with reference to the components of the audit that form a series of linked steps in the process.

An institutional audit is important because it is considerably broader than the accountancy approach and enables the organisation to respond to potential impact on a wider front. An institutional audit consists of the following components that form a series of linked steps in the process (UNAIDS 2002):

- Personnel profiling
- Critical post analysis

- Assessment of organisational characteristics
- Estimate of organisational liabilities
- Productivity
- Organisational context

Each of these steps is examined in turn.

Step1: Personnel profiling: What kinds of people are employed? This question is addressed in relation to two sub-questions: which groups among employees are most likely to be susceptible to infection? What different skill levels exist in the organisation; what are their characteristics and what is their strategic importance to the organisation (UNAIDS 2002)?

This is important and necessary in the context of the management of human resource planning. Human resource planning is concerned with systematically reviewing human resource requirements to ensure that the required number of employees with the required skills is available when needed. It is the process of matching the internal and external supply of people with job openings anticipated in the organisation over a specified period of time (Muller et al. 2006).

Personnel profiling will also assist in the development of human resource goals and objectives in line with the strategic business goals. Effective human resource planning considers change from both long- and short-term perspectives, corresponding with the typical cycles for business planning, always keeping in mind the strategic vision, mission and goals (Muller et al. 2006).

Step 2: Critical post analysis: Are there key personnel whom it will be particularly difficult to replace, and on whom a production or administrative process depends (UNAIDS 2002)?

This is very important in the management of human resource planning; specifically, in terms of succession planning to ensure that the 'institutional memory' is not lost should the key personnel decide to leave the organisation.

Step 3: Organisational characteristics: Size of organisation and flexibility of employees.

This would be critical to the human resource manager in the sense that it would allow him/her to assess the following in the context of the management of human resource planning, recruitment and selection and placement (UNAIDS 2002):

- How easy it would be to replace or retrain within the organisation?
- Are there sufficient people to allow for internal training?
- Should the organisation introduce 'shadowing' of key employees (i.e. employ an additional staff member for every critical post)?
- Does it have sufficient internal resources to be able to undertake replacement and/or training or replacement of personnel?
- Is it big enough to move people around to take over other people's jobs?
- What is the lead time for training or recruiting a replacement for different skill levels?

Step 4: Liabilities: The potential or actual liability of an organisation will be determined by the level and type of employee benefits and/or the level of labour value added (UNAIDS 2002).

There is relevance of this point to the management of human resource recruitment and selection and placement, in terms of the contracts of employment and the benefits package for permanent employees. The level of labour value added to the organisation could be influenced by the type and quality of casual labour recruited, selected and placed.

Step 5: Productivity: There may be a reduction in the quality of labour supply by employees who are sick or are caring for sick dependants. Absenteeism may result in a slow and barely detectable decline in output in any organisation. How is this going to be detected and managed (UNAIDS 2002)?

This is relevant in the context of human resource planning and recruitment and selection and placement. The human resource manager may have to consider recruiting larger numbers of casual labour to replace people who are sick or have died. The question is, could larger numbers of unskilled workers replace the lost skilled workers? It may be a possible solution to outsource non-core functions or to consider multi-skilling staff enabling them to do their own and others' jobs, should the situation demand it (UNAIDS 2002).

Step 6: Organisational context:

What is the legislative and industrial relations framework?

What must an organisation do for its workers in the way of invalidity benefit, keeping them at work while they are HIV-positive but are not ill, or when they have AIDS but are not too sick to work (UNAIDS 2002)?

This is important in the context of managing human resource planning, recruitment and placement. The company commits to the principle of non-discrimination, and as such, prospective employees will not be required to undergo an HIV test as part of the recruitment process. Furthermore, employees living with HIV/AIDS will fall under the normal rules of the Benefit Schemes. These may or may not have exclusions or specific rules for medical conditions, including HIV/AIDS. The rules of the scheme will always take precedence. Employees living with HIV/AIDS will be allowed to work for as long as they are reasonably capable of performing a full day's work.

Conclusion

The foregoing discussion highlights the importance of an institutional audit and the necessity of such an audit in the management of human resource planning, recruitment and selection and placement. Although an institutional audit may use some of the techniques of accountancy or economics, its concerns are much broader than these.

Restructuring of Employee Benefits

Introduction

The purpose of this paper is to determine if it is necessary to revise and restructure employee benefits to reduce HIV/AIDS-related impact on the organisation, and to establish what revision/restructuring to recommend.

Discussion

Managing benefits and costs is one of the five key areas to mitigate the effects of HIV/AIDS on the workforces. Benefits provided to public service employees have been a lasting attraction to the work. For many organisations, HIV/AIDS has made providing these benefits more difficult and expensive. Suggesting even small changes in benefit packages can lead to strong employee opposition or support. Engaging employee representatives early in the process is important (Rau 2004).

The following revision/restructuring would be recommended (Rau 2004):

- Encouraging early retirement of chronically ill employees
- Restructuring sick leave to limit the time an employee can be away from the job
- Expanding compassionate leave for women and men who are caregivers for people living with HIV/AIDS
- Designated guidelines for funeral attendance
- Consolidating medical aid schemes into a single scheme and defining the types of services to be provided and methods of cost sharing
- Providing bereavement counselling and legal assistance for affected employees
- Adding or increasing the co-payment borne by employees for medical treatment and drugs.

One other decision to be made is whether to cover the costs of antiretroviral drugs for employees and perhaps dependants (Rau 2004). People living with HIV/AIDS should fall under the normal rules of the Benefit Schemes. These may or may not have exclusions or specific rules for medical conditions, including HIV/AIDS. The rules of the scheme should always take precedence.

Employees' benefits may be significantly affected by HIV/AIDS claims. Such benefits should be structured to take cognisance of the disease, thus avoiding conflicting and inequitable situations arising in the future or different benefit packages existing for various classes of employees.

Conclusion

It can be concluded from the foregoing discussion that it is necessary to revise and restructure employee benefits to reduce HIV/AIDS-related impact on the organisation. With that in mind, the company should create a viable non-discriminatory approach to benefits, such as medical aid and health related benefits, pension, housing and bursaries, training and subsidies.

Debswana's Important Steps in the Development of their HIV/AIDS Strategy
Introduction

The purpose of this paper is to use Debswana as a case study and to point out the most important steps in the development of their HIV/AIDS strategy.

Discussion

It was vital that top management of Debswana took complete ownership of the HIV/AIDS problem. The commitment to the process at all levels of the company was also particularly important to ensure that the institutional audit's findings were implemented effectively. The best way to ensure that a company 'owns' the results of the audit is for company personnel to undertake the work rather than management merely commissioning a report by outside consultants. This was particularly clear in the case of Debswana where the collection and analysis of information involved widespread participation by people throughout the company. This meant that when the audit revealed particular problems (for example, in relation to the company's Management Information Systems); the rationale for change was widely understood among middle-level management (UNAIDS 2002).

The institutional audit was quite important because it was this audit that identified the need to develop a separate strategy on HIV/AIDS in order to give the issue the attention it deserved. The process of carrying out a HIV/AIDS audit is almost as important as the results. In some cases, the process may be even more important than the outcome to the extent that organisational managers could not tackle the problems identified unless they had undertaken the audit together. Thus, the audit itself has important educational and team-building functions (UNAIDS 2002).

It was important that Debswana was able to adopt a generous policy towards antiretroviral drugs because the proximity of South Africa meant that the attendant costs were less than they would have been had the company been operating in a less favourable and less well-endowed environment. In practice, Debswana has been able to outsource antiretroviral treatment and supervision to the private sector in South Africa. Because of its size and influence, the company has also been able to negotiate good drug prices with some major pharmaceutical companies (UNAIDS 2002).

Another important step was the stakeholder engagement in order to evaluate the effectiveness of the strategy. It is worth mentioning that a company does not operate in isolation; it needs to look at its relationship with other companies, the government and the community and to consider how its decisions with regard to a HIV/AIDS response affect, and are affected by the wider environment (UNAIDS 2002).

Conclusion

The foregoing discussion highlights the most important steps in the development of Debswana's HIV/AIDS strategy. It can be concluded that the most important steps, include: top management taking complete ownership of the HIV/AIDS problem; widespread commitment at all levels of the company; the institutional audit;

generous policy towards ARVs; and stakeholder engagement in order to evaluate the effectiveness of the HIV/AIDS strategy.

Incentivising Employees Who Stay HIV Negative
Introduction

"What if we told you that if you stayed HIV negative for 20 years, we'd give you a BMW? Would it make a difference? We wouldn't care how you approached it – safe sex, monogamy, abstinence – you'd just need to stay negative" (McNally 2008).

The purpose of this paper is to discuss the possibility of incentivising employees to stay (or be) HIV negative.

Discussion

The premise of the following discussion is that it is possible to incentivise employees to stay HIV negative.

Charles Maisel is willing to stand outside clinics with handfuls of hard cash to give guys an incentive to get tested for HIV. He reckons that this is the cheapest and most effective way to grab the epidemic by the balls. The car is part of a lottery for long-term subscribers, but cash rewards are the backbone of Maisel's social marketing project to revolutionise the health system (McNally 2008).

Fresh notes crisp from an ATM is how he reckons HIV figures can be tipped back to how they were in the Seventies. He has a grant from overseas to pay unemployed men ZAR75 to get tested for HIV. After six months, if you're still negative, you get another R75. Another six months, another ZAR75. And so on (McNally 2008).

It means you can buy 18 loaves of bread or five cafe lattes, depending on your priorities. The catch is, if you're HIV positive the second time then you don't get the cash or the prizes. Maisel reckons from tests he's done so far that this simple reward system works. The question is, is it moral? Besides that, can ZAR75 (a labourer's daily wage) keep a man doing what massive billboard advertising has failed to do? What would be your price to change your habits and stay healthy? (McNally 2008).

He reasons that men, when deliberating over safer sex, are more likely to latch on to a tangible ZAR75 than the prospect of life or death. "We've got a welfare mentality of giving money to people who are HIV positive rather than rewarding people for staying negative," Maisel says. This he sees as the main crux of what needs to change – at least to start with (McNally 2008).

What most guys obsess about is work and money (how many hours they had to work for how much reward). So, to attach HIV to this ubiquitous, heavily discussed topic means these men in turn can talk more easily about the pitfalls of unprotected sex. It turns the taboo into a standard topic for discussion (McNally 2008).

Ironically, this is where behaviour is discussed and can be changed – and it's nowhere near a bed or a woman. Here in the cold, the mantra goes that a bit of money is better than nothing (McNally 2008).

As for the wads of cash Maisel needs as incentives, overseas investors are crucial because local groups are turned off by the concept. European investors have an approach that the cost is minimal compare to how expensive someone's drain becomes once they are HIV positive (from the drugs to other possible infections).

Maisel says the first question critics ask is: "What about the men once they turn positive?" And the answer is: "that's not our problem." It's a scheme dealing with incentivising people to stay HIV negative (McNally 2008).

The terrifying aspect of this study is it shows people know how to practise safe sex – or rather they understand that they could get AIDS and die – but need an extra push to commit. In this case, money. The education has sunk in but it's still not changing behaviour – without the cash, that is (McNally 2008).

Maisel's scheme hinges on exploiting what motivates us. "There are extrinsic and intrinsic motivators, explains Men's Health specialist psychology editor Rafiq Lockat – one based on other people's input and another based in personal pride. Here an extrinsic motivator is being applied, and hoping it gathers enough momentum, so, the person develops an internal motivation of what's "sensible" and no longer needs the money (McNally 2008).

The problem is the hierarchy of motivators. "Sex is primarily (along with food and water) while money is secondary," says Lockat. But sex tends to be satisfied quickly and once it's over you lose interest, while money, because it can be traded for literally anything, can hold our interest in unique ways (McNally 2008).

Maisel believes that the incentive of money is worth a shot, because the HIV situation has reached a point where we should be trying anything we can. "We know incentives work, but they have to be of sufficient scale to get people to change their behaviour," says Discovery's head of HIV strategy, Elaine McKay (McNally 2008).

Conclusion

It can be concluded from the foregoing discussion that it is possible to incentivise employees to stay HIV- negative.

Our messaging has to change to incorporate the fact that HIV infection is now much more of a lifelong, incurable, but still treatable disease, and that has implications about what the incentives are for staying negative, now that treatment is there (McElligott 2004).

5.7.17 Social Responsibility of Companies

Evaluating the Corporate Social Investment Response of a Company

Corporate Social Investment looks at what the business is doing for the community. Does the business work with the community to fix outstanding issues and social problems? How much of an investment does it make? What issues are they addressing? To what depth are the problems that they are working to fix? Are they trying to fix major issues? Is the problem they are working on fixing a large social problem with far-reaching consequences? Or is the problem a localised one that is area specific?

In his book From Corporate Social Investing: The breakthrough strategy for giving and getting corporate contributions (1998) Curt Weeden suggests certain steps to be taken when implementing a Corporate Social Responsibility Management Plan (du Toit 2008a, b).

The purpose of this paper is to evaluate the Corporate Social Investment (CSI) response of an organisation, using the Ten-Step Corporate Social Investment Management Model formulated by Curt Weeden.

Step 1:

In the first step Weeden suggests that traditional notions of corporate philanthropy should be replaced with a broader concept called corporate social investing (Weeden 1998). This implies that business should realise that by investing in society they are not engaging in welfare but in actual investment, for if the society has better living standards and education it will grow to a consumer society (du Toit 2008a, b).

The particular organisation (which is one of the major transport and logistics organisations in Southern Africa, with five operating divisions), has recently gone through a turnaround strategy. In terms of the new strategy, the organisation's Foundation is to lead the organisation's philanthropic activities whilst the operating divisions focus on strategic social investments (in other words, those activities that directly support each division's focus area).

Corporate Social Investment is viewed as an integral part of the organisation's business plan and a substantial contributor to the welfare of the people of South Africa. The organisation's real contribution to society is to stay in business, for it is when all are successful that the whole community benefits. The organisation's Corporate Social Investment seeks to use the resources and activities of the company – in the spirit of good corporate citizenship – for the social benefit of all South Africans. Hence the payoff line: "Positively touching the lives of all South Africans."

To illustrate this point, over the past year, the particular organisation's Health Train brought health and hope to thousands of rural South Africans in need of access to healthcare facilities. This 16-coach train with its 19 resident staff members, fondly known as the 'miracle train,' carries the most modern medical equipment on board. During the year it made 36 stops in four provinces. The train, with its highly committed, experienced staff and state of the art medical facilities, is now a training institution that is highly sought after by medical students. In June 2008, the pioneering work of the health train in bringing public services to poor communities was recognised with the United Nations Public Service Award for its excellence in public service delivery.

Based on Weeden's first step, it is evident that the particular organisation has not completely replaced the traditional notions of corporate philanthropy with a broader concept called corporate social investing; instead the particular organisation has decided to have both the traditional notion of philanthropy and the concept of corporate social investing running parallel to each other.

However, the bigger picture is that in hindsight the particular organisation does realise that by investing in society they are not engaging in welfare but in actual investment, for if the society have better living standards, better health and education it will grow to a consumer society. Therefore, the particular organisation's CSI approach is not far off from Weeden's first step.

Step 2:

In the second step the company should identify a significant business reason for every Corporate Social Investment and obtain as much business value from social investments as is allowable and practical. This would force companies to do a thorough research of where Corporate Social Investment is needed, but also to think how the company can benefit.

As a state enterprise, the particular organisation has a CSI programme whose initiatives are tied to the national goals of our primary shareholder, the government. Its unique position allows the Foundation to help the government achieve its goals faster through a grass-roots approach and quick mobilisation of resources. The particular organisation's CSI interventions are divided into five portfolio areas: education, health, arts and culture, under-utilised assets and sport.

Other than helping the government to achieve its goals faster, the particular organisation has not necessarily identified a significant business reason for every Corporate Social Investment. However, the recent turnaround or transformation that the organisation has just gone through, has allowed the particular organisation to reflect on a better way of engaging in Corporate Social Investment. Prior to the turnaround strategy, all the organisation's Corporate Social Investment activities were carried out by the Foundation.

As part of the new five-year corporate strategy, it has been decided that the Foundation is to lead the particular organisation's philanthropic activities whilst the operating divisions focus on strategic social investment. It is therefore expected that each of the operating business units will have identified a significant business reason for every Corporate Social Investment.

A highlight for the organisation's education focus was the Sharp Minds! Get Ahead in Life (Maths, Science, English and Technology) learner and educator programme initiated a few years ago. The project aims to build a sustainable stream of well educated, science, technology and engineering talent nationally, from which the organisation can recruit resources. While the Sharp Minds! Programme serves as an active intervention in the lives of both the learners and educators alike, it also addresses the critical skills shortage in the country.

Step 3:

In the third step Corporate Social Investment should be limited to non-profit organisations and exclusively public institutions.

The particular organisation's Corporate Social Investment is mainly targeted at rural communities. The particular organisation has recognised and acted on the need for critical intervention in rural and peri-urban areas where the needs are the greatest but yet the least support is currently provided. By putting the infrastructure in place, the particular organisation assists communities to access resources and therefore empower themselves socio-economically. The organisation supports projects in a vast number of isolated and less known communities.

Whether it is interventions in education, health, arts and culture, under-utilised assets and sport, our Corporate Social Investment is limited to non-profit and exclusively public institutions. Therefore, the particular organisation's Corporate Social Investment programme is in agreement with Weeden's third step mentioned above.

Step 4:

In the fourth step an open statement should be made that endorses corporate social investing or supports a broader concept that allows for social investing to be developed. Once this is done the company should however realise that this accompanies accountability. Once they have made an open statement the public can hold them accountable.

A statement that endorses corporate Social Investment has been made through various reports including the internet that our Corporate Social Investment strategy seeks to use the resources, and activities of the company – in the spirit of good corporate citizenship – for the social benefit of all South Africans. Hence our payoff line: 'Positively touching the lives of all South Africans.' Therefore, the public can hold the particular organisation accountable for that statement, especially with regard to corporate governance.

Step 5:

In the fifth step a clear message should be sent to employees and other stakeholders that the CEO endorses corporate social investing. It should also be taken into account that critique against corporate social investment are that companies are often so focused on corporate social investment and on publicity that accompanies this that they neglect their own workforce.

There is a message to employees and other stakeholders that our CEO endorses Corporate Social Investment. However, one has to admit that this message is not clear to all employees and other stakeholders, because there is no proper communication about it, except that it is found in the organisation's annual report.

The message is that the particular organisation's Corporate Social Investment initiatives are driven by the need to plough back into our communities, in particular our employee community. Several major projects are directed at employees, such as the Internal Choir Competition, which enjoys the support of over 2000 employees. Furthermore, it is recognised that increased employee involvement in projects has the potential to make a difference in their communities. Therefore, the Corporate Social Investment programme aims at encouraging employees to serve in a number of hands-on ways, including providing time, skills and expertise.

Perhaps, the only improvement required is to ensure that a clear message is sent to new recruits when they are inducted, and that the broader concept of Corporate Social.

Investment and the CEO's endorsement of it should be explained and communicated more often to all employees and other stakeholders.

From my perspective, the main danger is that statements issued through reports without follow-through with proper communication and implementation often end up collecting dust on the shelves, and they are often not clearly explained to employees and other stakeholders. Very often, employees and other stakeholders see activities happening, without being aware that these were endorsed by the CEO.

Step 6:

In the sixth step is to produce a written corporate social investment report that includes a review of social investments at least once a year. Even more important however is that the review should be evaluated, for quite often companies are involved in corporate social investment without doing the necessary research beforehand which might lead to investment in society where it is not needed most or most efficiently.

The particular organisation does produce a written corporate social investment report that includes a review of social investments at least once a year. In this report each of the five portfolio areas (that is, education, health, arts and culture, underutilised assets and sport) are well discussed and evaluated.

The organisation has established and is refining an evaluation and monitoring system which assists to gather information on the progress of projects and to make informed decisions regarding our Corporate Social Investment activities. The organisation is also in the initial stages of establishing a six-monthly provincial report to highlight how its Corporate Social Investment has contributed towards the organisation's overall strategy. Staff members regularly visit projects and keep in touch with beneficiaries. This adds the human touch as well as forming part of the benchmarking process to improve the Corporate Social Investment programme performance and to achieve the goal of creating a world-class Corporate Social Investment programme with 'best –in-class' initiatives.

Based on the foregoing explanation, the organisation's Corporate Social Investment is in agreement with Weeden's sixth step mentioned above.

Step7:

The seventh step is to commit now or by a specified date at least 2.5% (3.5% for manufacturing corporations that donate product) of an average of a company's last three years of pre-tax profits for corporate social investing.

The organisation commits a specific amount for corporate social investment during the budget month of October. The combined annual Corporate Social Investment budgets are greater than R100 million, with the bulk of this being spent through the Foundation.

The ZAR120 million committed for Corporate Social Investment for the current financial year far exceeds the 2.5% suggested in Weeden's seventh step. In fact, the organisation has committed approximately 10% of its pre-tax profits for Corporate Social Investing.

Therefore, the organisation's contribution for Corporate Social Investment exceeds the minimum of 2.5% by nearly 8%.

Step 8:

In the eighth step it should be suggested that some or all social investing should be postponed if projected business conditions warrant such action.

Over the past two years, the organisation has postponed social investing in the School of Excellence, as projected business conditions warranted such action. The conditions and management of the school was in a very bad shape and pouring money into such an institution did not make business sense. However, work to revive the School of Excellence has now been started. Simultaneously, the organisation, the founding donor and partner of the school, together with the South African Football Association, recently launched a maintenance programme aimed at improving the facilities, to make them conducive for learning for the stars of tomorrow.

Therefore, in agreement with Weeden's eighth step, it was suggested that some of the social investing should be postponed because projected business conditions warranted such action, as highlighted in the School of Excellence scenario mentioned above.

Step 9:

In the ninth step, influential line and staff leaders should be locked in as co-owners of the corporate social investment program. It should, however, be noted that there is often great discrepancy between the attitude of senior executives and that of their middle and lower management. To improve acceptance of corporate social investment initiatives, it is beneficial to include middle managers in the administration and formulation of policy.

Recognising the organisation's Foundation's mission to play a major role in the organisation's core business, senior management is deeply involved in guiding the strategic activities of the Corporate Social Investment programme. For line managers at all levels, up to the Chairman and the Group Chief Executive Officer, the Corporate Social Investment programme is welcomed and supported as a vital contributor to both the business and the community. Project launches are regularly officiated by high-ranking corporate representatives.

In agreement with Weeden's ninth step, it is therefore recognised in the organisation that influential line and staff leaders should be locked in as co-owners of the Corporate Social Investment programme. However, the only concern could be the non-involvement of middle managers in the administration and formulation of policy.

Step 10:

The last step is that day-to-day management responsibility should be assigned for corporate social investing to a position that is no more than one executive away from the Chief Executive Officer or Chief Operations Officer.

In one's organisation, the day-to-day management responsibility for Corporate Social Investment is assigned to the Executive Communication Manager of each operating division. The Executive Communications Manager is only one position away from the Chief Executive Officer.

However, there could be some teething problems and standardisation confusion across the organisation based on the organisation's new strategy that the organisation's Foundation is to lead the organisation's philanthropic activities whilst the operating divisions focus on strategic social investments. Having the philanthropic activities running parallel with the strategic social investment activities could pose a challenge in terms of the day-to-day management responsibility.

In the past (over many years) Corporate Social Investment was the key function of the organisation's Foundation. Therefore, handing over some of the functions including on-going projects to the operating divisions could create challenges of sustainability or continuity. Whilst the Foundation was very established regarding the day-to-day social responsibility, the operating divisions still need to adapt to their new social investment role.

Although on paper, the day-to-day management responsibility for Corporate Social Investment in the organisation is in agreement with Weeden's last step mentioned above, the newly appointed Executive Communications Managers for the operating divisions still need to adapt to their new Corporate Social Investment responsibility and ensure that the high standard is maintained and that the programme is sustainable.

The foregoing discussion evaluated the Corporate Social Investment of the organisation, using the Ten-Step Corporate Social Investment Management Model suggested by Curt Weeden. The evaluation indicates that nearly all aspects of the organisation's Corporate Social Investment are in agreement with the Ten-Steps suggested by Weeden.

However, it has to be emphasised that for Corporate Social Investing to be efficient there needs to be an awareness of what Corporate Social Investing requires and how it is implemented. Sustainability of the Corporate Social Investment programme is important, especially as part of the new business strategy of the organisation.

Involvement of companies in supporting HIV/AIDS programmes as part of CSI.

Social responsibility is an ethical or ideological theory that an entity whether it is a government, corporation, organisation or individual has a responsibility to society but this responsibility can be "negative" in that it is a responsibility to refrain from acting (resistance stance) or it can be "positive," meaning there is a responsibility to act (proactive stance).

Various definitions of Corporate Social Responsibility exist which display diversity of philosophical starting points, objectives and end results. After all, each business is trying to reach different goals. However, there are four areas that should be measured no matter what the outcome that is needed. Those measures are Economic function, Quality of life, Social investment and Problem solving. Social investment looks at what the business is doing for the community.

Taking into consideration the theory of Corporate Social Responsibility, the purpose of this paper is to explain why it is important for organisations to be involved in supporting HIV/AIDS programmes in organisations and communities, from a Corporate Social Investment (CSI) angle.

The involvement of organisations (especially the private sector) in the battle against HIV/AIDS cuts to the heart of Corporate Social Responsibility.

HIV/AIDS is arguably the greatest health crisis the modern world has ever faced. In the worst affected countries, one in four adults are now affected. More than 80% of people dying of HIV/AIDS are in their 20s. The disease is hollowing out economies and leaving entire communities composed only of the very young and very old.

As a result, within 20 years the total workforce in 15 of the worst-affected countries will have shrunk by 24 million. And already the total costs incurred are estimated at some $500 billion. And since it affects all, it is the responsibility of all to participate in this battle, with the kind of resources that are available (du Toit 2008a, b).

That is why AIDS is an issue which is ripe for a new form of public/private partnership stretching from the global level right down to individual communities. But this need for a dynamic new business response is not restricted to HIV/AIDS: the same is true for many of the other challenges faced by companies striving to be good corporate citizens in today's world. And responding effectively demands a new vision of global corporate social responsibility.

Businesses see themselves as part of a broader societal response to HIV/AIDS. Governments, non-governmental organisations (NGOs), unions, and business associations have expertise and skills in tackling the virus from which businesses can benefit. Businesses, particularly where governments lack the financial and human capacity to cope with the problem alone, have skills and funds to help plug the gap. Many of the most effective business HIV/AIDS policies have been developed in conjunction with public sector partners – there is rarely a need to go it alone (World Economic Forum 2005).

The challenge is now for corporations to move to the frontline of trying to help countries build more effective states that focus on reducing risk, providing stability and supporting human development of their citizens. And that means, using Corporate Social Responsibility interventions to strengthen rather than substitute for government capacity in areas like HIV/AIDS.

While local, community-focused projects still have a place, the real way forward for corporate social responsibility is broader public-private partnerships that confront these bigger issues across global networks and devote more energy and resources to cross-cutting social and economic issues such as HIV/AIDS. That is the best way for companies that operate everywhere but are strangers in most countries to build up a reputation as good citizens in a global neighbourhood (du Toit 2008a, b).

There is tremendous scope for more coherent and committed business support for the issue of development in general. Business needs to be at the forefront of the challenge.

That is also why joint action between governments, international agencies, civil society and business to tackle HIV/AIDS more effectively is so important. And the organisation is not operating in a vacuum. Already many businesses have undertaken innovative schemes that are paying real dividends: Anglo-American has begun exploring direct purchase of AIDS drugs for its employees in Southern Africa. Merck and the Bill and Melinda Gates Foundation have joined in an unusual public-private venture to channel $100 million in aid over a period of five years to Botswana (du Toit 2008a, b).

But, however encouraging these initiatives are, they are only the tip of the iceberg of what can and should be done. And while exact interventions will vary by company and country, there are three broad areas where real impact can be made (du Toit 2008a, b).

First is advocacy – being prepared as business leaders directly to address the issue of AIDS in public and private forums and using the organisation's communications operations to spread the message. Such statements not only help break the silence and stigma that is still all often associated with the disease but build positive brand-name rewards.

Second and more concretely, bosses can take direct action with their own organisations/companies – supporting and educating employees, particularly in developing countries, and working to ensure that their subsidiaries, suppliers and other partners across the world do likewise. And here there has been the business equivalent of an earthquake in recent months following the dramatic drop in costs of AIDS drugs thanks to efforts of the global pharmaceutical companies. And that leaves the private sector as the real new frontier where there is the best chance of expanding access to treatment, particularly given the fact that it is now more cost-effective to treat workers than to find and train new ones.

An organisation/business can help with financial and other support for broader initiatives. At one level the business can engage through the Global Business Council on HIV/AIDS as well as a number of National Business Councils being set up to help coordinate private sector inputs and responses in many developing countries (du Toit 2008a, b).

Even the most successful company HIV and AIDS prevention programme can become outdated in time or stand as a single effort in a surrounding wilderness, unless there is a concerted effort to build a united HIV and AIDS response. Businesses should seek opportunities to collaborate with each other, with their suppliers and with other organisations – locally, nationally, or globally – to offer AIDS programmes and services (UNAIDS Technical Update 1997).

Linking workplace programmes with public or private health services and other organisations in the community outside the workplace has resulted in effective programmes as well as benefits for the companies concerned. Such linkages are also useful when companies do not have adequate resources themselves: linking up, for instance, with an NGO or public health service can help create an effective programme (UNAIDS Technical Update 1997).

The sometimes-lengthy process of obtaining top and middle level management support in the workplace is critical to the long-term viability of a programme. A concerted effort to demonstrate the negative impact of HIV and AIDS on business, compared with a workplace programme established at reasonable cost, can prepare the way for a sustainable programme. Workplace HIV programmes should be constantly evolving. Knowledge of the employee culture – and of such factors as the incidence of Sexually Transmitted Infections (STIs), of violence (including rape) and of drug and alcohol misuse among employees and in their community – is essential for making programmes as relevant and effective as possible (UNAIDS Technical Update 1997).

The workforce is both the most accessible target audience for companies and the one that has the most immediate effect on the bottom line. Protecting staff through workplace activities is a natural first priority of programmes, followed by looking to the wider community (World Economic Forum 2005).

People infected with HIV will eventually need antiretroviral drug treatment to control AIDS (and, obviously, many already do). In some countries, governments have successfully taken on this responsibility and it is important that the work of businesses complements rather than duplicates that of governments. In others, firms have taken up some of the slack and ensured that their workers and their dependents have access to treatment, care and support (World Economic Forum 2005).

The driving force behind many HIV/AIDS prevention and care activities at the community level is provided by non-governmental and community-based organisations. In many countries, the community response has preceded the government response. In almost all cases, it has proved essential to successful national response, particularly in the areas of awareness-raising, prevention, advocacy, policy and legal changes, and family or community care and support. When addressing HIV/AIDS, where the culture of denial and social attitudes towards prevention and care take on such importance, it is extremely difficult to change attitudes and practices in the workforce in isolation from the community as a whole. Effective prevention and care in the world of work therefore has to be aimed at the community, through the workforce (ILO 2000).

The foregoing discussion highlights the importance for businesses to be involved in supporting HIV/AIDS programmes in organisations and communities from a CSI angle. HIV/AIDS continues to be a major concern (Implats 2008) for organisations and the community. While interventions will vary by company and country, there are three broad areas where real Corporate Social Investment impact can be made: advocacy, direct action within the organisation, and help with financial and other support for broader initiatives.

References

Animaw, W., & Seoum, Y. (2017). Increasing prevalence of diabetes mellitus in a developing country and its related factors. *PLoS One, 12*(11), e0187670. https://doi.org/10.1371/journal.pone.0187670.

Anstey, M. (1999). *Managing change – Negotiating conflict* (pp. 129–178). Sandton: Juta & Co, Ltd.

Arora, J., Chauhan, K., John, S., & Mukhopadhyay, A. (2011). Multi-sectoral action for addressing social determinants of non-communicable diseases and mainstreaming health promotion in national health programmes in India. *Indian Journal of Community Medicine, 36*, s43–s49.

Barnett, T., & Whiteside, A. (2002). *AIDS in the twenty-first century: Disease and globalisation.* New York: Palagrave MacMillan.

Baum, F., & Harris, L. (2006). Equity and the social determinants of health. *Health Promotion Journal of Australia, 17*(3), 162–276.

Birn, A., Pillay, Y., & Holtz, T. H. (2009). *Textbook of international health: Global health in a dynamic world.* New York: Oxford.

Brink, B. (2003). *Response to HIV/AIDS in South Africa: A business perspective. Anglo American Corporation of South Africa Limited.* Labour markets and social frontiers: number 4 South African Reserve Bank.

Brookman-May, S. D., et al. (2017). Challenges, hurdles and possible approaches to improve cancer in developing countries – A short breakdown of the status quo and future perspec-

tive. *Advances in Modern Oncology Research, 3*(5), 205–212. https://doi.org/10.18282/amor.v3.i5.221.
Brown, T., Franklin, B., MacNeil, J., & Mills, S. (2001). *Effective prevention strategies in low prevalence settings*. Arlington: Family Health International.
Business Report. (2003). *Business is doubling the cost of HIV/AIDS by managing it incorrectly.*
Carvallo, M. S., Coeli, C. M., Chor, D., Pinheiro, R. S., Fonseca, M. D., & Carvallo, L. C. D. (2015). The challenge of cardiovascular diseases and diabetes to public health: A study based on qualitative systemic approach. *PLosS ONE, 10*(7), e0132216. https://doi.org/10.1371/journal.pone.0132216.
Centers for Disease Control and Prevention. (2010). *Where malaria occurs* [Online]. Available from http://www.cdc.gov/malaria/about/distribution.html
Classen-Hoskins, B. J. (2005). *The impact of Human Immunodeficiency Virus & Acquired Immunodeficiency Syndrome in the department of Agriculture: Western cape: A human resource management planning strategy*. Unpublished master's thesis, University of Stellenbosch, South Africa.
Colagiuri, S., Kent, J., Kainu, T., Sutherland, S. & Vuik, S. (2015). Rising to the challenge: Preventing and managing type 2 diabetes. Report of the WISH Diabetes Forum.
Crawshaw, P., & Newlove, C. (2011). Men's understanding of social marketing and health: Neo-liberalism and health governance. *International Journal of Men's Health, 10*(2), 136–152.
Daimler Chrysler. (2002). Workplace policy on HIV/AIDS.
De Zulueta, J. (1998). The end of malaria in Europe: An eradication of the disease by control measures. *Parassitologia, 40*(1–2), 45–46.
Dennill, K., & Vasuthevan, S. (2005). *The health of southern Africa.* Cape Town: Juta.
Department of Health. (2003). *Operational plan for comprehensive HIV and AIDS care, management and treatment for South Africa.*
Dooris, M. (2009). Holistic and sustainable health improvement: The contribution of the settings-based approach to health promotion. *Perspectives in Public Health, 129*(1), 29–36.
du Toit, J. (2008a). *Social responsibility of companies.* Africa Centre for HIV/AIDS Management, Stellenbosch University.
du Toit, J. B. (2008b). *Community/organization mobilization.* University of Stellenbosch.
du Toit, J. B. & Freeman, A. (2002). *Community mobilization.* Unpublished manuscript, University of Stellenbosch.
Ellis, L. & Terwin, J. (2004). *The impact of HIV/AIDS on selected business sectors in South Africa.* Bureau for Economic Research and South African Business Coalition on HIV & AIDS (SABCOHA).
Eriksson, M., & Lindstrom, B. (2008). A salutogenic interpretation of the Ottawa charter. *Health Promot International, 23*(2), 190–199.
Fountaine, T., Lembong, J., Nair, R. & Dyckerhoff, C. S. (2016). *Tackling Indonesia's diabetes challenge: Eight approaches from around the world.* Center for Healthcare Research and Innovation. McKinsey & Company.
Global AIDS Learning & Evaluation Network (2002). International Association of Physicians in AIDS Care. Module No. 9.
Global Business Coalition on HIV/AIDS (GBC) (2005). *HIV/AIDS management in the oil and gas industry.* New York: GBC.
Government of Malaysia. (2001). *Code of practice on prevention and management of HIV/AIDS at the workplace.*
Government of South Africa. (2000). *HIV/AIDS/STD strategic plan for South Africa 2000–2005.* Pretoria, South Africa.
Graham, H. (2004). Tackling inequalities in health in England: Remedying health disadvantages, narrowing health gaps or reducing health gradients? *Journal of Social Policy, 33*(1), 115–131.
Graham, H. (2009). Health inequalities, social determinants and public health policy. *Policy and Politics, 37*(4), 463–479.
Green, J. (2000). The role of theory evidence-based health promotion practice. *Health Education Journal, 15*(2), 125–129.

Grier, S., & Bryant, C. (2005). Social marketing in public health. *Annual Review of Public Health, 26*, 319–339.
Harden, A., Peersman, S., Oliver, M., Mauthner, M., & Oakley, A. (1999). A systematic review of the effectiveness of health promotion interventions in the workplace. *Occupational Medicine, 49*(8), 540–548.
Hazelle, R. 2002. *Consideration of reports of state parties in Uganda*. Committee on the elimination of discrimination against women, exceptional session 5–23 August 2002. Uganda.
Health and Development Networks. (2006). *HIV and people on the move*: Risk and vulnerabilities of migrants and mobile populations in southern Africa. Summary report of the structured discussion on AF-AIDS eForum, April–August 2005.
Health24.com. (2008). *Sociocultural aspects of HIV/AIDS*. Retrieved April, 10, 2008, from http://www.health24.com
Hunger Project. 2002. *Gender inequality fuels the spread of HIV/AIDS*. The Kampala commitments on AIDS and gender inequality. HIV/AIDS and gender inequality: Action at the grassroots conference, Kampala, Uganda. Retrieved April, 17, 2008, from http://www.thp.org/aids/302.
ILO. (2000). *HIVAIDS: A threat to decent work, productivity and development*. Document for discussion at the Special High-Level Meeting on HIV/AIDS and the World of Work. Geneva, 8 June 2000.
ILO Code of Practice on HIV/AIDS and the World of Work. 2001.
ILOAIDS. A *Workplace Policy on HIV: putting it into practice*.
Implats. (2008). *Corporate Social Responsibility Report*. Retrieved October, 14, from http://www.implats.co.za/annual_report/2000/corp_responsibility.html
International AIDS-Economics Network. (2002). State of the art: AIDS and Economics. Shared risk factors. Amsterdam.
International Federation of Medical Students' Association. (2018). *Noncommunicable diseases and the 4 most common*.
International HIV/AIDS Alliance. (2003). *Working with men, responding to AIDS*. USAID.
International Labour Office. (2000). *HIV/AIDS: A threat to decent work, productivity and development*. Geneva: International Labour Office.
International Labour Office. (2006). *HIV/AIDS and work: Global estimates, impact on children and youth, and response*. Geneva: ILO.
International Labour Organisation (ILO) (2005). *Workshop on developing strategies for implementing HIV/AIDS policy and programmes in the coal mining sector in India*, 22 November 2005.
International Monetary Fund. (2004). *The Macro-economics of AIDS* (edited by M. Haacker).
International Organization for Migration. (2003). *Mobile populations and HIV/AIDS in the Southern African region: Recommendations for action. Desk review and bibliography on HIV/AIDS and mobile populations*, May 2003.
International Organization for Migration. (2005). *HIV/AIDS, population mobility and migration in southern Africa. Defining a research and policy agenda*, June 2005.
Johnson, L. & Budlender, D. (2002). *HIV risk factors: A review of the demographic, socio-economic, biomedical and behavioural determinants of HIV prevalence in South Africa*. Centre for Actuarial Research, University of Cape Town, South Africa.
Joubert, G., & Ehrlich, R. (2007). *Epidemiology: A research manual for South Africa*. New York: Oxford.
Judd, J., Frankish, C. J., & Moulton, G. (2001). Setting standards in the evaluation of community-based health promotion programmes – A unifying approach. *Health Promotion International, 16*(4), 367–380.
Keates, A. K., Mocumbi, A. O., Ntsekhe, M., Sliwa, K., & Stewart, S. (2017). Cardiovascular disease in Africa: Epidemiological profile and challenges. *Nature Reviews Cardiology*. https://doi.org/10.1038/nrcardio.2017.19.
Kirigia, J. M., & Barry, S. P. (2008). Health challenges in Africa and the way forward. *International Archives of Medicine, 1*(27), 1–3.

Mabuza, M. P. (2018a). *Epidemiology and statistics for public health research: Concepts, applications and critical perspectives*. Beau Bassin: Lambert Academic Publishing.
Mabuza, M. P. (2018b). *Health and society: Critical and contemporary perspectives*. Beau Bassin: Lambert Academic Publishing.
Mabuza, M. P. (2018c). *Health promotion: Approaches, concepts, methods and critical perspectives*. London: Kindle Publishing.
Mabuza, M. P. (2018d). *Management of health systems: Critical perspectives*. Beau Bassin: Lambert Academic Publishing.
Mabuza, M. (2018e). Efficacy of calendula officinalis as an antibacterial agent for in vitro pseudomonas aeruginosa. *Eurasian Journal of Medicine and Oncology, 2*(2), 55–60. https://doi.org/10.14744/ejmo.2017.18.189.
Mabuza, M. P., & Shumba, C. (2018). A qualitative exploration of doctors and nurses' experiences on the management of TB and HIV coinfection in a TB-HIV high burden community in northern KwaZulu-Natal, South Africa. *Journal of Public Health in Africa, 9*, 770. https://doi.org/10.4081/jphia.2018.770.
Maharaj, B. (2004). Immigration to post-apartheid South Africa. *Global Migration Perspectives 1*, June 2004. Global Mission on International Migration. Geneva, Switzerland.
Management Sciences for Health. (2003). *Human Resource Management Rapid Assessment Tool for HIV/AIDS Environments: a guide for strengthening HRM systems*. Cambridge.
Manser, C. (2005). Leadership in the management of HIV/AIDS. *The Healthcare Journal, 9*, 17.
Marais, L. & Venter, A. (2006). Hating the compound, but ...: Mineworker housing needs in post-apartheid South Africa. Centre for Development Support, University of the Free State, South Africa. *Africa Insight, 36*(1), March 2006.
Mayosi, B. M., Flisher, A. J., Lalloo, U. G., Sitas, F., Tollman, S. M., & Bradshaw, D. (2009). The burden of non-communicable diseases in South Africa. *The Lancet, 374*(9693), 934–947.
McDermott, L., Stead, M., & Hastings, G. (2005). What is and what is not social marketing: The challenge of reviewing the evidence. *Journal of Marketing Management, 21*, 545–553.
McElligott, M. (2004, June 11). *Working group recommends integrative approach to HIV*. Health Systems Trust.
McNally, P. (2008, August). Blood money. *Health*, p. 178.
Merson, M. E., Black, R. E., & Mills, A. J. (2012). *Global health: Diseases, programs, systems, and policies*. London: Jones & Bartlett.
Metcalfe, M. (2004). *HIV/AIDS: A strategic business imperative*. Retrieved October, 29, 2008, from www.foundation-development-africa.org/africa_hivaids/strategic_business_imp
Ministry of Health and Social Welfare of the Kingdom of Swaziland. (2003). *National HIV/AIDS Clinical Care Guidelines*.
Mohan, V., Seedat, Y. K., & Pradeepa, R. (2013). The rising burden of diabetes and hypertension in southeast Asian and African regions: Need for effective strategies for prevention and control in primary health care settings. *International Journal of Hypertension*. https://doi.org/10.1155/2013/409083.
Morhason-Bello, I. O., Odedina, F., Rebbeck, T., Harford, J., et al. (2013). Challenges and opportunities in cancer control in Africa: A perspective from the African Oranisation for research and training in Cancer. *Lancet Oncology, 14*, e142–e151.
Muller, M., Bezuidenhout, M., & Jooste, K. (2006). *Healthcare service management*. Cape Town: Juta.
Naidoo, J., & Wills, J. (2009). Concepts of health. In *Foundations foe health promotion* (3rd ed.). Edinburgh: Bailliere Tindal Elsevier.
Narayan, V. (2016). The mysteries of type 2 diabetes in developing countries. *Bulletin of the World Health Organization, 94*, 241–242. https://doi.org/10.2471/BLT.16.030416.
National Code of Practice for HIV/AIDS in the Workplace. 2007.
Nel, P. S., Van dyk, P. S., Haasbroek, G. D., Schultz, H. B., Sono, T., & Werner, A. (2005). *Human resources management* (6th ed.). Oxford University Press.
Njobe, T. & Smith, G. (2004). *HIV/AIDS: The costs to SA business*. Deutsche Securities. South Africa.

Noblet, A. (2003). Building health promoting work settings: Identifying the relationship between work characteristics and occupational stress in Australia. *Health Promotion International, 18*(14), 351–359.

Noblet, A., & Lamontagne, A. D. (2006). The role of workplace health promotion in addressing job stress. *Health Promotion International, 21*(4), 346–353.

Noe, R. A., Hollenbeck, J. R., Gerhart, B., & Wright, P. M. (2008). *Human resource management: Gaining a competitive advantage* (6th ed.). Singapore: McGraw Hill.

Novo Nordisk. (2013). *Where economics and health meet: changing diabetes in Indonesia*. The blueprint for change Programme. Indonesia.

Nutbeam, D. (1998). Evaluating health promotion – Progress, problems and solutions. *Health Promotion International, 13*(1), 27–44.

Plath, S., Kohler, T., Krause, H., & Pfaff, H. (2008). Prevention, health promotion and workplace health management in German banks: Results from a nationwide representative survey. *Journal of Public Health, 16*, 195–203.

Prata, N., Morris, L., Mazive, E., Vahidnia, F., & Stehr, M. (2006). Relationship between HIV risk perception and condom use: Evidence from a population-based survey in Mozambique. *International Family Planning Perspectives, 32*(4), 192–200.

Quattek, K. (2000). *Economic impact of AIDS in South Africa*. Available from www.ingbarings.com

QUICK MBA 2008. *Strategic management*. Retrieved September, 15, 2008, from http://www.quickmba.com/strategy/strategic-planning/.

Randolph, M. E., Pinkerton, S. D., Bogart, L. M., Cecil, H., & Abramson, P. R. (2007). Sexual pleasure and condom use. *Archives of Sexual Behaviour, 36*(6), 844–848.

Raphael, D. (2000). The question of evidence in health promotion. *Health Promotion International, 15*(4), 355–367.

Rau, B. (2002). *Workplace HIV/AIDS programs – An action guide for managers*. Arlington: Family Health International.

Rau, B. (2004). *Workplace HIV and AIDS programs*. Arlington: Family Health International.

Ricci, F. (2012). Social implications of malaria and their relationships with poverty. *Mediterranean Journal of Hematology and Infectious Diseases, 4*(1).

Sampson, D. (2004). *AIDS guide*. Cape Town: Uhuru Communications.

Schapink, D., van Poelje, R., Reerink, I. H., Delion, J., & Gurung, D. (2000). *Strategy to involve rural workers in the fight against HIV/AIDS through community mobilisation programs*. Amsterdam: Royal Tropical Institute.

Stoppacher, R., & Adams, S. P. (2003). Malaria deaths in the United States: Case report and review of deaths, 1979-1998. *Journal of Forensic Science, 48*(2), 404–408.

Swanepoel, B. J. (1999). *The Management of Employment Relations – Organisational level perspectives* (pp. 324–338). Durban: Butterworths.

Swart, S. J. & Kotze T. (2003). *Standard for HIV/AIDS management system specification document*. NOSA.

Tan, K. K., Vehvilainen-Julkunen, K., & Chan, S. W. (2014). Integrative review: Salutogenesis and health in older people over 65 years old. *Journal of Advanced Nursing, 70*(3), 497–510.

Tandon, A. (2005). *Macroeconomic impact of HIV/AIDS in the Asian and Pacific region*. ERD Working Paper Series No. 75.

Taute, F. (2007). *A life skills training program as part of employee assistance programs in South African companies*. Retrieved August, 20, 2008, from http://h08.cgpublisher.com/proposals/154/index_html

Tawfik, L., & Kinoti, S. N. (2003). *The impact of HIV/AIDS on health systems and the health workforce in sub-Saharan Africa*. Washington, DC: USAID, Bureau for Africa, office of sustainable development.

The Gender and HIV/AIDS Technical Sub-Committee. (2002). *Mainstreaming gender into the Kenya national HIV/AIDS plan 2000–2005*.

The Healthy Employee. (2008). *Stress management*. Available from http://thehealthyemployee.typepad.com/beproactive/stress_management/

Thompson, A. A., Strickland, A. J., & Gamble, J. E. (2007). *Crafting & Executing Strategy: The quest for competitive advantage*. New York: McGraw Hill.
UNAIDS. (2000). *The Economic impact of AIDS in Africa Country by Country: An update*. Geneva: UNAIDS.
UNAIDS. (2002). *The Private Sector Responses to the Epidemic: Debswana – a global benchmark*. UNAIDS case study, September 2002. Geneva.
UNAIDS. (2006). *AIDS epidemic update*. Available at http://data.unaids.org/pub/EpiReport/2006/2006EpiUpdate en.pdf
UNAIDS. (2007). *AIDS epidemic update*. Retrieved April, 17, 2008, from http://www.unaids.org/en/KnowledgeCentre/HIVData/EpiUpdate/EpiUpdArchive/2007default.asp
UNAIDS Technical Update. (1997). *Community mobilization and AIDS*. Geneva: UNAIDS.
United Nations. (2005). *Population development and HIV/AIDS with particular emphasis on poverty*: The concise report. department of economic and social affairs. Geneva: United Nations.
USAID. (2010). *AIDS impact: HIV and AIDS projections for policy dialogue, planning, and advocacy. Futures group health policy initiative*. USAID, Washington, DC.
USAID Health Policy Initiative. (2008). *Developing an HIV and AIDS policy: Content, process, challenges and implementation*. Stellenbosch University, South Africa.
Van den Heever, A. M. (2002). *Review of economic impact studies of HIV/AIDS on South Africa: Preliminary analysis*. Washington, DC: USAID, Bureau for Africa, Office of Sustainable Development.
Victorian Government Department of Human Services. (2008). *Planning for effective health promotion evaluation*. Melbourne: Victorian Government Department of Human Services. Available from http://www.health.vic.gov.au/healthpromotion/downloads/planning_may05.pdf. Accessed 16 Feb 2013.
Viswanathan, V., & Rao, V. (2013). Problems associated with diabetes care in India. *Diabetes Manage, 3*(1), 31–40.
Walley, J., & Wright, J. (2010). *Public health: An action guide to improving health*. New York: Oxford.
Weeden, C. (1998). *From corporate social investing*. San Francisco: Berett-Koehler Publishers.
Wellbeing: HIV and AIDS, Prevention and Care. (2008). *The role of senior management*. Retrieved June, 27, 2008, from http://www.genderdiversity.cgiar.org/inclusiveworkplace/wellbeing/hiv-aids/
Whitehead, M. & Dahlgren, G. (2006). *Levelling up (part 1): Concepts and principles for tackling social inequities in health*. Studies on social and economic determinants of population health, 2, pp. 1–34. Copenhagen, Denmark: World Health Organization, Regional Office for Europe [Online]. Available from http://www.euro.who.int/document/e89384.pdf. Accessed 13 Feb 2013.
World Economic Forum. (2005). *A global review of the business response to HIV/AIDS 2005–2006*. Geneva: World Economic Forum.
World Economic Forum. (2006). *Business and HIV/AIDS: A healthier partnership. A global review of the business response to HIV/AIDS 2005–2006*. Geneva: World Economic Forum.
World Health Organization. (2009). *Interventions on diet and physical activity: What works: Summary report*. Geneva: WHO.
World Health Organization. (2011). *Global status report on noncommunicable diseases 2010*. Geneva: WHO.
World Health Organization. (2018a). *NCDs and youth*. Available from http://www.who.int/global-coordination-mechanism/ncd-themes/ncd-and-youth/en/. Accessed 22 Nov 2018.
World Health Organization. (2018b). *Global Health Observatory (GHO) data*. http://www.who.int/gho/hiv/en/

Chapter 6
Adolescents, Sexual Reproductive Health (SRH) and Equity

Abstract In this chapter we see how the different aspects of adolescents' lives affect their health and wellbeing. They face comparatively high levels of unprotected sexual activity, suicide, substance abuse, road traffic accidents and malnutrition, and in some regions, violence through homicide and armed conflict are major problems. It is of concern that data from national surveys of many low- and middle-income countries demonstrate that the unmet need of adolescents is over two times higher than that of the general population in these countries. By strengthening national strategies and programmes to address sexual and reproductive health in adolescents, will directly and indirectly enhance the achievement of development goals. Since many of the public health issues affecting adolescents are further exacerbated by cultural, ethnic, religious, socioeconomic and educational inequalities already operating in many low- and middle-income countries, we need to make the case for both male and female adolescents as a public health strategy by opening the dialogue and reaching a consensus rather than impose what we believe and know from a medical perspective.

Keywords Adolescents · Circumcision · Complex emergencies · Conflict situations · Cultural norms · Educational inequalities · Ethnic inequalities · Gender-based-violence · Gender inequalities · Genital mutilation · Humanitarian crises · Medical perspective · Religious inequalities · Sexual and reproductive health · Sexual violence · Socio-economic · Strategies for sexual and reproductive health · Teenage pregnancy · Vulnerable groups

6.1 Sexual and Reproductive Health Issues Affecting Adolescents

It is so unfortunate that young people especially children and adolescents are often left out when it comes to public health programmes, investments and policymaking, and yet global trends show that the young face serious challenges pertaining to

M. P. Mabuza, *Evaluating International Public Health Issues*,
https://doi.org/10.1007/978-981-13-9787-5_6

sexual and reproductive health, and this has a huge bearing on the Sustainable Development Goals (SDGs).

> *Young people, especially adolescent girls and young women in sub-Saharan Africa, are being left behind at all points on what is known as the HIV treatment continuum, evidenced by still rising infection rates (adolescents and young women represent 40% of all new infections, with eastern and southern Africa the 'epicentre' of adolescents living with HIV, making up 60% of all adolescents living with HIV globally).*
>
> *In addition, the calculus of future infection rates emphasizes a demographic 'youth bulge', meaning that the size of the adolescent population, especially in Africa, is set to increase, and already, says UNICEF, adolescents and young people represent a growing share of people living with HIV worldwide.*

Such challenges faced by the young became apparent to one policymaker after having been involved in a research survey aimed at exploring family planning methods in the rural, urban and industrial settings of one of the southern African countries. There was realisation that in some sectors of society the subject of sexual and reproductive health is often seen as taboo, particularly with regard to adolescents/children. In some low- and middle-income countries, adolescents/children are often perceived as not mature enough to understand issues of sexual and reproductive health.

The reality is that there is such a big concern about teenage pregnancies in low income countries, and this suggests that a number of teenagers are engaging in unprotected sex which also puts them at high risk of contracting sexually transmitted infections including HIV. Interestingly, Seamark and Lings (2004), report that there are positive experiences of teenage motherhood. Perhaps, it remains a question of the affected adolescent's background or whether the unprotected sexual activity was consensual or forced, but the bottom line is that adolescents/children are vulnerable. Birn et al. (2009) observe that girls are at heightened risk of exploitation, forced to get married early and denied or disrupted of their education.

In parts of low- and middle-income countries affected by humanitarian crises, it is disturbing to get news of adolescents/children and even babies being raped almost on a daily basis. Some studies suggest that such a high rate of children being raped is because of the myth that having sex with a virgin will cure HIV and AIDS (Meel 2003). Is that the only reason for raping children and adolescents? It is unlikely. Sexual violence affects a significant proportion of youth, with 3–24% of women surveyed in the World Health Organization (WHO) multi-country study on women's health and domestic violence reporting that their first sexual experience was forced, in a majority of cases while they were adolescents (Merson et al. 2012).

The current strategies and priorities for addressing the issue of sexual vulnerability of adolescents, particularly girls in South Africa, is that in addition to the South African Youth and Adolescent Health Policy guidelines which include the prevention of unhealthy lifestyles, each provincial health department should develop policies and strategies that address their specific priorities such as adolescent reproductive health issues (Dennill and Vasuthevan 2005). The decentralisation approach makes sense because it acknowledges the unique challenges of the different settings pertaining to adolescent sexual and reproductive health and that there is increased funding to address this issue.

On the other hand, it is of concern that the decentralisation has resulted in a disjointed approach. It is worrying that the focus is only on the positive potential of young people as opposed to the real problems that manifest. Sexual and reproductive health issues affecting adolescents and children are more than just a health issue. As such, a multi-sectoral approach that also involves empowerment and active participation without victimisation of the adolescent girls would ensure effective prioritisation, implementation and sustainability in terms of addressing the issue.

6.2 Female Genital Mutilation and Male Circumcision

Female genital mutilation is regarded as another kind of violence against women, and this is a practice that has been reported in more than 40 low- and middle-income countries and has followed immigrants from these areas to high-income countries (Merson et al. 2012). Although any type of genital cutting carries a risk of infection, the implications of genital cutting for long-term reproductive health differ according to the severity of cutting, conditions of delivery, and socio-demographic factors.

While it is widely perceived that female genital mutilation is carried out by lay people under unsterile conditions in the communities, it is interesting that in some countries, evidence suggests that a growing proportion of these procedures are being carried out by medical personnel (Yoder et al. 2004). Could the carrying out of this procedure by medical personnel be a strategy to reduce the risk of complications or a way of making this procedure more acceptable from a modern medical perspective? As far as one is concerned, even the medical personnel who carry out these procedures are also violating the women's or girls' rights even if this procedure is carried out under sterile conditions.

An observation is that some of the ethnic groups or tribes do carry out circumcision for cultural reasons. However, in recent times there has been an outcry because of the large numbers of boys who die as a result of this procedure or ritual. As such, there has been a recommendation in the health strategy that circumcision be carried out only by medical personnel. This has been met with challenges as the circumcision is much more about the cutting, but it is a ritual that involves many other activities that are carried out as part of the rights of passage from boys to men. Most of the South African tribes that practise this culture feel that having the procedure done by medical personnel would be like an insult because it undermines their being.

The strategy should be aimed at improving awareness and motivation rather than simply dismissing or banning what people believe in and are so attached to. There should be focused programmes for example with the traditional leaders, religious leaders, parents and children of the target population so that there could be awareness and consensus to ensure sustainability. There has to be a case made for both male and female circumcision as a public health strategy by opening the dialogue and reaching a consensus rather than impose what is believed and known only from a medical perspective (Castro et al. 2010).

6.3 Sexual Violence/Gender Based Violence

The issue of sexual violence is indeed a matter that needs urgent intervention as it seems to be getting out of hand. It has reached a stage where communities have now decided to take the law into their own hands because of the frustration that arrests and convictions of perpetrators are very low despite the fact that the rates of sexual violence against babies and adolescent girls have spiralled out of proportion, such as in South Africa. Maybe the fact that the might of the law does not seem to be decisively punishing the perpetrators has resulted in victims of sexual violence being discouraged to report cases anymore, and this exacerbates the issue even further.

The issue is much deeper than meets the eye, and the reasons for not reporting are very complex and cannot be generalised. As such, interventions should be well planned and targeted at addressing the root cause or causes in that particular setting and for that particular individual, family, group or population, as generic interventions may sometimes cause more harm than good, in certain settings.

It is possible that the root causes may be due to one or a combination of factors such as social, cultural, economic, or political factors. In that sense, a more comprehensive intervention strategy may be suggested. For example, the socio-ecological model is balanced and does not only consider the individual factors but it also looks beyond those individual factors and also takes into cognisance of the relationships, community and societal factors as well as the uniqueness of the particular setting (Dahlberg et al. 2002).

However, it cannot be denied that there are lessons to be learned from scientific research as it can provide a guide or a point of reference on how to effectively address challenges of sexual violence based on results obtained from various settings. Merson et al. (2012) suggest that the following interventions are crucial and effective in terms of addressing sexual violence:

- Reducing the availability and harmful use of alcohol
  - Regulating sales of alcohol
  - Raising alcohol prices
- Promoting gender equality to prevent violence against women
  - School-based programs to address gender norms and attitudes
- Changing cultural norms that support violence
  - Social marketing to modify social norms
- Victims identification, care, and support programs
  - Psychosocial interventions

Sexual violence is becoming a growing cause for concern as it puts many adolescents at high risk such as the risk of contracting sexually transmitted infections, pregnancy, disrupted schooling, social exclusion and mortality. In this regard, well planned and effective interventions could enhance the achievement of a number of public health goals.

6.4 Conflict as a Key Factor in Health Outcomes for Adolescents and Other Vulnerable Groups

Because of their powerlessness, adolescent girls in refugee situations are more vulnerable to forced marriage, sexual slavery and forms of gender-based violence, among other abuses. They are also the least likely to be offered education and reproductive health care, putting them at greater risk for HIV/AIDS, unwanted pregnancy and unsafe abortions. (**Mary Diaz, in a letter to the New York Times**).

Conflict situations have been there for time immemorial, but, in recent times, the growing complexity of conflict situations has attracted so much focus. It is hardly surprising that some authors have even adopted the term 'complex emergencies' to acknowledge that there is a growing realisation that many of the conflict situations combine a number of features such as their political antecedence, their deep embedment in socio-cultural and economic cleavages, their protracted duration, and their occurrence within and across borders (Merson et al. 2012).

In conflict situations, children, women and people with disabilities are often ignored and yet these groups are usually the most vulnerable and therefore the most affected, regardless of whether the conflict situation is short-lived or protracted. In fact, these vulnerable groups bear the brunt of the conflict situation as reports indicate that there is often high mortality, abuse and suffering among children, women and people with disabilities during and after conflict situations (Merson et al. 2012). This situation is often exacerbated by the fact that conflict situations are often characterised by displacement of people, diseases outbreaks due to collapse of clean water supplies and sanitation, in general (Birn et al. 2009). Sometimes, children are used as targets and instruments of war, and they also suffer from collateral violence. Out of sheer desperation to make ends meet, some of the affected children allow their bodies to be used.

My sister is only 15 years old but every night she goes out to have sex with humanitarian workers and peacekeepers for money. I tried to stop her before, but I have given up since I do not have anything to give her. We all rely on the money she gets to support the family. (**17-year-old young man, Liberia**).

I am sleeping every night with a hungry stomach. I choose to sleep with a soldier who is HIV-positive who provides me with food. I know eventually I would contract HIV but at least I continue to live another few years with food in my stomach. (**Young woman, northern Uganda**).

One boy tried to escape [from the rebels], but he was caught... His hands were tied, and then they made the other new captives, kill him with a stick. I felt sick. I knew this boy from before. We were from the same village. I refused to kill him, and they told me they would shoot me. They pointed a gun at me, so I had to do it. The boy was asking me, "Why are you doing this?" I said I had no choice. After we killed him, they made us smear his blood on our arms. They said we had to do this so we would not fear death and so we would not try to escape…I still dream about the boy from my village who I killed. I see him in my dreams, and he is talking to me and saying I killed him for nothing, and I am crying. (**Susan, 16, girl soldier abducted by the Lord's Resistance Army**).

According to the Women's Refugee Commission (2012), the displacement of people may lead to a growing number of refugees and asylum seekers, and some of the destination countries often use detention as a response to deal with the influx of asylum seekers and immigrants, and there have been reports of women being highly vulnerable to sexual abuse in these detention facilities. Sometimes, the populations most in need are unable to flee, and the situation of the trapped populations becomes dire as they are subjected to different aspects of abuse, lack of or poor resources, lack of or poor access to healthcare services, deteriorating living conditions, and overcrowding which may result in disease epidemics (Merson et al. 2012). What makes this even more complicated is that the 'trapped' vulnerable groups may be at on-going risk from violence perpetuated by the state and other powerful local actors and have their needs more hidden than those persons who are displaced across borders (Merson et al. 2012).

Everyone says "yes, yes, yes" [about including the girls in resettlement], but then no one has taken any significant action. (**U.S. government official, speaking about how few Sudanese girls have been resettled in the United States**).

Sometimes, criminal elements also take root as women and children particularly girls may be subjected to trafficking and forced prostitution. There are already intensified campaigns against human trafficking in South Africa, as this issue appears to be widespread throughout the world. Women, children and people living with disabilities are at highest risk of human trafficking and sexual slavery as conflict situations exacerbate their vulnerability to a number of risks.

All the aforementioned are important factors that influence the health and well-being of the vulnerable groups such as women, children and the disabled in conflict situations. It would therefore be important to urgently address the health problems of these vulnerable groups in an equitable manner. It would be important to focus on how to address the health problems of those living with disabilities, as they are often the most forgotten in the context of conflict situations, globally.

First and foremost, one would advocate for change of global health policies, national health policies and humanitarian policies to ensure that people living with disabilities have increased access and also included in the healthcare programs. There is need to conduct research or assessments to determine the magnitude of the problem, but more importantly, the people living with disabilities have to be actively involved in the research so that we can get a better understanding of the challenges that they go through in conflict situations. It is encouraging to see the active involvement and partnerships between the United Nations High Commission for Refugees (UNHCR) and the Women's Refugee Commission in this regard in countries such as Thailand, Bangladesh, Nepal and Ethiopia (Women's Refugee Commission 2012). In fact, it is good that the legislation as pronounced by the UNHCR which is aimed at protecting refugees with disabilities and other people with disabilities as this will ensure that the health problems of this vulnerable group are addressed in an equitable manner (UNHCR 2010). Healthcare services should be adapted to suite the people living with disabilities, and healthcare workers should be properly trained to be able to understand and address health needs of people living with different types of disabilities.

Women, children and people living with disabilities are forgotten and yet these groups are exposed to heightened vulnerability in conflict situations. People with disabilities are even more forgotten.

6.5 Strategies and Programmes for Sexual and Reproductive Health

In some sectors of society, sexual and reproductive health strategies or programmes put strong emphasis on the integrity and strength of the family unit and overlook the aspect of directly addressing topics about sexual and reproductive health in adolescents (DeJong et al. 2005). The integrity and strength of the family unit has a protective effect, but the bottom line is that young people such as adolescents lack access to information about the subject of sexual and reproductive health and yet there are increasing challenges faced by adolescents, and these challenges include unwanted pregnancy and abortion, sexual violence, and sexually transmitted infections/HIV/AIDS (Merson et al. 2012).

> *Yatta, 17, was confused about family planning methods due to misinformation she received from her friends... [S]he did not use a family planning method and became pregnant. As a result, she had an unsafe abortion and consequently nearly lost her life.* (**Yatta lived in Sinje refugee camp, Liberia**).

It is encouraging that sexual and reproductive health has been introduced into the education curricula even at lower primary schools in countries such as the Kingdom of Eswatini. However, DeJong et al. (2005) observe that in some of the low-income countries education curricula that include sexual and reproductive health topics are rare and where they do exist, relevant sections are frequently skipped over by teachers, who are unprepared. Health service providers neither recognise the needs of this age group nor make young people such as adolescents welcome, particularly those who are unmarried. Taboos surrounding discussion of sexuality remain a key constraint, and data on unwanted pregnancy and abortion, violence against adolescents, and sexually transmitted infections such as HIV are limited (DeJong et al. 2005).

What is puzzling though is that while on the one hand adolescents are deprived of information about sexual and reproductive health, on the other hand the very same adolescents are sometimes forced to get married in some of the developing countries. Of course, one would expect that if adolescents are forced to get married, then it means they are also ready or mature enough to understand information about sexual and reproductive health. As such, the rhetoric and conflict in values does in a big way create a barrier when it comes to strategies for addressing sexual and reproductive health in this group.

> *Many girls are forced to marry at early ages by their parents because of poverty. Their husbands are much older than them .... Men marry many wives and have dozens of children and they cannot afford to care for them.* (**Abibatu, a teenager in Sierra Leone**).

Building on proven models and existing efforts, there is an urgent need for the development of national programmes to support the wellbeing of adolescents and to ensure that there is equitable access to quality health services and sexual and reproductive health information (Magnan and Reynolds 2006). Educational programmes are needed to help parents, teachers, and health professionals to overcome barriers to addressing adolescent sexual and reproductive health (Magnan and Reynolds 2006). More importantly the adolescents themselves should play an active role in the planning, implementation and evaluation of the strategies.

Interestingly, insights from developmental neuroscience emphasises the importance of understanding the adolescent brain. Such insights focus particularly on the social brain, prefrontal cortex, and emotional and reward processing regions.

Social brain: Adolescents are particularly susceptible to social influence. Opportunities for sexual and reproductive health interventions such as prevention of sexually transmitted infections, include peer-led teaching and interventions; positive role models. Vulnerabilities include self-discovery and rejection of self; the power of social exclusion; and greater peer influence on negative than positive behaviours.

Pre-frontal cortex: The prefrontal cortex is still developing, in adolescents. This part of the brain is the seat of executive functioning such as flexibility, inhibition, planning, multi-tasking, judgement or synthesis, and decision making. Opportunities for SRH interventions for adolescents include the fact that adolescents are capable of processing facts and making judgements; more open to new ideas; fewer concrete opinions. Vulnerabilities include the fact that in adolescents, judgement and decision making are more impacted by environment; long-term consequences are less influential on decision-making; planning susceptible is susceptible to changes in routine.

Emotional and reward processing regions: Opportunities for SRH interventions for adolescents include the fact that adolescents can be passionate, motivational, determined drivers of change; and susceptibility for reward-based interventions. Vulnerabilities include tendency towards rewarding/risky decisions in stimulating situations; and susceptibility to negative emotional responses.

As such, in terms of neurodevelopment and SRH interventions and management for adolescents, there is need to separate decision-making from stimulating situations linking long-term benefits with short-term benefits; enhancing positive, supporting environments and reducing stigma. By strengthening national strategies and programmes to address sexual and reproductive health in adolescents, will directly and indirectly enhance the achievement of development goals.

Lessons learned suggest that programs seeking to engage young men could consider combining health services with recreational opportunities, non-judgmental information and support within a private, youth friendly environment.

Gendered powerlessness in at-risk adolescent and young adult women was observed in terms of condom use behaviour. Prevention efforts targeting at-risk adolescent women would benefit from overturning sexual divisions of power and countering the structure of social norms and expectations that undermine young women's sexual agency.

Development of typologies for target populations may allow a more targeted approach for designing, marketing, and promoting HIV prevention products to adolescents and young women, and their partners.

The growing challenge of adolescents' poor adherence to antiretroviral treatment is largely because of lack of commitment and effort by policymakers and programmers to fully understand the developmental and sociological aspect of how individuals and communities construct disease and health, and to some extent the underlying challenge. The issue of adolescents and young people was a prominent feature during the 22nd International AIDS Conference held in Amsterdam, the Netherlands. It was clear that the "one-glove-fits-all" approach of interventions does not work. The voices of the different target populations such as adolescents should be heard and understood, and they should be meaningfully involved at all levels of the response.

References

Birn, A., Pillay, Y., & Holtz, T. H. (2009). *Textbook of international health: Global health in a dynamic world*. New York: Oxford.

Castro, J. G., Jones, D. L., Lopez, m., Barradas, I., & Weiss, S. M. (2010). Making the case for circumcision as a public health strategy: Opening the dialogue. *AIDS Patient Care and STDs, 24*(6), 367–372.

Dahlberg, L. L., Mercy, J. A., Zwi, A. B., & Lozano, R. (2002). *World report on violence and health*. Geneva: World Health Organization.

DeJong, J., Jawad, R., Mortagy, I., & Shepard, B. (2005). The sexual and reproductive health of young people in the Arab countries and Iran. *Reproductive Health Matters, 13*(25), 49–59.

Dennill, K., & Vasuthevan, S. (2005). *The health of southern Africa*. Cape Town: Juta.

Magnan, M., & Reynolds, K. (2006). Barriers to addressing patient sexuality concerns across five areas of specialisation. *Clinical Nurse Specialist, 20*(6), 285–292.

Meel, B. L. (2003). The myth of child rape as a cure for HIV/AIDS in Transkei: A case report. *Medicine, Science and the Law, 43*(1), 85–88.

Merson, M. E., Black, R. E., & Mills, A. J. (2012). *Global health: Diseases, programs, systems, and policies*. London: Jones & Bartlett.

Seamark, C. J., & Lings, P. (2004). Positive experiences of teenage motherhood: A qualitative study. *The British Journal of General Practice, 54*(508), 813–818.

UNHCR. (2010). *Conclusion on refugees with disabilities and other persons with disabilities protected and assisted by UNHCR*. Available from: http://www.unhcr.org/4cbeb1a99.html

Women's Refugee Commission. (2012). *Research. Rethink. Resolve*. Available from: http://www.womensrefugeecommission.org/resources/annual-reports/955-annual-report-2012/file

Yoder, S., Abderrahim, N., & Zhuzhuni, A. (2004). *Female genital cutting in the demographic and health surveys: A critical and comparative analysis*. Calverton: ORC Marco.

Chapter 7
Globalisation, Climate Change, and Disasters

Abstract A holistic and critical approach to the disaster cycle/disaster-development continuum may provide a better opportunity to address the root cause of vulnerability, but an uncritical strategy may do more harm than good. The concept of vulnerability or vulnerable groups should not inadvertently create the risk of group discrimination but paying attention to the root causes of the dynamism and vulnerability of certain groups could provide us with lasting solutions for disaster management. Recovery, mitigation and preparedness are essential, but planning, leadership and coordination are crucial to ensure that there is effective and sustainable disaster reduction. Climate change has an influence in extreme weather events resulting in disasters, and this needs urgent interventions in the context of disaster management, while also bearing in mind that there are constraints and challenges with regard to addressing the issue of climate change and its influence on disasters. There needs to be prioritisation of psychological consequences for disaster preparedness and response, while at the same time we also need to be cautious of instrumentalising decisions because managing disaster may be complex, multidimensional and individually unique. The health sector can best contribute to mitigation against and preparation for possible future food shortage crises by influencing political decision-making and facilitating multi-stakeholder partnerships to ensure that there is adequate resource allocation and capacity to address the issue of food shortages. The known strategies and frameworks of mitigation against and preparation for future food shortage crises are all important, but we need to be aware that nutritional concerns in low-income and middle-income countries are diverse, and the burden of diseases can complicate the whole picture and create a novelty of food shortage. Early warning systems can be more useful if they are linked to and complemented by timely response mechanisms.

Keywords Behavioural hazards · Biological hazards · Chemical hazards · Climate change · Complex humanitarian emergencies · Demographic shift · Disaster cycle · Disaster risk management · Early warning systems · Epidemic · Ergonomic hazards · Exposure · Food shortages · Globalisation · Industrial hazards · Industrialisation ·

M. P. Mabuza, *Evaluating International Public Health Issues*,
https://doi.org/10.1007/978-981-13-9787-5_7

Mitigation · Occupational hazards · Physical hazards · Pollution · Preparedness · Radiological hazards · Recovery · Risk perception · Socioeconomic hazards · Sudden onset natural disasters · Technological hazards · Vulnerability

7.1 Globalisation and Climate Change

According to Walley and Wright (2010), globalisation is the increasing interconnectedness between countries which opens doors for information exchange, movement of people, trade and markets, technology advancement, financial and infrastructure development.

Globalisation in terms of industrialisation and urbanisation can be seen as a boost to the national economy and also creates employment opportunities, thereby addressing poverty (Hill 2009). On the other hand, this creates problems because as more and more people flock to the industrial and urban centres, there is often the creation of mega cities and the proliferation of informal settlements.

The informal settlements in many parts of low- and middle-income countries are often characterised by overcrowding, poor sanitation, and poor living conditions in general. This situation creates environments where there is increased vulnerability to risky sexual behaviour, alcoholism, and drug dependency, which may perpetuate the spread of sexually transmitted infections such as HIV. Poor drainage systems may provide breeding ground for malaria spreading mosquitoes particularly in the warmer regions. Merson et al. (2012) observe that children and pregnant women are even more vulnerable to recurrent malaria. As more and more economically active individuals get ill or die from diseases such as AIDS-related conditions, the poverty situation of households is exacerbated as there is no one to provide for the affected households.

This situation puts more strain on the national budget as more money needs to be spent on the public health sector to cater for the increasing burden of disease (Davies and Lam 2001). Some South African firms have even considered opting for downsizing or automation due to the high morbidity of the workforce. Mohr and Fourie (2004) observe that while automation may increase productivity, it may worsen unemployment, thereby exacerbating the poverty situation. As such, hunger and malnutrition complicate the whole picture and negatively impacts on households' health and wellbeing.

Climate change is one of the major challenges of the twenty-first century and adds considerable stress to societies and the environment (United Nations 2018). In fact, in October 2018, the Intergovernmental Panel on Climate Change (IPPCC) issued a special report on the impact of global warming, highlighting the likelihood that global warming will reach 1.5 °C between 2030 and 2052 if it continues to increase at the current rate (United Nations 2018). The understanding the human, social and ecological implications of climate change is complex and challenging as it involves a study of at least three uniquely complex and multi-dimensional systems which interact with one another. Such systems include the climate system, the biophysical system of natural environment, and the social system of humans (McCoy 2016).

In recent times, climate change has resulted in severe weather events such as droughts, flooding, landslides and environmental degradation, which makes it difficult for rural households to make ends meet (Coppola 2011). The impacts of climate change on health are varied and occur through many different pathways which span the full breadth of the immediate and underlying determinants of health, including: the direct impacts of heat and extreme weather events; access to the essentials of life such as clean water, nutritious food and shelter; forced migration, conflict and societal disruption; and loss of biodiversity (McCoy 2016). As such, this worsens the poverty situation. The deepening poverty situation in rural South Africa has resulted in more and more people flocking to urban or industrial areas in search for employment.

It is observed that discussions on the effects of climate change are often focused on its impacts on the environment and the general population, but there has been very little focus on its repercussions on occupational health and safety, yet workers can be affected both directly and indirectly by climate change (Adam-Poupart et al. 2013).

The current economic boom in many sub-Saharan African countries is accompanied by an unprecedented increase in non-communicable diseases (NCDs) due to industrial pollution, including pesticides. While local and international mobilisations call for more stringent pesticide control measures, African governments often refrain from adopting and enforcing strict regulations – considered as potential obstacles to "development". There is need to explore the trade-offs between production and prevention that underlie the expansion of chemical-intensive agriculture on the continent, to understand the relationships between technique, knowledge and power that condition the inclusion of African populations in the globalised economy, and to grasp the resulting health and environmental inequalities.

As in other areas with intensive use and poor regulation and/or implementation, pesticide-related health risks are exacerbated in Africa by the inadequacy of regulatory frameworks, and the weakness, or inexistence of surveillance and control systems. As a result, the import, production, trade and use of pesticides take place without the legal safeguards and institutional counterweights ensuring that public health concerns receive adequate attention in a political context where "development", narrowly defined as economic growth, and "food security", with a single dominant focus on increased agricultural production, are the overriding priorities. Facing strong activism denouncing the adverse effects of industrial agriculture and corporate influence over pesticide-related public policy making, some European governments have started to backpedal at home – at least in their declarations of political intent. African governments and Western development agencies are less challenged, however, when – backed by private foundations and transnational corporations – they are calling for an "African Green Revolution", still essentially based on the much-contested model of chemical-intensive agriculture, with pesticides as the cornerstone. In parallel, foreign agro-companies and governments are making large-scale land acquisitions in a new "scramble for Africa", transforming the continent into the new frontier of global agro-industrial expansion.

The observation that the chemical-based intensification of agricultural production in sub-Saharan Africa, which is likely to be aggravated by climate change, bears new occupational and environmental health hazards, which are exacerbated by the use of highly toxic pesticides (often banned in Europe), by informal trade, by dysfunctional control systems, by *lack of access to risk information, by the inexistence of protective gear appropriate for tropical climates, and by the diversity of exposed populations (approximately 80% of the active population has an agricultural activity – mostly on family farms, potentially exposing vulnerable populations such as women and children). As rapid population growth and trade liberalisation boost domestic and international demands, these hazards confront African governments with technically and politically intricate regulatory and public policy choices. While international donors, industry players and environmentalist groups try to influence pesticide legislation and its implementation, the underlying trade-offs between productive and preventive considerations become a major political stake, and the way these trade-offs are formulated becomes an important field of scientific enquiry. (**Tropical Pesticide Research Institute, 2018**)*

Similar to climate change, discussions on the effects of globalisation have largely not focused on its impacts on occupational health and safety, yet workers are directly and indirectly affected by globalisation. As rapid economic growth is often characterised by an increasing demand for goods and services, the logistics in the supply chain and pressure on businesses to increase production and profits, many workers may be exposed to a number of occupational hazards, in the process. Such occupational hazards may include biological hazards; behavioural hazards; ergonomic hazards; physical hazards; and radiological hazards. The exposures to occupational hazards may occur across a broad spectrum of sectors or industries, such as agriculture, healthcare, manufacturing, mining, transport and logistics, among others, particularly if there are no control measures in place. For example, if overseas markets have a high demand for bulk or break-bulk cargo such as coal, chrome, copper, manganese, or sulphur, this may expose workers to hazards such as disease-causing inhalable dust, while commodities such as phosphate rock and zircon may expose workers to disease-causing inhalable dust and radiological hazards, particularly if there are no effective controls in place (Kolo 2014).

At global level, market forces may speed up health reforms, thereby, improving the health and wellbeing of households (Edwards 2005). However, this can cause more harm than good in certain settings, as no 'one glove fits all'. Globalisation and climate change are global phenomena that may hamper food security, water resources and health, and they call for collective response in terms of global partnerships (Merson et al. 2012). International organisations such as the World Health Organization (WHO) are better positioned to provide leadership, coordination, advocacy, and global standards in terms of public health goods (Ruger and Yach 2005).

Climate change is fuelling disasters across the globe, and globalisation is a huge factor that is accelerating climate change. In many low- and middle-income countries, there are growing numbers of 'hot spots' where there are increasing levels of air pollution, water pollution, and general environmental degradation due to the rapid increase in the number of mines, industries, construction and the development of infrastructure. There is likelihood that the extreme weather conditions and severe drought experienced by many parts of southern Africa between 2015 and 2016, was certainly influenced by climate change phenomena, mass deforestation, rapid industrialisation of towns and cities and the increasing number of air pollution 'hot spots.'

Studies show that global climate change will increase the probability of extreme weather events, and such events create significant public health needs that can exceed local capacity to respond, resulting in excess morbidity or mortality and in the declaration of disasters (Keim 2008). Such adverse effects of climate change on human health will result in a greater burden on the healthcare system, in addition to other coexistent increases in demand (Weaver et al. 2010). This shows that urgent interventions are required to address the serious challenges posed by climate change, especially in the context of disaster preparedness, mitigation, response and recovery.

According to Keim (2011) vulnerability reduction programmes can reduce susceptibility or the degree of exposure to hazards and increase resilience or the capacity to cope with or recover from disaster consequences. It is worth highlighting that human vulnerability is a complex phenomenon that comprises social, economic, health, and cultural factors.

It is believed that by addressing the factors that cause changes in climate, the effects of climate change can be mitigated; and by addressing the factors that make society vulnerable to the effects of climate, there can be adaptation to climate change as local public health agencies are uniquely placed in the communities to build human resilience to climate-related disasters (Keim 2008). Other authors observe that training of healthcare professionals about climate change and its effects will also be important in meeting long-term workforce demands (Weaver et al. 2010). Furthermore, the role of insurance as a mechanism for climate change adaptation has been explored, and the finding is that insurance is critical to disaster recovery but its role in preparedness remains poorly understood, under-developed and under-utilised (Booth and Williams 2012).

Climate change has an influence in extreme weather events resulting in disasters, and this needs urgent interventions in the context of disaster management. However, it cannot be denied that there are constraints and challenges with regard to addressing the issue of climate change and its influence on disasters. From a low- and middle-income countries' context, some of the challenges include the influence of rapid globalisation, relatively moribund air quality governance, and financial implications associated with the complete phasing out of ozone-depleting substances.

7.1.1 Case of a 19-Year-Old Unemployed Widow in Mozambique

A 19-year-old unemployed widow in the remote rural areas one of Mozambique is in a dire situation as she is left to take care of her 2-year-old girl child and younger siblings. Both her parents died when she was still a toddler. She and her younger siblings were brought up by her aunt who recently died, due to complications of the prevailing severe drought in the sub-Saharan African region. The 19-year-old window's extended family structures are no longer there, and, as such, this puts her in a precarious position as she is left to fend for herself, her baby and younger siblings, under challenging circumstances. The fact that she had to drop out of school, due to pregnancy, increased her vulnerability. The severe drought has worsened the situation as the household lost their source of livelihood as they can no longer cultivate any crops, due to the severe drought. Even if there was no drought, the household could no longer afford to buy grain seeds, due to the worsening poverty situation. In the past, the household used to obtain seeds from their organic grain harvest, but this is no longer possible, because they have been using genetically modified grain seeds, recently, which they had to buy with the little money they had. The use of genetically modified grain seeds has perpetuated the cycle of poverty, because even poor households have to buy the seeds, as they cannot obtain seeds from the genetically modified grain harvest.

The case highlights that globalisation and climate change have influenced the poor household's health and wellbeing. It is so unfortunate that the young widow is literally left to care for herself, her child and younger siblings under such difficult and poor conditions.

One could propose initiatives/strategies which may help to positively improve the household's chance of health and wellbeing and to reduce the impact of globalization. While the approach is to try and address this at community, national and global levels, one should also be wary of the fact that this issue should not be viewed in isolation, but it calls for coordinated actions that interlink the community, the national and global spheres.

At local/community level, it is proposed that there be collective community partnerships to improve health. It has been impressive to see initiatives such as the 'Gone Rural' initiative implemented in the Kingdom of Eswatini. The 'Gone Rural' initiative is multifaceted, and it embraces the vitality and artistic potential of rural women, gives all rural households a chance for a livelihood through various income generating projects, provides easily accessible mobile healthcare, and empowers rural communities on holistic health and wellbeing and also addresses the issue of stigma. Such an initiative is equitable as a strategy/approach because all the rural women have an equal opportunity to sustain their household's health and wellbeing. The reality is that most of the men seek employment in the urban and industrial settings.

At national policy level, health system strengthening strategy should be informed by the root causes that increase people's vulnerability such as poverty, gender inequality and inequitable access to healthcare, and by efficient mobilization of funds and management of resources (Hecht et al. 2010). Addressing these root causes of vulnerability through public private partnerships and community involvement will ensure that there is livelihood, food security and equitable access to quality healthcare for all. As such, this will not only improve household health, but it will also improve national health and wellbeing. In that sense, this is a highly equitable strategy as long as it is well planned, well implemented and sustained.

At global level, the Universal Declaration of Human Rights should be espoused by all countries. The monopoly of the big international pharmaceutical companies should be broken so that the already highly indebted developing countries can also be able to locally produce therapeutic drugs such as ARVs at a low cost. Coupled with political will, effective prevention methods and structural changes, this will be an equitable strategy to improve the health and wellbeing of the household because it will address the challenge of transport, poor adherence and frequent shortages of therapeutic drugs in the public health sector which is accessed mainly by the poor majority population of many part of the developing countries, particularly in sub-Saharan Africa.

7.1.2 Case of a 37-Year-Old Man Who Migrated to the City in Thailand

A 37-year-old married man with one wife and five young children, is forced to migrate to the city in Thailand, due to inevitable circumstances such as his household's worsening poverty and prolonged heavy flooding which rendered their piece of land un-farmable. He realized that he urgently needed to find a job in the city to try and support his family. Luckily, he managed to get employed by one of the big firms in the city and was paid a good salary. As a responsible man, he always made sure that he went back home every month-end to provide for his family, as his wife was unemployed. As the 37-year-old man stayed in the city, he from time to time engaged in unprotected casual sexual intercourse with a few women. A couple of years later, the man fell ill, and could not go to work. He was then referred to hospital where it was confirmed that he had contracted HIV and had complications of cryptococcal meningitis. The man subsequently disclosed to his wife that he had been unfaithful to her as he had engaged in unprotected casual sexual intercourse with a few women in the city, and he suspected that he had contracted the HIV through such acts. It also transpired that the wife also engaged in unprotected sexual intercourse with a secret lover, while her husband was away working in the city. Both parties were devastated, as the man could no longer provide for his household, due to illness and loss of a job. This had dire consequences for the household as it sunk them deeper into poverty.

Climate change is the root cause of the whole issue, in the sense that climate change may have resulted in extreme weather events such as the serious flooding that rendered the 37 year-old man's land un-farmable thereby forcing him to migrate to the urban area for employment purposes so that he could be able to provide for his family back home. It is so unfortunate that the 37-year-old man's migration to the urban area or large city in Thailand had exposed him to risky behaviour, which had negative consequences in terms of the health and wellbeing of his household. As such, it would be imperative to put initiatives/strategies in place to ensure that the issue is effectively addressed at local/community level, national policy level, and at global agreement level. All these three levels are interlinked.

At local level, an initiative/strategy that would be suggested is a community participatory approach to determine exactly why the land is un-farmable, and to come up with alternative solutions that will reduce the community's vulnerability to disasters such as flooding. Who knows, may be the land that was considered un-farmable was on low-lying ground which is highly susceptible to flooding. An alternative would be to reach a consensus with the community that they should consider moving their farmlands to higher ground in order to reduce the risk of flooding, or come up with a solution of how their farmland should be rehabilitated so that it could produce yields (Coppola 2011). Once the land is farmable, it is unlikely that people like the 37-year-old man would be compelled to migrate to urban areas to seek employment, and this would enhance social cohesion, family cohesion, and livelihood. As a result, this may help to positively improve the household's health and wellbeing. After all, globalisation-induced changes in social cohesion such as migration of breadwinners to urban areas for employment purposes can be detrimental to the health and wellbeing of households (Huynen et al. 2005).

At national level, the government should have policies in place to ensure that the farmers are provided with subsidies, insurance and training as means of motivating and supporting them to derive maximum benefits from their farms (Mohr and Fourie 2004). This will encourage people to remain in the rural areas, as they will have productive farms, be able to provide for their households, and this may help to positively improve the household's health and wellbeing.

At global level, the higher international political and public profile of climate change adaptation might generate additional impetus for innovation in international financing frameworks and international institutional structures for disaster risk reduction with a development framework (Schipper and Pelling 2006). Such climate change adaptation may enhance sustainability of the farming practice and help improve the household's health and wellbeing.

There is need for foresight when designing the strategies at local, national and global level. The reality is that there has been so many reactive and hastily designed public health strategies being implemented at local, national and global level where so much money and resources were spent, and yet no effectiveness in terms of health outcomes or improvement of the health and wellbeing of households.

According to Janes (2010), globalization (including climate change) has created newly vulnerable poor who are at higher risk of poor health and malnutrition such as in the context of men who migrate from their farmland to seek employment in urban areas, leaving their wives and children behind.

At local/community level, there is need to build local resilience and adaptive capacity with active participation of the community members, reducing the need for poor people to migrate away from affected areas (Black et al. 2008). This initiative/strategy is equitable because people in the rural areas may not be at a disadvantage, as they will be self-sustained. This may help to positively improve the household's chance of health and wellbeing.

While the government of Thailand has begun framing policies to both adapt to and mitigate climate change, its response so far has been limited due to shortcomings in both the planning and implementation processes, and the fact that Thailand has the practice of giving higher priority to economic growth than environmental protection, due to the demands of globalization (Marks 2011). It is therefore imperative that at national level, Thailand should have proactive climate sensitive development policies that will put higher priority to environmental protection and the strengthening of the country's social safety nets which will soften the shocks of the impacts of climate change on the poor (Marks 2011). Such a strategy is equitable and may help to positively improve the household's chance of health and wellbeing.

At global level, there is need for agreements or treaties that will enforce commitment from all countries, particularly dealing with developed countries against exploiting the natural resources of low- and middle-income countries. It is encouraging that there is a legal obligation under the United Nations Framework Convention on Climate Change (UNFCCC) for developed countries to help developing countries adapt to the consequences of climate change (Atapattu 2010). This strategy is equitable because it encourages the levelling of the playing field between the developed and developing countries in terms of environmental protection, even though the reality is that the damage has already been done in the low-income countries, and the damage still continues to be done due to the market forces of globalization. Foresight is required to recognize the need for both mitigation and adaptation, and the international community must be quick to act on this, so that this strategy may help to positively improve the household's chance of health and wellbeing.

Crucially, it needs to be acknowledged that globalisation is a clear sign that the world is changing, and that 'change always brings risks and/or opportunities, and that the faster the change, the higher the risk, or bigger the missed opportunity'. Change can be regarded as any variation of the status quo (Muller et al. 2006). Change is inevitable in every aspect of life, and it is influenced by change agents, the most powerful of which are called drivers or driving forces which may create risks and/or opportunities (Thompson et al. 2007). According to Coppola (2011), risk can be regarded as the probability that fatalities and/or injuries and/or damage will occur, whereas opportunity can be regarded as a good chance to do better. There are different levels of change, and the drivers of change do not necessarily happen in isolation, but they are often interlinked, and the major ones may include climatic and environmental change, demographic and social transition, and economic and geopolitical transition (Coppola 2011).

Sometimes, change happens very fast, and such change can be regarded as transformational or chaotic, and this may result in serious risks or even missed opportunities especially if such change is unanticipated (Muller et al. 2006). The impact of the risks may be profound especially if the affected individuals or communities are vulnerable, such as in the low-income countries (Merson et al. 2012).

The consequences of the devastating effects of fire and floods in the informal settlements of some of the low- and middle-income countries have been more pronounced because of the rapid overcrowding in urban areas. McMichael (2002) highlights that globalisation has a great influence on the rapid social and economic changes.

In some of the low- and middle-income countries National Disaster Task Teams are formed immediately in the aftermath of the devastating effects of disasters. A National Disaster Task Team is a huge opportunity for putting measures in place to be better prepared for disasters that could occur in the future. There could be other direct and indirect benefits, such as greater public awareness of such risk, new technologies and creation of jobs during the reconstruction (Coppola 2011).

However, Kent (2002) observes that there could still be further unintended consequences due to decision-makers' inability to plan or implement the measures properly. For instance, victims of disaster may be forced to relocate as part of mitigating the risk, but the consequences of the relocation may be overlooked, especially with regard to the demographic, social and political factors pertaining to the new comers being integrated with the locals who will have to compete for the same resources. There is no doubt that the magnitude of the risk of global climate change may require adaptation and international intervention (Coppola 2011).

If change is deliberate and happens slowly or gradually, such change can be regarded as transitional, and the magnitude of the risks is usually minimal because there is possibly an opportunity to properly anticipate and manage the consequences or outcomes during the course of the change process. Change happens in a number of ways and at different rates in particular places, and the rate of change has greater impact than the direction of the change (Muller et al. 2006).

Another aspect of change is rapid demographic transition, in this regard. Rapid demographic transition influences the ability to manage disasters. According to Merson et al. (2012), rapid demographic transition is the rapid change in birth and death rates that is historically associated with the shift from a traditional society to a modern society.

According to classic theory, it is postulated that all societies start with a high birth rate and a high death rate, and as a result population growth is low because the birth and death rates balance each other out (Merson et al. 2012). It is also postulated that as the population gets modernised and is exposed to better healthcare and better standard of living, mortality rates fall, and as a result there is a sharp or explosive population growth because birth rates far exceed death rates, until at some point birth rates also start to fall, and a new equilibrium is reached (Merson et al. 2012).

This influences our ability to manage disasters in the sense that during the explosive population growth, more and more people are likely to settle in risky areas in the urban centres. The rapid population growth may result in rapid overcrowding, rapid proliferation of informal settlements, and intense competition for scarce resources as often seen in the urban areas of many parts of middle- and low-income countries where more and more people search for employment and other opportunities. Coppola (2011) observes that human settlement has always been directed by the needs of individuals and societies, such as the need for food, water, defence, and access to commerce.

Overcrowding due to explosive population growth can lead to conflict over land, hunger and malnutrition, and also health, education, and other services do not keep pace with population growth (Walley and Wright 2010). If a disaster happens in the overcrowded settlements or risky areas, the risk is more pronounced or magnified, and therefore, our ability to manage disaster may be hampered if the underlying cause is not addressed (Coppola 2011). Addressing the underlying cause may not be a health issue, but it may require a multidisciplinary approach, such as the involvement of economists, town planners, civil engineers, and architects. However, it is argued from some quarters that the foregoing postulation does not hold water, because societies differ, and the process of demographic transition is quite varied and does not always follow the path suggested by classic theory (Merson et al. 2012).

It is indeed important to anticipate and plan for change well in advance, and such planning should be collaborative in such a way that there is buy-in from all stakeholders. In fact, disaster management should be more proactive rather than reactive.

"Risk should not be defined solely by pre-determined, supposedly objective criteria that enable its various levels to be gauged through quantification. It is also a social construct, interpreted differently by all of us. Some find certain events or situations unacceptably risky and will do their utmost to avoid being involved, while to others the same events may offer exhilaration and thrills that stimulate their whole purpose of living. There may even be others to whom the particular event is a non-issue, something to be totally ignored. These differences in perception and response, coupled with differences in people's socio-economic characteristics and circumstances, result in a wide range of vulnerability in any community. Social aspects of risk interpretation must be recognised if risk is to be effectively managed, and community participation in the practical management of the problem faced is a vital component of this approach.

When disaster managers perform the hazards risk management process, they take many steps during the process that require the use of both qualitative assessments and personal experience and opinions. Because of differences in risk perception, the hazards risk management process can be flawed if risk managers do not accommodate inconsistencies between their own and their constituents' perceptions.

Risk perception may have the opposite, compounding effect for disaster managers. For instance, it is possible that a risk that is essentially harmless or has extremely low likelihood or consequence, is perceived to be much greater than reality by a manager or by the public. Such faulty perceptions on the part of the disaster management team could result in time or funding wasted in mitigation and preparation for a risk that may never happen at the expense of neglecting a more severe risk that threatens the population to a greater degree. Only effective public education and risk communication can counter the effects of public misperception of the risk" (Coppola 2011).

7.2 Sudden Onset Natural Disasters

Looking at the main causes of death in an earthquake, a cyclone, floods, and wildfires, it would be important to prioritise financial investments in the health sector for purposes of mitigation or minimisation of the risk and preparedness or precautionary measures vis-à-vis each hazard. In some parts of the world, such priorities are usually not sustained because some of the hazards are very rare in those countries.

Earthquake

An earthquake is caused by sudden movement of the earth, due to abrupt forces and faults in the constantly moving earth's plates (Coppola 2011). This may directly or indirectly cause death through trauma, drowning, landslides and collapse of buildings and infrastructure which may severely hamper lifelines such as intensive care units (Kohl et al. 2005).

Financial investment would be prioritised in capacity for disaster needs assessment; public's education and awareness to ensure prompt evacuation; health facilities that are resilient; backup power supplies; medical supplies; capacity for casualty care, hospital care and primary healthcare in temporary community shelters to ensure prompt emergency medical care as survival of victims largely depends on early interventions (Ashkenazi et al. 2005).

Cyclone

A cyclone is a spinning storm related to atmospheric weather patterns that mainly affect coastal areas, and, rarely inland areas (Coppola 2011). Although the direct cause of death by a cyclone may be due to drowning and direct trauma, its major causes of death are indirect and they are largely due to the extensive devastating effects of landslides and flooding resulting in spread of diseases due to contaminated water and also damage to infrastructure which compromises access to lifelines (Coppola 2011).

It would be important to prioritise investment in health facilities that are resilient to the devastating effects of cyclones, capacity and personnel to conduct needs assessment, evacuation programme, and education and awareness of the public to ensure sustainability of the preparedness and mitigation plan.

Floods

Floods can be regarded as a hydrologic hazard because they are related to the water cycle (Coppola 2011). Although the direct causes of death due to floods can be as a result of direct trauma and drowning, most of the causes of deaths due to floods are as a result of indirect effects such as landslides, and environmental changes which may result in waterborne diseases such as cholera, and vector borne diseases such as malaria (Merson et al. 2012).

It would be important to invest in flood resistant health facilities; equipment and personnel for adequate casualty care; environmental health such as vector control, hygiene and supplies of portable toilets and clean water to prevent water-borne diseases; education and awareness of the public would also be a priority to ensure prompt evacuation (Fundter et al. 2008).

Wildfires

These are fires that burn out of control and they usually cover wider geographical areas and may damage buildings vegetation and directly or indirectly cause death, through burns, asphyxiation, and trauma (Coppola 2011).

It would be key to invest in capacity for fire risk assessment, education of the public to enhance prompt evacuation, capacity for casualty and hospital care, as well as capacity for provision of primary healthcare in temporary community shelters (Coppola 2011).

It is crucial to prioritise financial investment for the purpose of mitigation and preparedness vis-à-vis each hazard. However, investment in excess resources could create further challenges.

In certain parts of the world, many fatalities are caused as a result of the direct and indirect effects of hazards such as cyclones. Coppola (2011) defines a fatality as a death due to an accident or a disaster, and believes that since the number of fatalities may surge during a disaster, and that established systems of fatality management may be quickly overwhelmed, it therefore becomes the responsibility of government to manage fatalities.

In addition to the large numbers of fatalities, the large numbers of injured people who would require emergency care may also surge, and this may also overwhelm disaster response healthcare efforts of certain settings as there may be insufficient personnel and facilities for effective handling of the situation especially if the disaster was of sudden onset and caused extensive devastation. Merson et al. (2012) observe that although many low income countries' healthcare systems are ill prepared to deal with massive disasters, even established disaster management systems of developed nations may be overwhelmed in disaster situations caused by cyclonic storms such as what happened during Hurricane Katrina in the United States of America.

There was a time when the continued surge of large numbers of people who had sustained extensive burn injuries overwhelmed the disaster response, due to lack of leadership and command during the wildfire disasters of 2010 and 2011. The "flooding" of the southern African hospital with healthcare personnel and other experts from different places created confusion, as almost each and every individual was making suggestions about how to handle the situation. This suggests that the healthcare response to the disaster was uncoordinated, as many of the healthcare professionals felt so helpless and overwhelmed by the confusion.

Romundstad et al. (2004) suggests that command and control could have been the possible solution to preventing such uncoordinated efforts and confusion. This implies that a framework needed to be established whereby a single leader or committee could manage the overarching disaster response and this is also applicable to casualty care in a hospital setting (Coppola 2011).

There is an urgent need for more Southern African health personnel to be trained in disaster management and disaster medicine to ensure that they know exactly what to do in situations where they are faced with large numbers of disaster victims, based on previous trauma scenarios. The reality is that many parts of Southern Africa are faced with persistent brain drain, and the few remaining healthcare personnel that are specialised in disaster medicine are also specialised in other medical fields, and only episodically dedicate their professional life to disaster medicine (Ashkenazi et al. 2005). Mass "flooding" of disaster victims into health facilities could create confusion if there is no leadership and command among the disaster response healthcare team.

The emotional toll on survivors of disasters must also be addressed. In fact, some researchers even admit that the field of emotional trauma in disaster situations has been far less studied (Hafstad and Haavind 2012). In most instances, so much focus is paid on dealing with the physical trauma, whereas, the emotional or psychological aspect is not given much attention during and after disasters. For example, during the heavy floods and wildfire disasters that hit parts of the South African province of KwaZulu-Natal, many people lost everything, many were displaced, many suffered severe injuries, some died, and in fact there was mass trauma. No one in the disaster management team seemed to pay particular focus on the emotional or psychological aspects of the victims as many families were severely affected by the disaster. Even if the emotional and psychological aspect was mentioned in some of the protocols, it was merely glossed over.

There needs to be an integrative approach to mass trauma around the world, and the emotional aspect cannot be overlooked, because it is unlikely that there would be complete healing after a disaster if the emotional aspect is not properly addressed Travis (2011). This should also take into account the emotional vulnerabilities of different groups such as children, and the fact that parenting after a disaster has its challenges. Studies suggest that the degree of actual threat in terms of children's proximity to the disaster, physical injury, and witnessed experiences is proportional to the risk of developing post-traumatic stress disorder (Hafstad and Haavind 2012).

While information for the medical aspects of disaster surge is increasingly available, there is little guidance for healthcare facilities on how to manage the psychological aspects of large-scale disasters that might involve a surge of psychological casualties (Meredith et al. 2011). In addition, no models are available to guide the development of training curricula to address these needs (Meredith et al. 2011).

Emotional or psychological aspects need to be seriously addressed in the context of disaster situations. There needs to be prioritisation of psychological consequences for disaster preparedness and response. However, some authors argue that most people exposed to potentially traumatic events are resilient, even though research about the factors that may promote or deter resilience has been limited (Bonanno et al. 2007). Travis (2011) observes that in situations of mass trauma, some people perform rituals and practices for resilience and meaning making. As such, there is need for caution in instrumentalising decisions, because managing disaster may be complex, multidimensional and individually unique.

7.2.1 A 90-Day Operational Plan for the Myanmar-Cyclone Nargis Flash Appeal

According to Coppola (2011), a flash report is quickly released to ensure that there is recognition that the disaster did happen, and, the report or appeal also serves to ensure that there is wider coverage about the magnitude of the disaster, revealing exactly what has happened, the current situation, the requirements and what needs to be done to address the situation within specific short-term, mid-term and long-term time-frames (Table 7.1). The purpose of this section is to choose one of the health sector projects in the Myanmar-Cyclone Nargis Flash Appeal of 2008, and to use the following worksheet to design a 90-day operational plan based on that particular chosen health project as shown in Table 7.2. The health project is titled: "Emergency Health Response" whose main objectives are to prevent and effectively manage diarrhoea and measles, to prevent water-borne and food-borne diseases, and to prevent and manage the malaria (United Nations 2008).

Table 7.1 Point of the situation and objectives

Function		Desired level of performance	Current state of things	Desired status after 90 days
1. Assessment and monitoring	1.1. Assessment	Health needs, health system delivery capacity and operational constraints known; information consolidated, arranged, and displayed in a manner that facilitates consensus and decisions	Urgent need for water receptacles and water-purifying tablets; Need for emergency health kits; Need for mosquito nets (United Nations 2008). Damaged transportation infrastructure is an operational constraint (Merson et al. 2012). Information is not consistent because it comes from different sources.	Adequate provision of clean water, mosquito nets, and rehabilitated transportation infrastructure. Coordinated and consistent information to prevent confusion (Coppola 2011).
	1.2. Surveillance and early warning	Priority health threats and system's critical capacities monitored regularly with possibility of early warning	Potential outbreaks of malaria because 70 per cent of the population lives in malaria endemic areas, Potential outbreak of measles due to low vaccine coverage; Risk of diarrhoeal diseases such as cholera due to poor sanitation and a lack of drinking water (United Nations 2008).	A fully functional emergency health response surveillance program
2. Support to coordination	2.1. Health coordination	Organised space and time for all health partners to discuss issues, decide upon action to take, and assign responsibilities; mechanisms for follow-up, evaluation, and readjustment established	Government plays the overall leadership role through the Emergency Committee and there is an operational national disaster management plan. Humanitarian coordinator through the Humanitarian country team plays the supportive coordinating role. Cluster Leads responsible for assessments, monitoring, evaluation, and management of information to ensure effectiveness (United Nations 2008).	Health cluster Lead effectively playing the leadership role regarding health coordination including organised space for all health partners to discuss issues, action to be taken, and mechanisms for follow-up.
	2.2. Coordination with other sectors	Work in all other sectors geared to the survival and healthy and sustainable livelihoods of the population	Cluster leads collaborate with counterparts in other sectors to ensure sustainability of efforts.	Sustainable clean water and nutritious food supplies.

(continued)

Table 7.1 (continued)

Function		Desired level of performance	Current state of things	Desired status after 90 days
3. Identifying and filling gaps	3.1. Filling the life-threatening gaps	Life-threatening conditions prevented or promptly addressed, with CFR maintained within international norms	Measles vaccination coverage is poor. Rehydration salt and clean water to prevent diarrhoeal diseases especially among children (United Nations 2008).	Effective prevention measures, early diagnosis and treatment of measles, malaria and water-borne and food-borne diseases.
	3.2. Filling gaps that are critical to effective delivery of health care	Appropriate means applied to improve equitable access to health care in a sustainable way and according to international standards (e.g., SPHERE)	Many places are still inaccessible due to the damaged infrastructure, and therefore equitable access to healthcare is more compromised (United Nations 2008).	Rehabilitated and reconstructed infrastructure to ensure sustainable and equitable access to healthcare.
4. Strengthening and repairing systems, and building capacities	4.1. Building national capacities	National health partners fully integrated in, and supportive of the delivery of humanitarian assistance	There appears to be lack of full integration between government relief agencies and non-governmental agencies (United Nations 2008).	Fully integrated partnership between government and non-governmental agencies.
	4.2. Building capacities of international partners	International health partners effectively complementing national efforts	The capacity is there, as 10 United Nations organisations and 9 non-governmental organisations are willing to assist the government's efforts. But it is a concern that some of the United Nations' assistance seems to be bilateral and skewed towards governmental agencies (United Nations 2008).	A more balanced coordinated complementary partnership between international and national efforts.
5. A safe and strong programme	5.1. Programme administration	Programme staff and assets are safe, properly administered, and accounted for, with no rupture in the pipeline; there is real-time exchange of information	Real-time exchange of information seems to be hindered by the disruption of communication systems (United Nations 2008).	Well administered program, with no rupture in the pipeline. Fully functional information systems for effective and efficient real-time exchange of information
	5.2. Programme direction and management	The program has overall direction, is represented as needed, and gets backstopping from HQ; management is informed on progress	Update on progress may take some weeks (United Nations 2008).	Well managed and well represented program with clear direction. Management should be updated on progress at least daily.

Table 7.2 The "90 days plan"

Function		Desired status after 90 days	Measures for improving the situation		
			What must be in place in 30 days	What must be in place in 60 days	What must be in place in 90 days
1. Assessment and monitoring	1.1. Assessment	Adequate provision of clean water, mosquito nets, and rehabilitated transportation infrastructure. Efficient and effective healthcare delivery	Capacity to enhance healthcare delivery and better coverage (Coppola 2011)	Information system that reflects consensus so that this could prevent any confusion and ambiguity (Merson et al. 2012).	Rehabilitated and reconstructed infrastructure to prevent operational constraints (Coppola 2011).
	1.2. Surveillance and early warning	Fully functional surveillance and early warning system	Health risk assessment and needs analysis	Statistics and updates on incidence of measles, malaria, diarrhoeal diseases, water-borne and food-borne diseases	Full capacity for surveillance and early warning
2. Support to coordination	2.1. Health coordination	Health cluster Lead effectively playing the leadership role regarding health coordination including organised space for all health partners to discuss issues, action to be taken, and mechanisms for follow-up.	Health coordination plan	Full implementation of the health coordination plan.	Mechanisms for follow-up of the health coordination
	2.2. Coordination with other sectors	Effective and sustainable coordination between the health cluster, water and sanitation cluster, food cluster, and logistics cluster	Coordination plan between the health cluster, water and sanitation cluster, food cluster, and logistics cluster	Full implementation of the inter-sectoral coordination plan	Mechanisms for follow-up of the inter-sectoral coordination

(continued)

Table 7.2 (continued)

Function		Desired status after 90 days	Measures for improving the situation		
			What must be in place in 30 days	What must be in place in 60 days	What must be in place in 90 days
3. Identifying and filling gaps	3.1. Filling the life-threatening gaps	Effective and sustainable healthcare, including prevention, early diagnosis and treatment of measles, malaria, water-borne and food-borne diseases.	Provision of mosquito nets, portable drinking water, food, soap, mobile toilets, and medical supplies	Health promotion and awareness to ensure that the community also understands the importance (Walley and Wright 2010).	No new cases or recurrence of measles, water-borne and food-borne diseases, and malaria.
	3.2. Filling gaps that are critical to effective delivery of health care	Capacity and infrastructure to ensure sustainable and equitable access to healthcare (Merson et al. 2012).	Sufficient human resources and capacity for the delivery of emergency healthcare, particularly with regard to the management of diarrhoeal diseases, measles, water-borne and food-borne diseases, and malaria (United Nations 2008).	Rehabilitated and reconstructed causeways, waterways and jetties (United Nations 2008)	Rehabilitated and reconstructed water supply systems, sanitation, healthcare services and facilities (United Nations 2008)
4. Strengthening and repairing systems, and building capacities	4.1. Building national capacities	Fully integrated partnership between government and non-governmental agencies (United Nations 2008).	Integration of national partners through the Emergency Committee (United Nations 2008)	Designation of Cluster Lead to drive the national efforts regarding the Emergency Health response (United Nations 2008).	Coordinated efforts between governmental and non-governmental agencies
	4.2. Building capacities of international partners	A more balanced coordinated complementary partnership between international and national efforts to ensure sustainability of efforts (Coppola 2011).	Integration of international partners through the United Nations Humanitarian Coordinator (United Nations 2008)	Designation of inter-cluster Lead to drive the emergency health project with support from the global cluster Lead	A strong integrated international partners' emergency health response to complement the national response

5. A safe and strong program	5.1. Program administration	Well administered program, with no rupture in the pipeline. Fully functional information systems for effective and efficient real-time exchange of information	The humanitarian country team to be responsible for the overall administration of the programme, and to ensure safety of staff and programme assets	Appointment of a competent and qualified administrator to be specifically responsible for the administration of the emergency health response project.	Information systems to ensure real-life information exchange
	5.2. Program direction and management	Well managed and well represented program with clear direction. Management should be updated on progress at least daily.	Full representation of key stakeholders in the program to ensure ownership and sustainability (Walley and Wright 2010).	Implementation of program guidelines to give a clear direction to the program	Information system to ensure daily updates on progress

7.3 Biological Hazards

An epidemic is characterised by the occurrence of cases of disease in a community or region at a level that is clearly in excess of the background incidence of disease for this defined group during a particular time period (Joubert and Ehrlich 2007). It cannot be denied that there are a number of instances where epidemics have occurred after a disaster, and as such, it is hardly surprising that disasters often strike fear of epidemics in many quarters. It is observed that the fear of epidemics after a disaster appears to be a constant media and political issue because of the mere fact that epidemics are difficult to control and that they are statistically considered to be the greatest killer of human beings (Coppola 2011).

Natural disasters such as the earthquake that devastated Haiti in 2010, often result in damage to infrastructure, water supplies and sanitation. This poses a risk, because cholera epidemics could arise if the situation is not promptly managed through safer water and better sanitation to prevent transmission (Tappero and Tauxe 2011).

Sudharsanam and Gautam (2012) argue that sometimes the media can unjustifiably fuel the fear of epidemics after a disaster such as what happened after the media misinformation which associated the South Asia tsunami disaster of 2004 with the outbreak of measles in some parts of India. It is further added that the fear that unburied corpses could fuel the spread of epidemics after a natural disaster such as after the South Asia tsunami of December 2004, is a myth because it is not based on scientific evidence (Morgan and de Ville de Goyet 2005). However, it is acknowledged that scientific evidence alone is not enough to bring about public health action, but it is suggested that there needs to be clear practical standards and guidelines to be communicated to communities on how bodies of victims of natural disaster need to be managed (Morgan and de Ville de Goyet 2005).

Sometimes, the threat of epidemics is sensationalised, politicised and blown out of proportion, especially if the political system of the affected country is not favoured by the volatile and influential political opposition. It appears as if there is an element of hypocrisy and double standards at times as often seen by the deterioration of disasters due to the influence of so called "super powers" such as during the civil wars in countries such as Iraq, Afghanistan, Libya, and Syria, in recent times. In some countries, it is not uncommon to witness the politicisation and sensationalisation of epidemics by the government's ruling political party and by the main opposition political party whenever there is a disaster in a territory or province that is not governed by them.

The risk of epidemics after a disaster is negligible, but at the same time such a risk should not be ignored (Floret et al. 2006). There needs to be practical guidelines of communicating to the public about how corpses and carcasses should be managed, and how the spread of epidemics can be prevented after a disaster. Sometimes alarmist warnings and reporting have fuelled the fear of epidemics and yet studies show that this fear which appears to be a constant media and political issue is not justified, as epidemics are not always a constant feature following a disaster.

Sometimes, there is chaos that ensues after a disaster and this contributes to the outbreak of communicable diseases. As such, the challenge of poor immunisation coverage, poor sanitation, poor shelter, and proliferation of diseases vectors are pertinent issues regarding the perpetuation of epidemics especially after a disaster.

It is pity that there is often a delay in response to the outbreak of epidemics, particularly in low- and middle-income countries and rather more so during periods of economic crisis as what happened during the outbreak of Konzo in the Democratic Republic of Congo where many of the worst affected areas were remote and inaccessible (Bonmarin et al. 2002). In such instances, lack of resources and lack of reliable information appears to be a big challenge in implementing a prompt and effective public health response after a disaster. As such, it becomes difficult to provide accurate information about the magnitude of the epidemic in the affected areas.

This calls for countries to have effective surveillance systems for specific diseases or programme areas such as maternal death notification system, expanded immunisation programme and the statutory notifiable diseases system, among others (Walley and Wright 2010). In a nutshell, disease surveillance can be described as a state of watchfulness to detect trends or changes in disease patterns which require an active public health response. The functions of a disease surveillance are: to estimate the magnitude of a problem; determine the geographic distribution of illness; portray the natural history of disease; detect epidemics and define a problem; generate hypotheses and stimulate research; evaluate control measures; monitor changes in infectious agents; detect changes in health practices; and to facilitate planning (Joubert and Ehrlich 2007).

In fact, the disease surveillance should be part and parcel of routine health information systems, and this should be up to date because out-dated information may not be of much help especially in the context of a disaster as this requires urgent public health response. Specifically, in a country with significant health problems and limited resources, there is need to know what diseases are currently responsible for the main burden on healthcare services and how well health services are running so that resources can be used effectively and efficiently. For that reason, it is hardly surprising that the World Health Organization has proposed the implementation of integrated disease surveillance programmes at country level to achieve synergy and sharing of resources (Joubert and Ehrlich 2007).

The incompleteness of routine data, and the fact that data are often obtained from different sources, are the main problems or limitations of the routine health information systems of many of the low- and middle-income countries. The chaos about the perpetuation of epidemics after a disaster may be compounded by the lack of effective disease surveillance systems. After all, a strong disease surveillance system with early warning mechanisms will enable effective rapid response to disease outbreaks (Coppola 2011).

There is no doubt that advancement in medical scientific research has made it possible to produce antimicrobial agents and vaccines that have prevented the spread of epidemics and pandemics, and to a large extent this might have resulted in the widely held global assumption that infectious diseases will be contained and diminished over time. However, the emergence and re-emergence of infectious disease threats which are diseases caused by microbial agents that were previously not known to cause disease in humans, has come with realisation that several distinct phenomena can produce unexpected and urgent infectious diseases threats (Merson et al. 2012).

In recent times, there has been a few of such unexpected and urgent infectious disease threats, including the 2009 influenza H1N1 virus of swine origin, which by the time it was detected, it had already undergone several mutations and widespread dissemination among humans which suggested that efforts to contain it would be futile. It is hardly surprising that the World Health Organisation immediately issued a global alert of an inevitable H1N1 influenza pandemic.

The 2009 influenza H1N1global alert caught many by surprise because at that time, public health officials and vaccine manufactures were still busy preparing for another possible influenza pandemic caused by the highly pathogenic avian influenza A (H5N1) of which human cases first appeared in 1997 (Merson et al. 2012). After the 2009 influenza H1N1 global alert, there was so much panic in Southern Africa as the media continuously provided hourly updates about precautionary measures to take and about the number of human cases of H1N1 that were detected per specific Southern African location.

Ports of entry and workplaces had to quickly develop guidelines about how to deal with the threat of the spread of the H1N1 influenza. In one of the major seaports of southern Africa, the biggest challenge was that there was a higher because of the frequent entry of cargo ships and sea fearers from different parts of the world. During that period, the seaport's productivity was severely affected because many employees decided to be absent from work either because they had influenza symptoms or because they feared that they would get infected with the H1N1 influenza A virus because of their frequent interaction with the sea fearers. Fraser et al. (2009) observe that even though there was limited data and uncertainty about the virulence and pandemic potential of the H1N1 influenza virus, it is very likely that international travellers from endemic countries, such as Mexico, at the time, may have contributed a great deal to the rapid spread of the HI1N1 influenza A virus, across the globe.

Despite the uncertainty about the pandemic potential of the H1N1 influenza virus, the 2009 H1N1 influenza global alert was warranted because the emergence or re-emergence of infectious diseases should never be taken lightly because the outcome could be dire if there is no concerted and quick response. Although it ultimately turned out that the H1N1 influenza virus was not as virulent as was initially anticipated, global alerts such as the 2009 H1N1 influenza could enhance a shared responsibility among nations which could help strengthen the fabric of the global public health response and security (Khan et al. 2009). After all, there is still a possibility that a pandemic of such influenza may occur sometime in the future (Walley and Wright 2010).

It cannot be denied that the 2009 H1N1 global alert was probably over-exaggerated, of which the media and public health policies played a big part and that so much money and resources were spent as part of the global, regional and in-country preparedness, mitigation and response to the potential threat of the H1N1 influenza. Schwarzinger et al. (2010) observe that alarmist public health policy messages were countered with public dissonance because the general public's daily experiences did not confirm the widely publicised threat of H1N1 influenza, and as such, even the mass vaccination campaigns in countries such as France encountered challenges and resistance because of the general public's fear of the safety of such a vaccine. In that sense, other urgent public health priorities might have been compromised and overlooked as more attention and energy was channelled towards the H1N1 influenza threat which turned out to be not such a huge threat even though it still produced widespread morbidity and mortality.

7.4 Technological and Socioeconomic Hazards

Given the staggering list of hazards in the world, it would be beneficial for disaster managers to be acquainted with the different categories and different classification systems of hazards, to ensure that hazards that are most likely to cause the most devastation are easily recognised, identified, evaluated and controlled (Coppola 2011). Looking at the concept of man-made hazards and their different categories, and may be interesting to determine whether man-made hazards, specifically technological hazards by human failure and by intention should be classified under the same heading as social, economic, or political hazards.

A hazard is the capacity of a natural or man-made agent or activity to cause a particular adverse effect to the population, environment, infrastructure, and built structure. Man-made hazards are due to the intentional or unintentional actions of humans or human innovations, and such hazards are generally categorised into technological hazards and socioeconomic hazards (Coppola 2011). Technological hazards may be sub-divided into transportation hazards, infrastructure hazards, industrial hazards, structural fires and failures, and intentional, civil and political hazards (Coppola 2011).

Given the growing number of disasters that occur as a result of transportation by road, railways, airways, and to some extent by sea; transportation can be considered as a major technological hazard of our time (Coppola 2011). Judging from the Express Railway disaster in Amagasaki, transportation hazards pose a huge risk to life, property and the environment, and have social, economic and political consequences (Nagata et al. 2006).

Infrastructure hazards include power facilities, telecommunication systems failure, computer network failures, critical water or sewer systems failure, major gas distribution line breaks, dam failures (Coppola 2011). Failure of such infrastructure may hamper critical life systems, communication systems, business systems, access, food supplies, health and hygiene systems; and this has social, economic and political consequences (White 1999).

Industrial hazards include hazardous material storage processing and storage accidents, and raw material extraction accidents such as mining accidents (Coppola 2011). An observation is that the people who die in mine disasters are usually bread winners who support extended families from the poverty-stricken rural areas such as in Southern Africa. This really magnifies the social, economic and political consequences of mining disasters.

Exposure to the risk of structural fires and failures is extreme because of the high number of casualties that this may cause, and such a risk cuts across all countries of the world, and damage of built structures through fires or human failure may have negative socioeconomic and political consequences, as employment, commerce and government services may be affected (Coppola 2011).

Technological hazards by human intention may include deliberate attacks through biological agents, nuclear weapons, civil unrest, stampedes, crime and wars (Coppola 2011). For example, the atomic bombing of the Japanese cities of Nagasaki and Hiroshima during World War II, caused tremendous socioeconomic-political disaster, the effects of which lasted for many decades (LaDou 2007).

Many of the technological hazards by human failure and by intention have social, economic or political implications. While classifying such technological hazards in the same group as social, economic or political hazards may seem feasible, this should be avoided or done with caution to prevent confusion and ambiguity.

It appears as if some of the technological hazards' risks have somehow been accepted by society due to their perceived benefit. There is no doubt that technological innovation has made life somewhat convenient and easier to some extent especially now that the world has become a global village. Globalisation appears to drive the fast pace of technological innovations including transportation, infrastructure, industrialisation, and built structures (Hill 2009).

Transportation by roadway, railway, airway, and by sea has made it a lot convenient and quicker for the movement of people and goods from one point to another, and yet the risk posed by such transportation hazards can be enormous. The astronomical figures of transportation fatalities throughout the world, are spine chilling, despite the numerous campaigns and transport policies aimed at preventing transportation disasters (Walley and Wright 2010). It is hardly surprising that Coppola (2011) regards transportation hazards as having become a norm or such a common part of global society.

Technological innovations such as mobile phones seem to be contributing, at least in part, to the high number of roadway accidents in many countries, as it has somewhat become a norm to see drivers using their mobile phones and even sending text messages while driving.

Industrialisation comes with opportunities for employment, and society often perceives such opportunities as beneficial towards addressing challenges such as poverty, and yet the industrial hazards that come with such development tend to be overlooked or not regarded as an issue. The most common political argument in many of the low-income and middle-income countries is that it is necessary to protect jobs and industries, and this seems to give a licence to the proliferation of poorly regulated industries, in such areas (Hill 2009).

Sometimes, it is not about society embracing the risks posed by the technological hazards, but there is a possibility that society, or at least, a large segment of society is not aware of the risks posed by such technological hazards. Kasperson and Pijawka (1985) observe that lack of familiarity with technological hazards, generally low levels of community awareness and preparedness, the rapid onset of the hazard event, and the potential for larger secondary consequences present critical problems for emergency and disaster managers.

While it may appear as if society has embraced the risks posed by technological hazards, it is also possible that a segment of society is not familiar with the risks because many of the technological innovations are still relatively new. Managing technological hazards requires the simultaneous goals of enlarging social benefits and reducing risks of such hazards (Kasperson and Pijawka 1985). Society should be familiarised with the risks of technological hazards and should be protected in accordance with set standards and legislation, and at the same time society should also take responsibility (LaDou 2007).

7.5 Food Shortages and Slow Onset 'Natural' Crises

Food shortage or the situation whereby food supplies cannot meet the energy and nutrition requirements of people, does not necessarily translate into a crisis, but there are times where it can spiral into mass incidence of food shortage, and possibly famine (Coppola 2011). Mass incidence of food shortage is a humanitarian crisis because it threatens the health and life of a large number of people, and as such, the health sector in collaboration with other stakeholders has a key role to play to address the situation (Coppola 2011).

Mitigation against and preparation for possible future food-shortage crises can be complex because food shortage can be as a result of the complex interaction of a number of acute and chronic factors such as food production crises, socio-cultural factors, politico-economic factors, and environmental factors (Coppola 2011).

Therefore, mitigation against and preparation for possible future food-shortage crises requires concerted effort from various stakeholders such as the public sector, private sector, non-governmental organisations, and donor agencies, among others. The health sector or health professionals are better positioned to influence political decision-making by providing research evidence, tools and frameworks about mitigation against and preparation for future food shortage crises. Such influence of the health sector can provide the impetus and influence for multi-stakeholder partnerships for the purpose of planning, assessing, and analysing the situation to ensure that appropriate and relevant interventions are implemented as different settings may differ with regard to the causes and effects of food shortages.

Proper planning, situational assessment, early warning systems and on-going full-country monitoring and analysis are important as long as it is known what to monitor and what not to monitor, and reference should be made to a baseline situation bearing in mind that such monitoring and analysis should not be limited to the confines of food security or food crisis, but should be holistic.

Judging from its very low gross national income per capita compared to the regional and global average, the chronic food insecurity issue in Niger is much deeper and insidious, because it is linked to chronic poverty (World Health

Organization, n.d.). Hence the need to look deeper and wider beyond the health sector with regard to mitigation and preparedness for future food-shortage crises relevant to such situations. Empowerment of the community, such as in community-based therapeutic care ensures that there is strengthening of local capacities as the community takes ownership of the mitigation measures and preparation for future food-shortage crises.

In many low- and middle-income countries such as in parts of sub-Saharan Africa, Asia and the Americas, issues of food shortage are well addressed on paper, but in practice, the mitigation against and preparation for future food shortage crises tend to fall short because the health sector does not seem to play an influential role, and some authors regard this as health sector gap.

Some of the strategies to deal with food shortages are aimed at building coping mechanisms at individual, community and local levels when crises occur. There is no doubt about the importance of resilience in times of crises. The main reason why the Southern Africa region was able to avert the food shortage crisis after the devastating drought of the early 1990s was because of the effective coping mechanisms of the affected people, despite the fact that the region was economically and politically less well prepared to withstand such a crisis than nowadays.

In recent times, some of the low- and middle-income countries have been facing food crises of surprising scale and novelty. What happened to the coping mechanisms of the affected people? Well, the answer may not be that simple because food shortage crises may be due to a complex combination of many factors, and therefore interventions to deal with such a challenge have to take cognisance of that complexity (Coppola 2011).

While the familiar culprits of drought and mismanagement of national strategies were implicated in some of the recent food shortage crisis faced by the Southern Africa region, it is purported that the complexity of the challenge is compounded by poverty and the burden of disease in the region. It is observed that the HIV and AIDS epidemic has created a new category of highly vulnerable households, and has resulted in reduced viability of farming livelihoods, increased sensitivity of rural communities to external shocks, and has thus decreased their resilience. This suggests that the Southern Africa region is facing a new variant food shortage crisis that needs to be conceptualised and addressed through more innovative approaches, bearing in mind the importance of political will.

In parts some of the affected low- and middle-income countries, the magnitude of the challenge of the food shortage crisis is not really clearly understood, or maybe it is not taken seriously. There is currently a wave of high morbidity and high mortality, mainly due to the multiple burden of HIV and AIDS, cardiovascular diseases, diabetes mellitus, and cancer, among others, which is largely due to fragility of health systems, poor nutrition, lifestyle, behaviour, and poor adherence to treatment. Some of these issues are compounded by the fact that the affected people do not get the minimal nutrition requirements, particularly in the rural areas where people used to rely on farming for their livelihoods. Clearly, the burden of HIV and

AIDS, TB, Malaria, and the emerging epidemic of non-communicable diseases also contributes to the high morbidity and mortality. Without innovative interventions, and political will, food shortage crises can become a vicious cycle (Walley and Wright 2010).

The known strategies and frameworks of mitigation against and preparation for future food shortage crises are all important. However, there needs to be awareness that nutritional concerns in low- and middle-income countries are diverse, and the burden of TB, HIV and AIDS, Malaria, and non-communicable diseases can complicate the whole picture and create a novelty of food shortage (Merson et al. 2012).

There is urgent need for early warning systems to be robust, and the need for strengthening health systems to ensure that social determinants of health are addressed so that the cycle of issues such as food shortages can be broken. The continent of Africa is one of the most challenged continents in terms of cycles of issues such as food shortages, and this cycle needs to be broken. While considerable achievements in global reduction of food shortage and strengthening of health systems have been made, progress in Africa has been very limited as it is estimated that a third of the African population faces hunger and chronic malnutrition.

The speed and a host of crises have caught many countries unprepared, and therefore early warning systems represent one of the instruments of preventive disaster management. In the Southern Africa Development Community (SADC) region where, most of the SADC countries have operational early warning systems which make them aware of impending food shortfalls, even though timelines and accuracy of reporting varies across countries. However, as an early information system, a famine early warning system alone does not contribute much to food security, but it contributes to the higher systems such as food security systems, as long as those higher systems are linked with response mechanisms.

It is observed that while early warning systems may be sufficient to warn of impending food shortages, in most cases the information and analysis is insufficient to actually guide response planning. For example, in some of the SADC countries, governments were slow to acknowledge the impending production shortfalls of the year 2002. As such, it cannot be denied that while early warning systems have their advantages, especially in the context of the Southern Africa region which is prone to cycles of issues such as drought and food shortages, early warning systems also have their limitations.

It is argued that food shortage or famine early warning systems using socio-economic data suffer from several problems which include the following: they cannot, and do not attempt to, distinguish between qualitatively different kinds of food shortage or famine; they cannot predict these accurately or early enough because all the socio-economic indicators produce both false positives and false negatives, and the indicators themselves are late and because interpretation of the data is complex and time-consuming; within the context of a famine that is occurring, these indicators cannot predict excess mortality. Early warning systems can be more useful if they are linked to and complemented by timely response mechanisms.

7.6 Complex Humanitarian Emergencies

It would be interesting to assess whether the Responsibility to report initiative influences or hampers humanitarian work in complex emergencies. According to Merson et al. (2012), "complex emergencies" is a relatively new term that was recently coined after the new millennium by merging the terms "complex humanitarian emergencies" and "complex political emergencies" in order to maintain simplicity and consistency. While the term "complex humanitarian emergencies" attributes the cause and effect of significant humanitarian crisis to a combination of factors such as food shortages, war, and population displacements, among others; the term "complex political emergencies" locates the cause and effects of such significant crisis in the political sphere (Merson et al. 2012).

Coppola (2011) adds that complex emergencies appear to occur only in the poorest countries because the impact of dramatic and significant disruptions in the political, economic and social situation may seriously overwhelm the coping abilities of the population and seriously hamper or paralyse the ability of the government or local authorities to respond to the complex situation, and as a result, this may require a coordinated multi-sectoral international intervention such as military action.

International interventions such as those guided by the Responsibility to Protect came about in order to give directives as to whether interventions such as military action would be necessary, and also how such interventions should be executed in the event of a sovereign state failing or ignoring to protect its citizens from a major catastrophe such as civil war or insurgency, among others (Evans and Sahnoun 2001). Since security for the population of the affected country, region or society, as well as those involved with humanitarian work may be an issue in the event of complex emergencies, initiatives such as the Responsibility to Protect can address that security issue.

After all, the Responsibility to Protect initiative embraces prevention, response and rebuilding, and these specific responsibilities can influence humanitarian work in complex emergencies (Evans and Sahnoun 2001). For example, after military intervention, the Responsibility to Protect would support the affected place with regard to recovery, reconstruction, and reconciliation; and as such, this can influence humanitarian work as many humanitarian organisations would like to get involved at this stage.

The challenge though is that it is possible that military action and peacekeeping can also create tension and worsen the situation by creating more instability, as issues of security can deteriorate to such an extent that it may not be safe for humanitarian workers to be onsite. It is therefore important to realise that each society, country or region is unique, which implies that military intervention may not be relevant in all situations of complex emergencies. At the same time, it is reported that the situation may also deteriorate out of control if military intervention is not executed early enough as a form of prevention, which will ensure that the root causes and risks of complex emergencies are identified and promptly dealt with (Williams and Bellamy 2005).

The Responsibility to Protect can influence or hamper humanitarian work. It is crucial to analyse and to consider the uniqueness of the affected area before executing the Responsibility to Protect, because sometimes humanitarian interventions can be a dilemma in complex emergencies (Bellamy 2006).

In some instances, it is possible that the Responsibility to Protect may go a bit too far, especially when the international armed response takes the side of the opposition to overthrow the ruling government. The irony is that it often happens especially in low-income countries that once the ruling government has been overthrown, the situation gets even worse in terms of unrest, conflict, displacement of large human populations, and civilian killings (Merson et al. 2012).

It is hardly surprising that the then United Nations (UN) Secretary General, Mr. Kofi Annan lamented about the dilemma of international interventions in the months following the contentious invasion of Kosovo by NATO forces, and asked: "is it legitimate for a regional organization to use force without a UN mandate? On the other hand, is it permissible to let gross and systematic violations of human rights, with grave humanitarian consequences, continue unchecked?" (Bellamy 2006). The never-ending civil war in Syria is a typical example where there is dilemma about what to do as civilians continue to be killed at the hands of both the ruling government and the rebel groups supported by the meddling of some of the superpowers.

International interventions that use force to overthrow a ruling government seem to set precedence and also set the scene for chaos and unprecedented instability in that part of the world, as the political opposition is often fragmented, sometimes along the lines of ethnicity or religion. A good example is that of the uncalled-for invasion of Iraq by the United States of America led international military intervention, which in itself has subsequently created a chronic complex emergency situation in Iraq. Humanitarian work has become an on-going challenge in Iraq because the country has been sunk into deep divisions characterised by the on-going suicide bombings, which puts the security of civilians and humanitarian workers at stake.

Is the international armed response genuinely meant to protect the civilians, or there could be other hidden interests by the international states or so-called "superpowers" that are behind such military 'intervention'? If the superpowers are at fault, to whom are they answerable to? Is there accountability and fairness?

What is even more worrying is that in practice, the Responsibility to Protect seems to be about responsibility to protect low-income countries by the Western or so-called superpower nations. This seems to suggest that the low-income countries are at the mercy of the so-called superpower nations.

There are nations where there has been significant mass killings of civilians and yet international military intervention was delayed or not even considered, such as during the 1994 genocide in Rwanda, whereas, international military intervention is executed quickly in certain instances, as has been seen during the relatively quick military intervention by NATO forces in Libya. Could this be about a clash of principles and interests? (De Waal 2010).

There are many question marks about the Responsibility to Protect, largely because of the inconsistency in its application. The terrain has changed, and there is need for international interventions to be adaptable and fair (Spiegel 2010).

Humanitarian space: The international community's choice of who to assist as there is an increase in the rate of complex humanitarian emergencies, globally, is thought-provoking. At face value, it may be easy to suggest that there should be prioritisation for public health action, both at local and international level, and to ensure that there is capacity, tools and systems to enhance or influence such prioritisation. The reality is that the landscape is changing very fast, and so is the situation of global crises.

When one looks at new developments in the world, there is more to just the number of complex emergencies and how to prioritise international interventions. Recent developments have introduced a great deal of complexity in complex emergencies, particularly because contemporary wars are of protracted duration, intrastate, fought by irregular armed groups, and fuelled by economic opportunities and ethnic rivalry (Merson et al. 2012).

The complexity about how and when the international community chooses to respond to complex emergencies is also influenced by the fact that some complex emergency situations are immediately on the spotlight even if fundamental political solutions are not sought. Whereas, in other instances, on-going crises causing massive disasters remain hidden and therefore not explicitly recognised as complex emergencies.

The media does play a role in drawing the attention of the international community by putting the complex emergency on the spotlight, while those complex emergencies that are not projected by the media remain as hidden complex emergencies. Merson et al. (2012) observe that the hidden complex emergency situations nevertheless pose fundamental challenges to the health and wellbeing of affected populations since they seem to attract little attention and resources: and such discrepancies are likely to result from geopolitical concerns, media interest, and economic factors (Merson et al. 2012).

The unfortunate reality is that the power of the media may influence the dissemination of inaccurate information, and as a result, this may cause the international community to channel resources towards a situation that does not really require so many resources (Coppola 2011). This is such a paradox in the humanitarian enterprise.

Much as there may be guidelines or initiatives such as the Responsibility to Protect, which determine how and when the international community should respond to complex emergencies, the role of the media may be particularly powerful in anointing a country as a complex emergency worthy of attention, and bring popular demand for action (Merson et al. 2012).

The association between the Responsibility to Protect and women's rights during complex humanitarian emergencies, has been drawing attention from various quarters. Complex humanitarian emergencies are characterised by social disruption, armed conflict, population displacement, collapse of public health infrastructure, and food shortages (Gasseer et al. 2004). The Responsibility to Protect entails the responsibility of each individual state to protect its population, and that the international community should, as appropriate, encourage and help countries to exercise this responsibility and support the United Nations in establishing an early warning capability (Cabellero-Anthony 2012).

Over the years, there has been particular spotlight on women and children affected during humanitarian crises or any kind of disaster anywhere in the world. Interestingly, some studies report that men, boys, women, and girls face new roles and vulnerabilities during complex emergencies, and this highlights that it is not just women's rights that are violated during complex emergencies, but it is human rights in general that are violated, and this together with the destruction of economic and political institutions combine to create almost permanent states of insecurity (Lautze et al. 2004). Much as human rights in general are violated, the consequences of conflict, war and systems of organised and violent predation are determined by sex and have serious repercussions for different elements of the population, particularly women (Lautze et al. 2004).

According to Merson et al. (2012), children and women, particularly pregnant women, have been repeatedly shown to be the most vulnerable members of the community especially in situations of crises, war, and displacement, and they tend to have much higher mortality especially during the emergency period. A critical service that must be provided during the earliest stages of a relief effort is the establishment of emergency obstetrical care to ensure that maternal mortality is to be kept low (Merson et al. 2012).

Complex emergencies pose many challenges to both the affected victims as well as the humanitarian workers, but despite all these challenges, it is of paramount importance to maintain the protection of human rights, particularly the rights of the most vulnerable people such as women and children.

7.6.1 Priorities for Mitigation, Preparedness and Response to Risk Factors of Humanitarian Crises and Disasters in the Southern Africa Region by the Year 2025

7.6.1.1 Introduction

The Southern Africa region continues to experience crisis situations, and the impact of these crisis situations and disasters largely depends on the vulnerability and coping mechanisms of the affected populations (Humanitarian Futures Programme 2007). But the bottom line is that the future does not look promising between now and 2025, because of the negative effects of climate change and the fact that the majority of the Southern African population lives in poverty which affects the coping mechanisms of these vulnerable populations (Humanitarian Futures Programme 2007).

There are five main drivers that trigger crisis situations in the Southern Africa region, and these five drivers are further exacerbated by the issue of climate change, and this is foreseen to continue to create serious problems up to the year 2025 and beyond. The five main drivers or triggers of crises situations in the Southern Africa region include demographic shifts, water dimensions; environmental degradation, persistent health threats, and intra and interstate instability (Humanitarian Futures Programme 2007).

Demographic shifts such as the issue of rapid urbanisation because such shifts result in the proliferation of informal settlements, overcrowding, poor sanitation, poverty, crime, and increased incidence and prevalence of diseases including communicable diseases. Demographic shifts are also characterised by the rapid increase in the number of young people, and due to the number of orphans is expected to bulge by the year 2025 of which HIV and AIDS will also be one of the main contributing factors (Humanitarian Futures Programme 2007).

Water dimensions may be considered as a very critical issue in the Southern Africa region in the sense that drought and heavy rainfall have often wreaked havoc in many parts of this region, and as such, the most vulnerable people have been those who live in poverty situations. The issue of drought and excessive rainfall is anticipated to worsen by the year 2025 as water stress and water scarcity could create more crises in the region (Humanitarian Futures Programme 2007).

Environmental degradation is accelerated by activities such as deforestation, poor agricultural practices, and pollution, poses a huge challenge for this region because it hampers livelihood especially in the rural areas, and could force migration of more people from the rural areas to the urban areas.

Persistent health threats such as chronic infectious diseases including HIV/AIDS and tuberculosis, among others, remain a significant cause of concern today, and the situation is expected to worsen by the year 2025 (Humanitarian Futures Programme 2007).

Intra and inter-state instability is currently a driver and a shock in terms of humanitarian crises and vulnerability in some parts of the Southern Africa region of the countries. Given the growing concern about corruption and poor governance in many parts of the region, intra and inter-state instability is anticipated to worsen by the year 2025 (Humanitarian Futures Programme 2007).

Given the persistent and projected spread of the crises and disaster situation in the Southern Africa region, exacerbated by a number of risk factors, and further complicated by the overarching challenge of climate change, national and regional authorities and international partners will need to take humanitarian actions to tackle such risk factors. There should be priorities for mitigation, preparedness and response to the current and anticipated challenges that could spiral to disasters or complex emergencies.

7.6.1.2 Discussion

This report will be based on the Southern Africa region. The purpose of the report is to identify a priority for the region – mitigation, preparedness, or response – between now and 2025. This will be supported by a rationale and definition of the main risk factors and an outline of the actions that national and regional authorities and international partners will need to take to tackle those risk factors.

Definition of the Risk Factors

Given the frequent rate and intensity of humanitarian crises and disasters that have occurred and are still occurring in the world, there can be no doubt that national and regional authorities and partners will have to tackle the risk factors and the hazards that augment such situations. The Southern Africa region is faced with various types of hazards and risks which could result in crises and disasters. Crises and disasters are rarely an outcome of one factor, but rather, there tends to be an interaction of two or more interrelated factors. Coppola (2011) defines a risk as the probability of an event occurring multiplied by the consequence of that event; whereas a hazard is a chance that an agent will cause a disaster.

According to Humanitarian Futures Programme (2007), the main five drivers or triggers of crises and disasters in the Southern Africa region include demographic shifts, water dimensions; environmental degradation, persistent health threats, and intra and interstate instability.

Demographic shifts involve the notable changes that happen within and between populations. With the socioeconomic situation becoming a worsening challenge in many parts of the Southern Africa region, populations end up shifting from one place to another in search for better opportunities or livelihood (Humanitarian Futures Programme 2007). As such, there is rapid urbanisation which ends up creating further problems such as overcrowding and the creation of informal settlements with very poor living conditions. The high birth rate in many parts of the Southern Africa region is expected to result in a high increase in the number of young people between now and 2025 (Humanitarian Futures Programme 2007). The high increase in the number of young people is coupled with the increase in the number of orphans which may be propagated by the high incidence and prevalence of infectious and chronic diseases such as HIV and AIDS. This with create more demands for the affected countries and the region (Humanitarian Futures Programme 2007).

Water dimensions are an issue of great concern between now and 2025 because of the growing water shortages and flooding that affects many parts of the Southern Africa region (Humanitarian Futures Programme 2007). There are often reports indicating that some parts of the Southern Africa region are going to run short of drinking water in the next two decades or so. This is very worrying, because people depend on water in order for their livelihood, as water is used for agriculture, cooking, and drinking, among some of the many reasons. The reality is that many parts of this region are already experiencing the effects of water shortages as there have been a number of episodes of serious drought in recent times, and the situation seems to be getting worse. This will really create a crisis of great proportions in terms of food shortages, starvation, sanitation, water-borne diseases, morbidity, mortality, and conflict as people will be scrambling for the little water supplies, they can get. Other than the issue of drought, some parts of the Southern Africa region will continue to experience extreme situations of drought and flooding, and this will really hit hardest on the most vulnerable populations who are already affected by extreme poverty (Humanitarian Futures Programme 2007).

Environmental degradation is another major issue as natural mechanisms exacerbated by human actions such as deforestation, overgrazing, and pollution from pesticides and herbicides have caused an accelerated and irreversible destruction of the environment (Hattingh and Acutt 2003). This will render many parts of the region as permanent drought areas by 2025, and food insecurity will be a burning issue, thus putting more strain on the already weakened economies of many parts of the Southern Africa region. Environmental degradation will exacerbate situations of starvation, conflict, and migration of people from rural areas to urban areas, thus creating more problems (Humanitarian Futures Programme 2007).

Persistent health threats are another issue that could lead to crises of great proportions (Humanitarian Futures Programme 2007). The emergence and the re-emergence of serious infectious diseases will lead to very high morbidity and mortality. For example, the HIV and AIDS pandemic has already given us an idea of the magnitude that such diseases can cause as the Southern Africa region carries the highest burden of HIV and AIDS in the whole world. Persistent health threats such as HIV and AIDS, Tuberculosis, and other emerging and re-emerging infectious diseases, as well as the growing challenge of diseases of lifestyle will continue to wreak havoc between now and 2025 in this region as increasing numbers of the economically active population will be affected, and therefore their income will be compromised, thereby pushing households into deeper poverty (Humanitarian Futures Programme 2007).

Intra and inter-state instability is currently a driver and a shock in terms of humanitarian crises and vulnerability in some parts of the Southern Africa region of the countries (Humanitarian Futures Programme 2007). Given the growing concern about corruption and poor governance in many parts of the region, intra and inter-state instability is anticipated to worsen by the year 2025.

Over the next decade or so, the Southern Africa region will have to contend with or deal with the effects of climate change. Although it is still a subject of much debate as to whether climate change is induced by human action or is just part of a natural cycle, the bottom line is that climate change is happening at an alarming speed and intensity, and this is not only happening in the Southern Africa region, but it is also happening on a global scale (Coppola 2011). Climate change can be defined in different ways by different authors and organisations. With reference to the United Nations Framework Convention on Climate Change (UNFCCC), climate change is attributed to the direct and indirect human activities that alter the composition of the global atmosphere (Cromar et al. 2006).

Even though detecting the influence of observed and predicted changes in global climate on infectious disease transmission is not straight forward, a growing body of evidence has linked global climate change and the epidemiology of infectious diseases such as malaria, yellow fever, and dengue fever (Merson et al. 2012).

Climate change can lead to a number of disasters or crisis situations including the following: extreme heat; large scale spread of infectious diseases such as malaria; drought and subsequent food insecurity, spread of wild fires; excessive rainfall which can lead to flooding, landslides, waterborne diseases, and famine due to damage of crops as the majority of people in the rural areas of the Southern Africa region depend on small scale farming for their livelihoods (Merson et al. 2012). It is hardly surprising that climate change is regarded as probably the biggest global health challenge of our time and will affect billions of people in terms of health and wellbeing (Costello et al. 2009).

Actions to Tackle the Risk Factors

Given the foreseeable crisis and disaster situation between now and 2025, it would therefore be crucial for the Southern Africa region to identify priorities for mitigation, preparedness and response with regard to the deleterious consequences of such crises and disasters.

Mitigation is more about a sustained effort to minimise, reduce or prevent the capacity of a hazard from producing an adverse effect (Coppola 2011). The outline for mitigation should be based on the goals set for that particular mitigation. Regulatory measures such as land use management will serve to address the issues of environmental degradation, prevent and control the proliferation of informal settlements in unsafe areas, control the use of common natural resources such as aquifers so that drought can be prevented, storm water management so that environmental degradation could be prevented or minimised; Community awareness may be important to ensure that the public is aware of the hazards; Behavioural modification may encourage collective action and enhance social ties to encourage environmental conservation and safe practices such as environmentally friendly farming, and it can also prevent conflict such as in instances of water rationing during periods of drought (Coppola 2011). It has to be borne in mind though that there could be formidable obstacles to mitigation, such as the issues of high cost, lack of political support and sociocultural issues, and risk perception (Coppola 2011).

Preparedness is more about taking precautionary measures to ensure a timely, appropriate and efficient response (Coppola 2011). This requires good coordination as different stakeholders may be involved and the government is better positioned to play a leading role, even though sometimes such a role may also be played by an international organisation such as the United Nations. Preparedness requires proper planning, and that those who will be involved be properly trained and practise how to deal with a crisis situation (Coppola 2011). Public preparedness in the form of education, awareness, and behaviour change should also be considered as important (Coppola 2011). Tools such as early warning systems in the context of the Southern Africa region would be effective if all stakeholders have the competency and the capacity to understand and implement. Like in mitigation, it has to be borne in mind that there may be obstacles to preparedness, and these include communication barriers due to literacy issues, language, lack of access to technology and the media, class structure, poverty or the effects of poverty, cultural understanding, lack of government sponsorship, conflicting interests of big business, and hostile or restrictive governments (Coppola 2011).

Response is the most visible disaster function, but it can be very complex, challenging and draining as it is more about knowing when to take action, what to do and when to do it to effectively deal with the crisis or disaster situation that is imminent or has already occurred, and timing here is of great essence as delays can be very tragic (Coppola 2011). As such, for response to be effective and efficient there should be proper coordination and information flow to ensure that everybody involved does the right thing in the right way and at the right time. It is during the response stage that assessments should be conducted, victims of crises or disasters will have to be rescued, provided with first aid treatment, and evacuated; emergency health care should be established; victims should be provided with water, food, and shelter; emergency social services should be established; donations should be managed; critical infrastructure problems should be addressed in the short term; and security issues should not be taken lightly as security issues can affect both the responders and the victims of crises or disaster situations (Coppola 2011). In some instances, it can happen that the response resources are overwhelmed, and in such instances, it is the responsibility of governments of the affected countries to declare the disaster to ensure that the necessary international response such as food aid is provided (Coppola 2011).

7.6.1.3 Conclusion

The Southern Africa region is faced with serious challenges as the majority of the populations that live in this region live in poverty situations. As such, this renders them vulnerable to hazards and risks which are largely triggered by demographic shifts, water systems, environmental degradation, persistent health threats, and intra and inter-state instability. National and regional authorities and international partners will need to take action to tackle these challenges, but these actions should be coordinated to ensure that there is sustainability of efforts. However, it should be borne in mind that there may be obstacles or barriers such as lack of political support, cultural issues, literacy issues, language issues, financial issues that could hamper the actions efforts.

7.7 Disaster Risk Management

In many instances, efforts are often channelled towards dealing with the symptoms, rather than the root causes, and, as a result, there is often a vicious cycle between disasters and development. Anderson (1994) observes that there is an urgent need to analyse what causes public health issues such as vulnerability to disasters and why some people are more vulnerable than others. Vulnerability is an inherent disposition to harm as a result of exposure to a destabilising phenomenon (Cardona 2004).

The new public health paradigm acknowledges the importance of collaborative efforts of society from within and from without the remits of the health sector in order to protect and improve the health and wellbeing of populations (Scambler 2008). In hindsight this underlies the importance of public health in the development agenda (Hunter 2007).

Similar to the new public health paradigm, there seems to be a realisation in disaster management about the importance of prevention and of addressing the underlying cause of disaster (Anderson 1994). Interventions that disregard the importance of addressing the root cause and the full participation of the public are bound to fail because they are unsustainable.

The term disaster cycle including preparedness, response, recovery and mitigation, may be relevant in theory, but the reality is that in many resource-poor settings, response could be the only means of addressing the effects of the disaster, and this could perpetuate vulnerability (Coppola 2011). The preparedness stage involves prior planning for disaster, the response stage involves immediate action in order to give warnings or to address the immediate needs immediately prior to a disaster and when the disaster occurs, the recovery stage mainly focuses on the long-term response, and the mitigation stage mainly focuses on ensuring that the negative effects of the disaster do not happen again (Coppola 2011).

Although disaster cycle gives us an in-depth insight of all the stages of disaster management which incorporates both proactive and reactive elements, the term disaster-development continuum is more useful because it enables paying more attention to the relationship between disaster and development in order to gain a better insight of the burning issue of people's vulnerability to disasters. There is a direct relationship between development and vulnerability, and development without the buy-in of social and political structures can be a costly mistake (Anderson 1985).

The shrinking resources of development aid seem to force a shift towards short-term responses to disasters, and, as a result, this creates a 'monster' because it increases the population's vulnerability to further disaster as the long-term focus of development is compromised (Anderson 1994). For example, an observation is that, in parts of low- and middle-income countries such as in sub-Saharan Africa, most of the aid that victims of disaster have been receiving has now been terminated because it could not be sustained. Moreover, there have been challenges about sustaining the supply of therapeutic drugs such as antiretroviral treatment in some parts of the low- and middle-income countries. As a result, most of the affected people have become more vulnerable to disaster, mainly because of poverty and marginalisation.

Development and the risk of disaster: Development can either increase or reduce the risk of disasters. Coppola (2011) observes that low-income or developing countries such as El Salvador are at high risk of suffering ruinous effects after disasters as compared to the developed or industrialised countries such as the United States of America where a robust economy absorbs such impacts. At the same time, Coppola (2011) is interesting when he highlights that there is no fixed formula to accurately project how the effects of disasters will pen out, regardless of the socioeconomic or political status of that particular country, because no country is immune to disasters.

Although studies show that development is an important measure for reducing the risk posed by disasters, some authors argue that development such as rapid urban development could also increase the risk of disasters (Macrae et al. 1997). For example, there is an upsurge of the development and industrialisation of some of the previously 'undeveloped' parts of sub-Saharan Africa, and the contractors or developers have to rush against time to meet deadlines for the completion of such projects. Unfortunately, some of the hastily built facilities and infrastructure have collapsed and caused fatalities and injuries. One of such incidents is that of the shopping mall which collapsed and resulted in fatalities and injuries in the South African town of Tongaat, in November 2013, and there are fears that many other recently built structures pose a risk. Rapid development creates many other problems such as the concentration of people in prone areas which may cause or exacerbate poverty, conflict and crime, thereby increasing the risk of disasters (Cardona 2004).

Another challenge observed was that there seemed to be a culture of dependency that had been created by the Reconstruction and Development Programme (RDP) through which houses have been built for people throughout the country as part of development and as means to eradicate the proliferation of informal settlements in South Africa. Many people have crowded the informal settlements because they expect the government to build houses for them. Instead of seeing a decline in the number of informal settlements, there is a proliferation, and this is a 'recipe' for disaster.

Such problems are an indication for urgent measures to reduce the risk of disasters which are a consequence of development. Risk reduction can be regarded as the interventions to deal with the causal factors, but this should follow a holistic approach that is both consistent and coherent and should integrate the complexity of the socio-economic, cultural, political, geographical and structural facets (Cardona 2004).

It has to be acknowledged that the South African Department of Social Development together with non-governmental organisations have put together some initiatives aimed at addressing or reducing the risk of disasters, and the emphasis is mainly on social integration and the eradication of poverty (Vermaak and van Niekerk 2004).

The disaster cycle and the disaster-development continuum should not be viewed as mutually exclusive entities. There is need for a holistic perspective if there is to be effective implementation and sustainability of efforts in the field of public health (Walley and Wright 2010). Specifically, there is need to take cognisance of the fact that disaster management or public health in general is not a 'silo', but it is very broad, and it needs coordination and involvement of many different stakeholders to ensure effective and sustainable interventions.

The reality is that there seems to be knowledge about what to do, and there are also comprehensive proactive and reactive strategies such as the disaster cycle/disaster-development continuum at the disposal. However, one of the biggest challenges is the lack of synergy or coordination of efforts, and this poses a bigger risk in terms of disaster management or public health interventions in general. In the event of a disaster, it is not uncommon to find that a number of different organisations or agencies descend upon the scene, but each is doing their own thing as per their field of expertise, and sometimes there is friction or infighting or turf battles or even decisions not to participate. This could lead to inefficient use and duplication of resources, and even greater disaster consequences (Coppola 2011).

Poor coordination of efforts had a devastating effect during the extreme drought of 2010 and 2015 which affected parts of Southern Africa. The question is who should take responsibility for ensuring that there is an official coordination mechanism? Should the host government take that responsibility? Could the perception of status of development be a factor here, as studies show that the impact of the disaster is dependent on the level of development of that country (Anderson 1985)?

Coppola (2011) posits that coordination could be informal or formal, and it may originate within the non-governmental organisations, the donor agencies, the government of the affected country, or international bodies such as the United Nations (Coppola 2011). However, it is possible that low-income countries could be found wanting in the event of an extensive disaster, and therefore, international coordination through the United Nations Office for the Coordination of Humanitarian Affairs and the United Nations Disaster Assessment and Coordination team, could be the likely option (Coppola 2011). Uncoordinated interventions have neither the allure of saving lives nor of guaranteeing sustainable development (Christoplos et al. 2001).

Typically, vulnerable groups such as children, women, the elderly, the poor, and people with disabilities, need to be taken into account in the context of disaster management, because they may suffer disproportionately during a disaster (Leitmann 2007). Some authors observe that women have been put in a place of vulnerability because of the societal arrangements in some areas (Anderson 1994).

In parts of low- and middle-income countries, it is still not uncommon, particularly in some of the rural areas to see households headed by women who are poor, unemployed, and marginalised. In most instances, socio-culturally, men are regarded as the breadwinners. As such, men tend to leave the rural areas and work in far-away places such as in the mines and other industries, and only to return home at least once in a while. In such instances, the women have to take care of the children, and make ends meet, sometimes under deplorable conditions.

Studies indicate that the migration of men puts both the migrants and their women partners at high risk of sexually transmitted infections such as HIV, and it has been reported that there is a higher prevalence of HIV among women, such as in sub-Saharan Africa. Women, particularly black women, are more vulnerable because socio-cultural arrangements have placed them in a position of no power. Lurie et al. (1997) add that black people suffer much higher HIV infection rates than any other group, and black women are even more vulnerable because they are often unable to negotiate safer sexual practices with their male counterparts.

Interestingly, in others in other parts of low- and middle-income countries, there are growing numbers of women who are bread winners, in the sense that they are educated, entrepreneurs, employed, and/or empowered. There is also a growing trend of women occupying very senior positions in these societies. This shows that at least women are slowly gaining the power, and the traditional societal arrangements of putting women in a position of vulnerability are slowly diminishing. Perhaps, there is need to adapt the disaster management strategy taking into consideration the changing dynamics of specific societies.

The concept of vulnerability or vulnerable groups should not inadvertently create the risk of group discrimination, but it should be an attempt to take into account how specific social contexts influence specific groups so that proactive intervention strategies could be developed (Moatti and Souteyrand 2000). After all, disaster is like any social concept, it will always be influenced by the dynamism of a number of factors that exist in that society, and paying attention to the root causes of the dynamism and vulnerability of certain groups could provide lasting solutions for disaster management (Deeny et al. 2010). A holistic and critical approach to the disaster cycle/disaster-development continuum may provide a better opportunity to address the root cause of vulnerability, but an uncritical strategy may do more harm than good.

7.7.1 Comprehensive Plan for Recovery, Mitigation, and Preparedness for Haiti

Looking at the history of Haiti, the socio-political instability, particularly due to the socio-political crisis, or the coup years of the 1990s, has resulted in public health issues such as traumatic stress, insecurity, the displacement of large numbers of people, and has exacerbated poverty and the vulnerability of this country to disasters (James 2004). In recent times, Haiti has further sunk deeper into crisis because it has repeatedly been hit by disasters, such as the cyclone of 2007–2008, and more recently by the earthquake of January 2010 which has had continuing effects which have further exacerbated the vulnerability in Haiti (Merson et al. 2012). The following is an outline of the essential elements for a comprehensive plan for recovery, mitigation, and preparedness for Haiti, covering the next 10 years.

Recovery

The recovery phase focuses on the shot-term and long-term intervention so that the damaging effects of the disaster could be reversed, but more importantly this requires good coordination to ensure effectiveness (Coppola 2011).

Planning and effective leadership would be essential from the start, and assessment of the damage would provide a realistic picture of the extent or the magnitude of the damaging effects of the disaster, and also to determine the required resources that would inform the long term recovery process (Piotrowski 2010).

There should be quick organisation and allocation of financial and other resources to ensure that there is sustainability in terms of rebuilding houses, rebuilding the economy, the education system, the health system, rehabilitation of individuals and families, rebuilding the socio-cultural and political structures (Coppola 2011).

Special consideration should be given to guarding against the inadvertent creation of an imbalance or inequalities in society as a consequence of the recovery process, because inequity could create groups that are more vulnerable than others (Berke et al. 1993).

Mitigation

Mitigation can be defined as sustained effort aimed at ensuring that the likelihood and consequence of the risk is reduced, and it should follow a structural and non-structural approach. Structural mitigation may be considered as putting engineering controls in place, and this may include aspects such as ensuring that all built structures do not easily succumb to the might of the hazards by ensuring that these structures are built according to the stipulated standards and legislated regulations, and this could also reduce the risk of fatalities and injuries to the population. Non-structural mitigation may include regulatory measures; Community awareness and education programs; Non-structural physical modifications; Environmental control; and Behavioural modification (Coppola 2011).

Special consideration should be given to assessing and selecting mitigation options bearing in mind the impact of the risk mitigating option on community risk reduction, and also the probability that each option will be implemented. Methods of assessing mitigation options, should take into account the Social, Technical, Administrative, Political, Legal, Economic, and Environmental aspects; and proper implementation of an emergency response capacity should also be considered as a very important risk mitigation measure (Coppola 2011).

Preparedness

Preparedness is considered as a phase of anticipation way before a disaster occurs, and the government should play a leadership role in terms of it being a statutory authority to inform the decisions taken regarding planning, training, and to ensure that the required equipment meets the legislated standards. Public preparedness is also important because the members of the public need to be educated about possible hazards that could lead to disaster in Haiti, there needs to be awareness about these hazards, there needs to be behaviour change, and there should be early warnings about possible future disasters (Coppola 2011).

Special consideration should be given to the literacy level of the Haiti population, the language used, access to technology and media, class structure, poverty or the effect of poverty, lack of government sponsorship, conflicting interests of business, and the hostility and restrictiveness of government because these factors could become obstacles to the preparedness process or the disaster management process for the next 10 years (Coppola 2011).

7.7.1.1 Conclusion

In conclusion, recovery, mitigation and preparedness are essential, but it is of paramount importance to ensure that there is planning, leadership and cooperation to ensure that there is effective and sustainable disaster reduction for the next 10 years in Haiti.

7.7.2 Coordination in Disaster Risk Management and Humanitarian Assistance

Coordination can be defined as the involvement of two or more units or participating agencies who agree to work towards common objectives through the dedication of resources and the development of a joint organisation and programme of action

(Merson et al. 2012). The leading role is played by one of the participating agencies, and such an agency is referred to as the coordination agency (Lorreti 2006).

Coordination is a critical function in any human endeavour because it increases the efficiency, impact and sustainability as the implementation plan sets out clearly the strategic, operational and technical dimensions for a common purpose (Lorreti 2009).

For example, after having realised that many individuals and organisations have been making a contribution aimed at improving the health and wellbeing of people in parts of southern African communities most affected by the crisis of HIV/AIDS and poverty, it was decided to bring together all the stakeholders so that there could be a coordinated approach. This coordinated approach has enabled the development of a profile and mapping of the vulnerable areas, and it is believed this will make a bigger impact as compared to individual and uncoordinated efforts.

Coordination is particularly critical in crisis management where needs are critical and urgent, and so many different actors are involved. Some authors observe that even the largest humanitarian organisation is incapable of effectively managing a major crisis situation on its own (Stoddard 2003). Coordination can enable a wider coverage of disaster management efforts because the resources from the different actors are pooled together, preventing the duplication of efforts, cutting costs and saving time, and can also become the foundation on which increased disaster capacity will be built.

The cluster system through the leadership of the coordination agency of each cluster, and the overall coordination by the United Nations as the coordination body, enhances better coordination because it creates more focus by grouping the organisations that work within a certain theme (Lorreti 2009). There should be some flexibility in the cluster system to recognise that there could be the possibility of overlaps between clusters and that the uniqueness of different nations should be respected. Sometimes, coordination can be extremely difficult because some or all the stakeholders may be unwilling to be involved with the coordinated efforts for a number of reasons such as conflict of interests and due to other political reasons (Coppola 2011).

The meaning and implication of coordination is sometimes misunderstood as it may seem as if there is coordination when different organisations communicate and work together in a disaster affected area, and yet each organisation has not adjusted its own objectives to suite the context of the larger collective objective. Such working together can be regarded as cooperation rather than coordination. Cooperation occurs when two or more organisations keep their own separate but compatible objectives and agree to help each other when possible and, at least, to avoid actions that would hinder the other organisation in achieving its objectives (Merson et al. 2012).

Coordination is a critical function in any human endeavour, particularly in crisis management, even though the meaning of coordination is sometimes misunderstood. Leadership is crucial in coordination efforts.

Given the complexity and challenges of establishing a coordinated effort through the involvement of different actors with their own unique ways of doing things and the possible conflict that may arise, there is need for efficient coordination mechanisms.

In 2010, there was a crisis situation whereby one of the prominent South African Humanitarian bodies tried to play a coordinating role after a large number of homesteads were gutted by wildfire in the north-eastern parts of the country. Unfortunately, most of the humanitarian agencies that landed on the scene preferred to go about the disaster management in their own way, and even some of those that got involved with the coordinated approach ended up having conflicts which compromised the disaster management efforts. The situation worsened because there was confusion, panic and no clear coordination mechanism to deal with such a disaster. This gave me the impression that there was an urgent need for implementation and adherence to interagency guidelines for humanitarian assistance (IASC 2007).

Jones and George (2008) observe that there is need to incorporate various integrating mechanisms into the organisational architecture in order to increase communication and coordination among functions or between the different actors so that the problems can be prevented from emerging. These mechanisms include liaison roles, task forces, cross-functional teams, and integrating roles (Jones and George 2008).

Liaison roles are when the one leader in each function or participating agency is given the responsibility for coordinating with the other; and as such, liaison roles provide a way of transmitting information across an organisation (Jones and George 2008).

When more than two functions or actors share many common problems, direct contact and liaison roles do not provide sufficient coordination, a more complex integrating mechanism, a task force, may be appropriate, whereby one leader from each relevant function or participating agency is assigned to a task force that meets to solve a specific, mutual problem (Jones and George 2008).

In many cases, the issues addressed by a task force are recurring problems; and to address recurring problems effectively, the use of permanent integrating mechanisms such as cross-functional teams might be required (Jones and George 2008). Functional teams have the responsibility of ensuring that there is clarity and agreement regarding the exact coordinated direction to be followed from a strategic, operational and technical dimension (Jones and George 2008).

An integrating role is a role whose only function is to increase coordination and integration among functions to achieve performance gain from synergies such as the role played by the United Nations as a coordination body of the clusters (Lorreti 2009).

Preparedness and a coordination mechanism are crucial, particularly so in crisis management. However, it is worth acknowledging that disaster response is becoming increasingly complex with each event, and as such, some flexibility might be necessary to effectively deal with certain disasters (Coppola 2011). After all, effective coordination can only be a voluntary exercise based on mutual agreement (Lorreti 2009).

The increasing recognition of the spate of disasters has resulted in exponential growth of the number of NGOs that are focused on humanitarian relief and development (Coppola 2011). Non-governmental organisations (NGOs) are local or international organisations that are independent of government, and they often work in the field humanitarian relief and development (Coppola 2011). Walley and Wright (2010) are interesting when they posit that in keeping with the principle of neutrality, NGOs should just do their work, keep a low profile and make sure that the credit for the work goes to the entire coordinated effort with other actors.

A growing number of critical assessments suggest that the operational impact of NGOs in community development and emergencies is less than was claimed. Such critical assessments could jeopardise the NGOs' chances of getting funding from donors because funders are becoming more and more particular about accountability and impact to justify the need for future funding. Given the spate of emergencies in recent times, NGOs may have stretched the private sector donor base and the increase in the clout of NGOs in the developing world have all presented new challenges in the traditional work of international NGOs. NGOs are faced with marginalisation as global institutions are reshaped by financial markets, new corporate investment patterns, and the impact of information and communication technologies.

Some NGOs while providing relief impartially to all those in need, believe that they should also speak out in the face of gross human rights abuses and have become advocates for more international responses (Merson et al. 2012). This action may sometimes jeopardise their ability to remain in the affected area and, therefore, is not taken lightly. As such, it is hardly surprising that in the past few years, several governments have tightened up regulations on NGO registration, NGO programmes, and even whether NGOs are welcome to work in the country. Each country has specific circumstances, but the overall trend is unmistakable.

It cannot be denied though that in the changing NGO landscape it is still a hotly debated issue within NGOs whether to provide humanitarian relief and remain silent about human rights abuses and the diversion of relief resources or to speak out and risk having to leave the area (Merson et al. 2012). If an NGO has to leave the area without having provided any humanitarian assistance would be violating the traditional principle of humanity. Sometimes, speaking out against the violation of human rights by certain groups would not be different from taking sides, and this implies that the traditional principle or standard of impartiality would be compromised.

The importance and challenges of information-sharing in the context of a multi-agency disaster response, is also worth highlighting, as it has a bearing on coordination. It has been observed that the local people play a huge role in the event of a crisis, and they usually come up with solutions during the information sharing. Studies show that the local people are better positioned to respond immediately when a natural disaster occurs; therefore, participating agencies should give importance to local information and cooperate with the local community structures, for the success of coordinated disaster management efforts (Perry 2007). Incentives for sharing information, understanding each other's work-processed and the usability of information systems have shown positive effects on information sharing and coordination (Bharosa et al. 2010). Recent advances in communication technology present an opportunity for faster information flow at all levels, and this could enhance better coordinated disaster management efforts (Coyle and Meier 2009).

There may be challenges and obstacles in sharing and coordinating information during multi-agency disaster response. Uncoordinated information could cause delays, disorder, inefficiencies and further exacerbate the crisis and result in more complications. It has to be borne in mind that information sharing is influenced by obstacles within and between the community, agencies, and individuals; and that in a non-disaster situation, many of the agencies operate independently of each other (Bharosa et al. 2010). In a disaster situation, complexities may arise from a variety of elements, systems, processes and actors, and it is hard to get a clear picture of the entire situation within the time frame of a crisis (Bharosa et al. 2010).

Since information sharing and coordination is influenced by obstacles and located within and between the community, agency and individual levels, and that all three levels contain institutional and technological levels; effective disaster management would be possible if the challenges and obstacles are addressed simultaneously at all three levels (Bharosa et al. 2010).

Given the increasing frequency of natural disasters recently, it would help to have information-sharing synergies at the community, agency and individual level way before the disaster happens. Information sharing should not be taken at face value but it should be considered that the information flow must be two-way to be effective, information will not be used unless it is trusted, and that information will only be helpful if it is accurate (Coyle and Meier 2009).

Coordinated information flow is critical in disaster management, but this is not without challenges and obstacles. Simultaneously addressing the challenges at the community level, agency level and individual level presents an opportunity for effective disaster management.

References

Adam-Poupart, A., et al. (2013). *Impacts of climate change on occupational health and safety*. Quebec: Institut de recherché Robert-Sauve.

Anderson, M. B. (1985). A conceptualization of the linkages between disasters and development. *Disasters, 9*(s1), 46–51.

Anderson, M. B. (1994). Understanding the disaster-development continuum. *Gender and Development, 2*(1), 7–10.

Ashkenazi, I., Isakovich, B., Kluger, Y., Alfici, R., Kessel, B., & Better, O. R. (2005). Prehospital management of earthquake casualties buried under rubble. *Prehospital & Disaster Medicine, 20*(2), 122–133.

Atapattu, S. (2010). Climate change, human rights, and forced migration: Implications for international law. *Wisconsin International Law Journal, 27*(3), 607–636.

Bellamy, A. J. (2006). *Whither the responsibility to protect? Humanitarian intervention and the 2005 world summit* [Online].

Berke, P. R., Kartez, J., & Wenger, D. (1993). Recovery after disaster: Achieving sustainable development, mitigation and equity. *Disasters, 17*(2), 93–109.

Bharosa, N., Lee, J., & Jansen, M. (2010). Challenges and obstacles in sharing and coordinating information during multi-agency disaster response: Propositions from field exercises. *Information Systems Frontiers, 12*, 49–65.

Black, R., Kniveton, D., Skeldon, R., Coppard, D., Murata, A., & Schmidt-Verkerk, K. (2008). *Demographics and climate change: Future trends and their policy implications for migration*. Available from: http://r4d.dfid.gov.uk/PDF/Outputs/MigrationGlobPov/WP-T27.pdf

Bonanno, G. A., Galea, S., Bucciarelli, A., & Vlahov, D. (2007). What predicts psychological resilience after disaster? The role of demographics, resources, and life stress. *Journal of Consulting and Clinical Psychology, 75*(5), 671–682.

Bonmarin, I., Nunga, M., & Perea, W. A. (2002). Konzo outbreak, in the South-west of the Democratic Republic of Congo, 1996. *Journal of Tropical Pediatrics, 48*(4), 234–238.

Booth, K., & Williams, S. (2012). Is insurance an under-utilised mechanism in climate change adaptation?: The case of bushfire management in Tasmania. *Journal of Emergency Management, 27*(4), 38–45.

Cabellero-Anthony, M. (2012). The responsibility to protect in Southeast Asia: Opening up spaces for advancing human security. *The Pacific Review, 25*(1), 113–134.

Cardona, O. D. (2004). *Mapping vulnerability, disasters, development and people* [Online] London: Earthscan. Available from: http://www.la-red.org/public/articulos/2003/nrcvrfh ago-04-2003.pdf

Christoplos, I., Mitchell, J., & Liljelund, A. (2001). Re-framing risk: The changing context of disaster mitigation and preparedness. *Disasters, 25*(3), 185–198.

Coppola, D. P. (2011). *Introduction to international disaster management*. Oxford: Butterworth-Heinemann.

Costello, A., Abbas, M., Allen, A., Ball, S., Bell, S., Bellamy, R., Friel, S., Groce, N., Johnsosn, A., Kett, M., Lee, M., Levy, C., Maslin, M., McCoy, D., McGuire, B., Montgomery, H., Napier, D., Pagel, C., Patel, J., de Oliveira, J. A. P., Redclift, N., Rees, H., Rogger, D., Scott, J., Stephenson, J., Twigg, J., Wolff, J., & Patterso, C. (2009). Managing the health effects of climate change. *The Lancet, 373*(9676), 1693–1733.

Coyle, D., & Meier, P. (2009). *New technologies in emergencies and conflicts*. Washington: United Nations & Vodafone Foundation.

Cromar, N., Cameron, S., & Fallowfield, H. (2006). *Environmental health in Australia and New Zealand*. Oxford: New York.

Davies, H., & Lam, P. (2001). *Managerial economics: An analysis of business issues*. Harlow: Prentice-Hall.

De Waal, A. (2010). The humanitarian's tragedy: Escapable and inescapable cruelties. *Disasters, 34*, 130–137.

Deeny, P., Vitale, C. T., Spelman, R., & Duggan, S. (2010). Addressing the imbalance: Empowering older people in disaster response and preparedness. *International Journal of Older People Nursing, 5*, 77–80.

Edwards, N. (2005). Using markets to reform health care. *The British Medical Journal, 331*, 1464–1466.

Evans, G., & Sahnoun, M. (2001). *The responsibility to protect*. ICISS: Ottawa.

Floret, N., Viel, J., Mauny, F., Hoen, B., & Piarroux, R. (2006). Negligible risk for epidemics after geophysical disasters. *Emerging Infectious Diseases, 12*(4), 543–548.

Fraser, C., Donnelly, C. A., Cauchemez, S., Hanage, W., van Kerkhove, M. D., Hollingsworth, T. D., Griffin, J., Baggaley, R. F., Jenkins, H. E., Lyons, E. J., Jombart, T., Hinsley, W. R., Grassly, N. C., Balloux, F., Ghani, A. C., Ferguson, N. M., Rambaut, A., Pybus, O. G., Lopez-Gatell, H., Alpuche-Aranda, C. M., Chapela, I. B., Zavala, E. P., Guevara, D. M. E., Checchi, F., Garcia, E., Hugonnet, S., & Roth, C. (2009). Pandemic potential of a strain of influenza A (H1N1): Early findings. *Science, 324*, 1557–1561.

Fundter, D. Q. P., Jonkman, B., Beerman, S., Goemans, C. L. P. M., Briggs, R., Coumans, F., Willem, J., & Bierens, J. (2008). Governmental decision-making and resilience of the citizens. *Prehospital & Disaster Medicine, 23*(4), S70–s73.

Gasseer, N. A., Dresden, E., Keeny, G. B., & Warren, N. (2004). Status of women and infants in complex humanitarian emergencies. *Journal of Midwifrey & Women's Health, 49*(1), 7–13.

Hafstad, G., & Haavind, H. (2012). Parenting after a natural disaster: A qualitative study of Norwegian families surviving the 2004 tsunami in Southeast Asia. *Journal of Child and Family Studies, 21*, 293–302.

Hattingh, S., & Acutt, J. (2003). *Occupational health: Management & practice for health practitioners*. Lansdowne: Juta.

Hecht, R., Stover, J., Bollinger, L., Muhib, F., Case, K., & de Ferranti. (2010). Financing of HIV/AIDS programmes scale-up in low-income and middle-income countries, 2009–31. *The Lancet, 376*(9748), 1254–1260.

Hill, C. W. L. (2009). *International business: Competing in the global marketplace*. Boston: McGraw-Hill.

Humanitarian Futures Programme. (2007). *Dimensions of crisis impacts: Humanitarian needs by 2015* [Online].

Hunter, D. J. (2007). *Managing for health*. London: Routledge.

Huynen, M. M. T. E., Martens, P., & Hilderink, H. B. M. (2005). The health impacts of globalization: A conceptual framework. *Globalization and Health, 1*, 14.

IASC. (2007). *Inter-agency contingency planning guidelines for humanitarian assistance*. Available from: http://www.humanitarianinfo.org/iasc/downloaddoc.aspx?docID=4454&type=pdf

James, E. C. (2004). The political economy of 'trauma' in Haiti in the democratic era of insecurity. *Culture, Medicine and Psychiatry, 28*, 127–149.

Janes, C. R. (2010). Failed development and vulnerability to climate change in Central Asia: Implications for food security and health. *Asia-Pacific Journal of Public Health, 22*, 236S–245S.

Jones, G. R., & George, J. M. (2008). *Contemporary management*. Boston: McGraw-Hill.

Joubert, G., & Ehrlich, R. (2007). *Epidemiology: A research manual for South Africa*. Oxford: Cape Town.

Kasperson, R. E., & Pijawka, K. D. (1985). *Societal response to hazards and major hazard events: Comparing natural and technological hazards*. Public Administration Review. Special issue.

Keim, M. E. (2008). Building human resilience: The role of public health preparedness and response as an adaptation to climate change. *American Journal of Preventive Medicine, 35*(5), 508–516.

Keim, M. E. (2011). Preventing disasters: Public health vulnerability reduction as a sustainable adaptation to climate change. *Disaster Medicine and Public Health Preparedness, 52*, 140–148.

Kent, R. (2002). Humanitarian futures and adaptive futures. *Conflict, Security, and Development, 2*(3), 67–92.

Khan, K., Arino, J. A., Hu, W., Raposo, P., Sears, J., Calderon, F., Heidebrecht, C., MacDonald, M., Liauw, J., Chan, A., & Gardam, M. (2009). Spread of a novel influenza A (H1N1) virus via global airline transportation. *The New England Journal of Medicine, 361*(2), 212–241.

Kohl, P. A., O'Rourke, A. P., Schmidman, D. L., Dopkin, W. A., & Birnbaum, M. L. (2005). The Sumatra-Andaman earthquake and tsunami of 2004: The hazards, events, and damage. *Prehospital & Disaster Medicine, 20*(6), 356–363.

Kolo, M. T. (2014). Natural radioactivity and environmental risk assessment of Sokoto phosphate rock, Northwest Nigeria. *African Journal of Environmental Science and Technology, 8*(9), 532–538.

LaDou, J. (2007). *Occupational & environmental medicine*. New York: McGraw-Hill.

Lautze, S., Leaning, J., Raven-Roberts, A., Kent, R., & Mazurana, D. (2004). Assistance, protection, and governance networks in complex emergencies. *Lancet, 364*, 2134–2141.

Leitmann, J. (2007). Cities and calamities: Learning from post-disaster response in Indonesia. *Journal of Urban Health: Bulletin of the New York Academy of Medicine, 84*(1), i145–i153.

Lorreti, A. (2006). *Coordination and humanitarian clusters*.

Lorreti, A. (2009). *Coordinating the cluster*.

Lurie, M., Harrison, A., Wilkinson, D., & Karim, S. A. (1997). Circular migration and sexual networking in rural KwaZulu/Natal: Implications for the spread of HIV and other sexually transmitted diseases. *Health Transition Review, 7*, 17–27.

Macrae, J., Bradbury, M., Jaspars, S., Johnson, D., & Duffield, M. (1997). Conflict, the continuum and chronic emergencies: A critical analysis of the scope for linking relief, rehabilitation and development planning in Sudan. *Disasters, 21*(3), 223–243.

Marks, D. (2011). Climate change and Thailand: Impact and response. *Contemporary Southeast Asia: A Journal of International and Strategic Affairs, 33*(2), 229–258.

McCoy, D. (2016). *Climate change: Health impacts and opportunities – A summary of the IPCC working group 2 report*. The Global Climate and Health Alliance.

McMichael, A. J. (2002). Population, environment, and survival: Past patterns, uncertain futures. *The Lancet, 359*(9312), 1145–1148.

Meredith, L. S., Eisenman, D. P., Tanielian, T., Taylor, S. L., Basurto, D. R., Diamond, D., Cienfuegos, B., & Shields, S. (2011). Prioritizing psychological consequences for disaster preparedness and response: A framework for addressing the emotional, behavioural, and cognitive effects of patient surge in large-scale disasters. *Disaster Medicine and Public Health Preparedness, 5*(1), 73–80.

Merson, M. E., Black, R. E., & Mills, A. J. (2012). *Global health: Diseases, programs, systems, and policies*. London: Jones & Bartlett.

Moatti, J. P., & Souteyrand, Y. (2000). HIV/AIDS social and behavioural research: Past advances and thoughts about the future. *Social Science & Medicine, 50*, 1519–1532.

Mohr, P., & Fourie, L. (2004). *Economics for South African students*. Pretoria: Van Schaik.

Morgan, O., & de Ville de Goyet, C. (2005). Dispelling disaster myths about dead bodies and disease: The role of scientific evidence and the media. *Pan American Journal of Public Health, 18*(1), 33–36.

Muller, M., Bezuidenhout, M., & Jooste, K. (2006). *Healthcare service management*. Cape Town: Juta.

Nagata, T., Rosborough, S. N., Van Rooyen, M. J., Kozawa, S., Ukai, T., & Nakayama, S. (2006). Express railway disaster in Amagasaki: A review of urban disaster response capacity in Japan. *Prehospital Disaster Medicine, 21*(5), 345–352.

Perry, M. (2007). Natural disaster management planning: A study of logistics managers responding to the tsunami. *International Journal of Physical Distribution & Logistics Management, 37*(5), 409–433.

Piotrowski, C. (2010). Earthquake in Haiti: The failure of crisis management? *Organizational Development Journal, 28*(1), 107–112.

Romundstad, L., Sundness, K. O., Pillgram-Larsen, J., Roste, G. K., & Gilbert, M. (2004). Challenges of major incident management when excess resources are allocated: Experiences from a mass casualty incident after roof collapse of a military command centre. *Prehospital & Disaster Medicine, 19*(2), 179–184.

Ruger, J. P., & Yach, D. (2005). Global functions at the World Health Organization: WHO must reassert its role in integrating, coordinating, and advancing the worldwide agenda on health. *The British Medical Journal, 330*, 1099–1100.

Scambler, G. (2008). *Sociology as applied to medicine*. Oxford: Edinburgh.

Schipper, L., & Pelling, M. (2006). Disaster risk, climate change and international development: Scope for, and challenges to, integration. *Disasters, 30*(1), 19–38.

Schwarzinger, M., Flicoteaux, M., Cortarenoda, S., Obadia, Y., & Moatti, J.-P. (2010). Low acceptability of A/H1N1 pandemic vaccination in French adult population: Did public health policy fuel public dissonance? *PLoS One, 5*(4), 1–9.

Spiegel, P. B. (2010). Health-care needs of people affected by conflict: Future trends and changing frameworks. *Lancet, 375*, 341–345.

Stoddard, A. (2003). Humanitarian NGOs: Challenges and tends. *Humanitarian Policy Group Briefing, 12*, 1–4.

Sudharsanam, M. B., & Gautam, R. (2012). An outbreak investigation of measles after the tsunami in Cuddalore district, Tamil Nadu. *Annals of Tropical Medicine and Public Health, 5*(4), 291–294.

Tappero, J. W., & Tauxe, R. V. (2011). Lessons learned during public health response to cholera epidemic in Haiti and the Dominican Republic. *Emerging Infectious Diseases, 17*(11), 2087–2093.

Thompson, A. A., Strickland, A. J., & Gamble, J. E. (2007). *Crafting and executing strategy*. New York: McGraw-Hill.

Travis, B. G. (2011). Review of mass trauma and emotional healing around the world: Rituals and practices for resilience and meaning-making. *Ecopsychology, 3*(2), 149–151.

United Nations. (2008). *Myanmar tropical cyclone Nargis: Flash appeal*. Available from: http://ochadms.unog.ch/quickplace/cap/main.nsf/h_Index/Flash_2008_Myanmar/$FILE/Flash_2008_Myanmar_SCREEN.pdf

United Nations. (2018). *Climate change*. Available from https://www.un.org/en/sections/issues. Accessed 22 Nov 2018.

Vermaak, J., & van Niekerk, D. (2004). Disaster risk reduction initiatives in South Africa. *Development Southern Africa, 21*(3), 555–574.

Walley, J., & Wright, J. (2010). *Public health: An action guide to improving health*. Oxford: New York.

Weaver, H. J., Blashki, G. A., Capon, A. G., & McMichael, A. J. (2010). Climate change and Australia's healthcare system – Risks, research and responses. *Australian Health Review, 34*(4), 441–444.

White, P. (1999). The role of UN specialised agencies in complex emergencies: A case study of FAO. *Third World Quarterly, 20*(1), 223–238.

Williams, P. D., & Bellamy, A. J. (2005). The responsibility to protect and the crisis in Darfur. *Security Dialogue, 36*(1), 27–47.

Chapter 8
Conclusions and Notes to the Reader

Abstract The book aimed to evaluate international public health issues, with a particular focus on diseases and disasters, policies and practices in low-, middle- and high-income countries. The magnitude of the disease burden is heavier in the low- and middle-income countries, and the picture is further exacerbated by resource constraints. While donor governments have committed funding and technical assistance to support low- and middle-income countries deal with the heavy burden of diseases, such support presents a threat to health systems in the context of sustainable leadership and sustainable financing in the recipient countries, if the donor funding is terminated or reduced. Inequality is a sore point, both internationally and intra-nationally, as it undermines the realisation of health as a human right for all people. Effective and sustainable disease control requires a holistic approach that goes beyond clinical medicine. The international public health impact of globalisation, climate change and disasters are key issues that need urgent attention in the context of a changing world.

Keywords Adolescents · Burden of diseases · Climate change · Colonial history of public health · Disasters · Diseases control · Globalisation · Health systems · High-income countries · International public health · Low-income countries · Middle-income countries · Millennium Development Goals · Public health equity · Sexual and reproductive health · Sustainable Development Goals

International Public Health and the Burden of Diseases:

- Tackling the global disease burden is paramount in the context of the burgeoning epidemic of communicable and non-communicable diseases, especially in low- and middle-income countries.
- While most high-income countries have successfully implemented cost-effective interventions to tackle their burden of non-communicable diseases, low- and middle-income countries have to prioritise cost-effective interventions to tackle the multiple burden of communicable and non-communicable diseases and to strengthen their efforts to effectively address other key issues of public health concern.

M. P. Mabuza, *Evaluating International Public Health Issues*,
https://doi.org/10.1007/978-981-13-9787-5_8

- The irony is that while low- and middle-income countries carry the heaviest burden of disease, such countries have a minor share of the total global health spending, yet their economies are severely challenged and their populations are the most affected by poverty which has a negative impact on health.
- The first step is to understand the magnitude of the disease burden.

Inequity in Low- and Middle- Income Countries and the Colonial History of Public Health:

- The political power and influence of the medical model and issues of ethnicity and socio-economic status continue to influence current attitudes to and practices in public health programmes and contribute to continuing health inequalities and inequities in low- and middle-income countries.
- Poverty is a major public health issue in many low- and middle-income countries and the inequalities and inequities that exacerbate it.
- The gap between the rich and the poor still gets wider and wider all the time and deepens the inequalities.
- Unlike the rich, those who live in poverty continue to bear the brunt of poor health and discrimination.
- A potential solution to address poverty is to have the highest calibre of political leadership that will show commitment and vision to meaningfully and sustainably address the issue of poverty.

Health Systems:

- Effective leadership and governance are the cornerstone and important entry point for discussions of health policy, design, implementation, and for raising performance in healthcare delivery.
- Notably, measures of performance are missing from the health agenda of many low- and middle-income countries, especially when it comes to measuring the impacts of health care investments. In such countries, it is a limitation that measures of performance are missing, as such a scenario makes it impossible to reflect whether the health system is meeting the objectives, whether public resources are appropriately used and whether government priorities are implemented.
- The common practice of measuring the impacts of health care investments only by inputs and general health outcomes, is a glaring deficiency, and it is not good enough as it perpetuates inefficiencies and lack of accountability.
- The distinctive good governance issues and challenges that must be faced in health care delivery are often neither fully recognised nor addressed, yet, governance can serve as a critical facilitator of, or a barrier to, achieving high performance in health care delivery.
- The question is, given the uniqueness of different settings, should different countries have their own set of indicators to monitor performance of health care delivery?
- It is a human right to address clients' needs through a health system that provides a continuum of quality care in an effective, responsive and respectful manner.

- The key role of the client or patient should not be underestimated, as the client or patient has an important influence in the framework of health care quality assurance.
- It is critical that quality assurance is not seen as a sole responsibility of health professionals or those trained in quality assurance.
- The client or patient should be involved and regarded as a definer of health care quality; evaluator of health care quality; informant of health care quality; co-producer of health care quality; controller of health practitioner behaviour; reformer of health care through direct participation in the health system, administrative support of health care, ability to choose health care services, and ability to advocate for health care reforms.
- There is need for policymakers to ensure that clients or patients are informed and involved in the decision-making process, particularly in low-income and middle-income countries where the clients generally feel they have no power to influence the quality of health care.
- Moving from a failing disease-focused programme to a sector-wide approach (SWAp) may seem attractive, but SWAps have their own inherent challenges largely because they vary in different contexts, and therefore very difficult to monitor and evaluate in terms of their population health impact.
- The bottom line is that it is time for heads of state and government to deliver.
- The shift in health/development policy since 1980 through to the current day has been largely influenced by the individual and/or collaborative role of the World Health Organization, and International Financial and Economic Institutions such as the World Bank, and lately by the emergence of new players and initiatives such as the Global Fund.
- Despite the history of financial largesse and the massive expansion in health project funding, the World Bank has come in for sustained criticism over its health work, from concern about the underlying economic assumptions it worked with, to criticisms that projects were failing to offer the promised outcomes.
- After all, market-led solutions have often undermined the poorest and most vulnerable communities. In recent times, total development assistance for health has multiplied, largely driven by the adoption of the Millennium Development Goals (MDGs) and the Sustainable Development Goals (SDGs).
- In pursuit and aid towards achievement of the set goals, disease-focused multi-billion-dollar health initiatives have emerged in the landscape of public health, and governments of many low- and middle-income countries have increased their spending on health.
- However, in the absence of systematic evidence, there is ongoing debate about the merits of the global aid architecture and aid effectiveness in health.
- The emergence of vertically funded health initiatives through international development agencies and international funding agencies, has had both positive and negative effects on recipient countries' attempts to strengthen health systems.
- While Technical Assistance (TA) has been a substantial component of development assistance and is considered an effective tool for building sustainable capacity, it is argued that TA is often tied to and driven by donors and is not appropriate for the local setting of low- and middle-income countries.

- Human resources for health are a vital building block of a health system, and they are central towards the attainment of better health outcomes.
- It is a challenge that many low- and middle-income countries are faced with "brain drain" of their human resources for health, as many of the health care professionals from low- and middle-income countries move to work in high-income countries, where they get better pay and better working conditions.
- A mix of financial and non-financial incentives is important as part of a strategy to attract, retain and motivate staff, including health workers in resource-poor settings.
- Recognising the reality of limited resources and flat-lining of international donor funding, it is not possible for most low- and middle-income countries to meet all the needs of their populations.
- As such, it is important for countries to be efficient by meeting priority health needs or follow the approach of defining and providing a context-specific minimum service package or essential health package (EHP) of high quality.
- More attention needs to be given to the mechanism of delivery of EHP, and removing the constraints of delivering effective medical laboratory services to support EHPs.
- Lack of knowledge and understanding of the functions of laboratory services by policymakers, health professional and patients can stifle progress towards delivering cost-effective and equitable health services.
- Implementation of new technologies that have been effective in delivering evidence-based essential health services best practice or innovation in one setting may not necessarily be effective in another setting.

The UN Millennium Development Goals (MDGs):

- It is notable that some of the goals were directly related to health while the others were lateral but had a great influence on health.
- As such, it is important that the MDGs should not be viewed in isolation because they were interlinked in some way, and therefore successful implementation would have required concerted effort from a multi-sectoral perspective.
- It is worth highlighting that due to a number of factors, there were variations across countries/regions in their success in meeting the targets of the MDGs.
- While it was good that the MDGs created impetus for commitment towards improving public health, blanket targets for the MDGs as well as vertical programmes aimed at achieving the MDGs were not helpful because they ignored the unique underlying challenges of each setting and issues of sustainability and ownership.

The UN Sustainable Development Goals (SDGs):

- The deliberately ambitious and transformational 2030 Agenda for Sustainable Development has at its heart a foundation for ensuring lives of dignity for all in terms of freeing humanity from poverty, securing a healthy planet for future generations, building peaceful, inclusive societies, and leavening no one behind.
- As the clock is ticking, and the rate of progress in many areas is not as fast as it should to meet the targets by 2030, there is need for injection of a sense of urgency, effective leadership and partnerships, efficiency, cohesiveness, account-

ability, capacity for reliable data to measure progress, sustained momentum, and a paradigm shift that goes beyond business as usual.

- Despite the clearly ambitiously envisaged positives of the SDGs, it is a loophole that the SDGs are not a legally binding treaty, just like their predecessors, the MDGs, and this presents a drawback as countries may skirt their commitments.
- There is scepticism about the SDGs commitment to reducing inequalities, as inequality is not clearly articulated and not embedded in a cross-cutting manner across all seventeen goals, as it should have been.
- The SDGs have an inherent disconnect between the language of true human rights and that of development. Unfortunately, the international development discourse focuses on global economic growth which takes a long time, thereby exacerbating poverty, homelessness, hunger, oppression, dependency, disease and premature death among those who are already in jeopardy, and in itself posing a threat to the realisation of human rights for all.
- The SDGs' lack of clear division of labour opens room for confusion and indecisive action and defers the realisation of human rights for all far into the future, thereby disrespecting the human rights of those who are in jeopardy at present.
- Using the same metrics to measure progress towards the SDGs is rather unfair, because, wealthy countries have better capacity to realise most of the goals than poor countries. The danger is that this may perpetuate poor countries' dependency on wealthy nations, thereby court a relapse of oppression and domination, and stifle sustainable development in the poor countries.

Disease Control and the Promotion of Public Health Equity:

- The main aim of disease (communicable and non-communicable diseases) control is to reduce the number of people who get diseases, who get sick from the diseases, and who die from the diseases.
- Globalisation and rapid urbanisation have resulted in a surge of non-communicable diseases (such as cancer, cardiovascular diseases, diabetes mellitus, among others) in low- and middle-income countries, adding to the already heavy burden of communicable diseases (such as malaria, tuberculosis, HIV and AIDS, among others).
- Current vertical disease control programmes have advantages and disadvantages which impact positively or negatively on equitable public health outcomes, particularly, in low- and middle-income countries.
- There is merit in not only looking at vertical diseases control approaches, but also having a deeper focus on socioeconomic and political dimensions to address issues of equity in public health.
- The issue of tuberculosis including multi drug resistant (MDR) tuberculosis, extensively drug resistant (XDR) tuberculosis, and tuberculosis-HIV coinfections pose a huge challenge, as it complicates the whole picture of the tuberculosis and HIV and AIDS epidemics.
- Malaria should be regarded as a major global public health priority and efforts should be scaled up in the malaria endemic area, more so with the complications of climate change, as studies project that the malaria agent, will be able to spread into new areas in the near future.

- Many of the issues of disease control and promotion of public health equity that were raised for HIV and AIDS, TB and malaria are also relevant to other infectious diseases affecting specific parts of the world, specific communities or emerge under certain conditions, but, because their spread is more local, they do not receive the same attention.
- The lessons learnt will be useful in the development of management approaches that would be appropriate to specific health problems and settings.

Adolescents, Sexual Reproductive Health (SRH) and Equity:

- It is highlighted that different aspects of adolescents' lives affect their health and wellbeing. They face comparatively high levels of unprotected sexual activity, suicide, substance abuse, road traffic accidents and malnutrition, and in some regions, violence through homicide and armed conflict are major problems.
- It is of concern that data from national surveys of many low- and middle-income countries demonstrate that the unmet need of adolescents is over two times higher than that of the general population in these countries.
- By strengthening national strategies and programmes to address sexual and reproductive health in adolescents, will directly and indirectly enhance the achievement of development goals.
- Since many of the public health issues affecting adolescents are further exacerbated by cultural, ethnic, religious, socioeconomic and educational inequalities already operating in many low- and middle-income countries, there is need to make the case for both male and female adolescents as a public health strategy by opening the dialogue and reaching a consensus for a holistic approach rather than impose only what is believed and known from a medical perspective.

Globalisation, Climate Change, and Disasters:

- The processes comprising globalisation affect access to social determinants of health (SDH) by way of multiple pathways as the effects of globalisation on SDH are almost never uniformly distributed across populations.
- Globalisation and climate change are global phenomena that may hamper food security, water resources and health, and they call for collective response in terms of global partnerships.
- Globalisation (including climate change) has created newly vulnerable poor who are at higher risk of poor health and malnutrition.
- Illness, all too often leads to "medical poverty traps", creating a vicious circle of poor nutrition, forgone education, and still more illness – all of which undermine the economic growth that is necessary. This situation puts more strain on the national budget as more money needs to be spent on the public health sector to cater for the increasing burden of disease.
- International organisations such as the World Health Organization (WHO) are better positioned to provide leadership, coordination, advocacy, and global standards in terms of public health goods.
- The underlying cause of rapid demographic transition may not be a health issue, but it may require a multidisciplinary approach, bearing in mind that societies differ, and the process of demographic transition is quite varied and does not always follow the path suggested by classic theory.

- Risk perception may have the opposite, compounding effect for disaster managers.
- Faulty perceptions on the part of the disaster management team could result in time or funding wasted in mitigation and preparation for a risk that may never happen at the expense of neglecting a more severe risk that threatens the population to a greater degree.
- Only effective public education and risk communication can counter the effects of public misperception of the risk.
- A holistic and critical approach to the disaster cycle/disaster-development continuum may provide a better opportunity to address the root cause of vulnerability, but an uncritical strategy may do more harm than good.
- While it is highlighted that low-income countries are at high risk of suffering ruinous effects after disasters as compared to high-income countries, it is also highlighted that there is no fixed formula to accurately project how the effects of disasters will pen out, regardless of the socioeconomic or political status of that particular country, because no country is immune to disasters.
- The question of who should take responsibility for ensuring that there is an official coordination mechanism in the context of a disaster, is an interesting one as coordination is perceived to differ in the context of the level of development of the affected country.
- The concept of vulnerability or vulnerable groups should not inadvertently create the risk of group discrimination but paying attention to the root causes of the dynamism and vulnerability of certain groups could provide us with lasting solutions for disaster management.
- Recovery, mitigation and preparedness are essential, but planning, leadership and cooperation are crucial to ensure that there is effective and sustainable disaster reduction.
- Coordination is a critical function in any human endeavour, particularly in crisis management, even though the meaning of coordination is sometimes misunderstood. Leadership, preparedness and a coordination mechanism are crucial, particularly so in crisis management.
- Disaster response is becoming increasingly complex with each event, and as such, some flexibility might be necessary to effectively deal with certain disasters, as effective coordination can only be a voluntary exercise based on mutual agreement.
- In terms of humanitarian assistance and the changing landscape of NGOs, it can be posited that the future of international NGOs is now linked to their ability to examine their purpose and goals in a rapidly changing world; and the reality is that the various strands of what is described as globalisation are helping NGOs into roles that will minimise their long-term impact.
- Coordinated information flow is critical in disaster management, but this is not without challenges and obstacles.
- As much as is it crucial to prioritise financial investment for the purpose of mitigation and preparedness, vis-à-vis each hazard, investment in excess resources could create further challenges.
- Mass crowding of disaster victims into health facilities could create confusion if there is no leadership and command among the disaster response healthcare team.

- There needs to be prioritisation of psychological consequences for disaster preparedness and response, while at the same time, there is need to be cautious of instrumentalising decisions because managing disaster may be complex, multidimensional and individually unique.
- Climate change has an influence in extreme weather events resulting in disasters, and this needs urgent interventions in the context of disaster management, while also bearing in mind that there are constraints and challenges with regard to addressing the issue of climate change and its influence on disasters.
- The risk of epidemics after a disaster is negligible, but at the same time such a risk should not be ignored. As such, there needs to be practical guidelines of communicating to the public about how corpses and carcasses should be managed, and how the spread of epidemics can be prevented after a disaster.
- Sometimes alarmist warnings and reporting have fuelled the fear of epidemics and yet studies show that this fear which appears to be a constant media and political issue is not justified, as epidemics are not always a constant feature following a disaster.
- The perpetuation of epidemics after a disaster may be compounded by the lack of effective disease surveillance systems.
- Owing to alarmist public health messages, it is possible that other urgent public health priorities might be compromised and overlooked as in 2009 when more attention and resources were channelled towards the pandemic influenza threat such as H1N1 which turned out to be not such a huge threat even though it still produced widespread morbidity and mortality.
- Many of the technological hazards by human failure and by intention have social, economic or political implications.
- While classifying such technological hazards in the same group as social, economic or political hazards may seem feasible, this should be avoided or done with caution to prevent confusion and ambiguity.
- While it may appear as if society has embraced the risks posed by technological hazards, it is also possible that a segment of society is not familiar with the risks because many of the technological innovations are still relatively new.
- Managing technological hazards requires the simultaneous goals of enlarging social benefits and reducing risks of such hazards.
- Society should be familiarised with the risks of technological hazards and should be protected in accordance with set standards and legislation, and at the same time society should also take responsibility.
- The health sector can best contribute to mitigation against and preparation for possible future food shortage crises by influencing political decision-making and facilitating multi-stakeholder partnerships to ensure that there is adequate resource allocation and capacity to address the issue of food shortages.
- The known strategies and frameworks of mitigation against and preparation for future food shortage crises are all important, but there needs to be awareness that nutritional concerns in low-income and middle-income countries are diverse, and the burden of diseases can complicate the whole picture and create a novelty of food shortage.

- Early warning systems can be more useful if they are linked to and complemented by timely response mechanisms.
- Most of the worst affected countries are those ill-prepared for an effective response to the food shortages. As such, it could be beneficial for countries to be part of regional bodies such as the southern African Development Community (SADC) because this has the potential to share and maximise its resources in terms of collaborative efforts for preparedness and response against impending crises such as food shortage emergencies within that region.
- In the context of complex humanitarian emergencies, the responsibility to protect can influence or hamper humanitarian work.
- It is crucial to analyse and to consider the uniqueness of the affected area before executing the responsibility to protect, because sometimes humanitarian interventions can be a dilemma in complex emergencies.
- There are many question marks about the responsibility to protect, largely because of the inconsistency in its application.
- The terrain has changed, and there is need for international interventions to be adaptable and fair.
- Much as there may be guidelines or initiatives such as the responsibility to protect, which determine how and when the international community should respond to complex emergencies, the role of the media may be particularly powerful in bringing popular demand for action.
- It should be borne in mind that there may be obstacles or barriers such as lack of political support, cultural issues, literacy issues, language issues, financial issues that could hamper the actions efforts.
- Complex emergencies pose many challenges to both the affected victims as well as the humanitarian workers, but despite all these challenges, it is crucial to maintain the protection of human rights, particularly the rights of the most vulnerable people.

Glossary

Acceptability The intervention strategy fits with the culture and social expectations of the community.

Access Living within reasonable distance of health services.

Adequate coverage Indicator used to monitor and evaluate the progress of health unit activities or services. It is the percentage of the target population receiving the activity or service according to standard guidelines. For example, adequate coverage for prenatal care can be defined as the percentage of pregnant women who made at least three prenatal visits, including one during the last month of pregnancy.

Allocation of costs Deciding how much of different inputs are involved in producing a given output, such as a specific treatment or diagnostic test. The purpose is usually to produce a realistic estimate of the full cost of providing the service, so that managers can identify efficiency improvements and prioritise between services or different delivery strategies.

Ante-natal The period between conception and birth (also called pre-natal).

Assessment A study of inputs, process, outputs of a project or programme, conducted to measure performance and ascertain readiness and capacity to perform roles and responsibilities or achieve objectives. It is linked to policies and systems under which the programme operates.

Barriers Conditions that prevent people from doing something. For example, lack of time, money, equipment, authority, or supplies might be barriers to doing a job correctly.

Behaviour Actions and practices by individuals that may affect their health.

Burden of disease Measurement of premature mortality (deaths) and morbidity (non-fatal illness) in a given area. The aim of the study is usually to define which illness or sick factors are most significant in causing death and disability and hence to inform decisions about which services should receive priority. On its own, however, it is inadequate as a decision tool as it limits the issue of effectiveness of prevention or treatment strategies and the cost of implementing them.

M. P. Mabuza, *Evaluating International Public Health Issues*,
https://doi.org/10.1007/978-981-13-9787-5

Coverage (rates) The proportion of the estimated target population which has been reached. These are often used in relation to preventive programmes, where target populations can be more easily estimated.

Crude Birth Rate This is the number of live births per 1000 total population per year. The denominator includes men, women and children.

Crude Death Rate This is the number of deaths occurring per 1000 total population year.

Disability-adjusted life year (DALY) Concept developed by the World Bank and the World Health Organisation to measure the burden of disease, in terms of both premature death and disability. With adequate data, it can be used to compare potential health gain from different disease control programmes and thus to prioritise resource allocation according to cost-effectiveness principles.

Effectiveness The degree to which desired outcome s are achieved.

Efficiency The maximum possible sustained output. From a given set of inputs, this is known as technical efficiency. By contrast, allocative efficiency is used to describe a situation in which either inputs or outputs are put in their best possible uses.

Elimination The reduction of the global prevalence to a negligible amount, as is being attempted for leprosy. Or it is the reduction of an infectious disease's prevalence in the population of a global region to zero; and this has occurred or is underway in malaria, lymphatic filariasis, measles, mumps and rubella, onchocerciasis and yaws.

Empowerment The process through which individuals or communities gain greater control over decision and actions affecting their health.

Epidemic A rapid increase in the levels of a disease.

Epidemiology Study of the health and disease in the community and the application of this information to promote health. Descriptive epidemiology is concerned with measurement of health and disease. Analytical epidemiology is concerned with determination of risk factors and cause of disease.

Equity Access to health care and resources according to needs without discrimination by gender, income, religion, and race.

Essential (or basic) package Given the shortage of resources for health in developing countries and the high burden of disease, it is suggested that public funds be concentrated on a defined range of highly cost-effective services. These are often called 'essential packages.

Evaluation An appraisal of something or a process of making value judgements over a level of performance or achievement

Globalisation The process of increasing economic, political and cultural interdependence of countries.

Health sector reform A substantial change to the structure or processes of health services with the intention of improving outcomes.

Implementation The act of actually undertaking an intended and planned course of action.

Incidence A measure of new cases of a disease in a specified period of time per total population.

Indicator A measure of progress towards objectives (e.g. impact on mortality or morbidity), strategies (e.g. coverage of vaccination) or activities (number of health workers trained).

International Monetary Fund (IMF) An international organisation set up by governments to monitor and smooth financial exchange on a global scale. Interventions by the IMF to help countries in difficulty are usually associated with rigorous criteria for financial solvency, including reductions in government spending and encouraging exports.

Insurance Pooling risks with others in order to spread costs of health care (or other commodity) over time and protect against catastrophically expensive illness.

Integration The relationship between public health officials and a healthcare organisation that aims to strengthen the connection between clinical processes or the delivery of health care, and public health prevention efforts.

Interventions Are the means to control disease. They are the solutions to health problems. Examples include vaccination, health promotion (e.g. by condom promotion), impregnated bed nets and oral rehydration for diarrhoea.

Legislation Laws controlling personal or companies' behaviour so as to improve the lives of the public. In health, for example, laws limiting pollution, tobacco advertising, drinking and driving or making the use of seat belts compulsory.

Millennium Development Goals (MDGs) These were agreed by the United Nations in September 2000. They set targets in poverty, education, access to clean water and sanitation, child mortality, maternal health, HIV/AIDS and other infectious diseases and the environment.

Missed opportunities A missed opportunity for prevention is when preventive interventions such as vaccination, vitamin A capsules and family planning services, are not offered to, for example, a mother attending with a sick child.

Pandemic An epidemic spread over many countries, e.g. the AIDS pandemic

Performance Level of fulfilment of operational capacity of a programme or person.

Policy A deliberate system of principles to guide decisions and achieve rational outcomes. It is a statement of intent and is implemented as a procedure or protocol.

Population A group of people sharing a common geographical (e.g. district) boundary or the same age or sex group (children under one year, women of childbearing age) or health risk group (e.g. tobacco smokers).

Practice The application of public health science at the delivery level

Prevalence The number of people with a disease per total population. This can be at a point in time (point prevalence) or over a defined period (period prevalence).

Primary Health Care (PHC) The first tier of health care based at the community level defined in the Alma-Ata Declaration of 1978 as 'essential health care made accessible at a cost a country and community can afford, with methods that are practical, scientifically sound and socially acceptable

Prioritise Putting things in a specific order according to certain reasons. For example, ranking problems according to their seriousness, frequency and concerns for the community.

Programme A systematically designed set of interventions and delivery strategies which will achieve high risk group coverage, e.g. the expanded programme of immunization (EPI) includes protocols for child vaccination, modules for training, cold chain equipment and delivery (strategies) through static and outreach health services

Quality-adjusted life year (QALY) A measure of health gain which aims to measure life years added but also the quality of life which is achieved in those years. This is one measure used in *cost-utility analysis*. Another is the DALY – a narrower definition, but easier to measure.

Resources Manpower, money and materials.

Risk behaviour Specific forms of behaviour which are proven to be associated with increased susceptibility to specific diseases or ill health.

Sector-wide approaches (SWAPs) A particular method of collecting and distributing aid money. Rather than funds being earmarked for a specific project, the money is distributed across the whole sector. In this way funds for the health sector, for example, are pooled and the Ministry of Health sets priorities for spending.

Strategy The solution to a problem. This may be an intervention (e.g. bed nets as a means to interrupt mosquito contacts) or a delivery strategy e.g. social marketing as a means to provide and distribute bed nets.

Sustainable Development Goals (SDGs) A collection of 17 global goals set by the United Nations General Assembly in 2015. The SDGs are part of Resolution 70/1 of the United Nations General Assembly "Transforming our World the 2030 Agenda for Sustainable Development." That has been shortened to "2030 Agenda."

Sustainability The ability to maintain a system over time, at a reasonable level of operation and using the resources that are likely to be available. Sustainability has various dimensions, including financial, institutional, and social.

Target A quantified level of specific a specific objective to be reached within a given time frame.

Vertical programme A programme which is organised and managed (mainly) separately from the general health services, e.g. the staff have different pay, per diem and/or reporting supervision, and planning systems.

World Bank A group of international financial institutions, with the member states as shareholders. The largest shareholder is the United States of America (USA). The mission of the World Bank is to make grants and loans to improve global economic growth and contribute to a stable world economy.

World Health Organisation (WHO) The United Nations specialised agency for health, governed by the United Nations member states through the annual world assembly. Its activities include the sitting of global norms and standards in health and stimulating research and development into health issues of international importance.

Index

M. P. Mabuza, *Evaluating International Public Health Issues*,
https://doi.org/10.1007/978-981-13-9787-5

MIX
Papier aus verantwortungsvollen Quellen
Paper from responsible sources
FSC® C105338

If you have any concerns about our products,
you can contact us on
ProductSafety@springernature.com

In case Publisher is established outside the EU,
the EU authorized representative is:
Springer Nature Customer Service Center GmbH
Europaplatz 3, 69115 Heidelberg, Germany

Printed by Libri Plureos GmbH
in Hamburg, Germany